Getting Started in Teaching for Nursing and the Health Professions

Getting Started in Teaching for Nursing and the Health Professions

JUDITH A. HALSTEAD, PhD, RN, ANEF, FAAN
Executive Director
Commission for Nursing Education Accreditation
National League for Nursing
Washington, DC;
Professor Emeritus
School of Nursing
Indiana University
Indianapolis, Indiana

DIANE M. BILLINGS, EdD, RN, ANEF, FAAN
Chancellor's Professor Emeritus
School of Nursing
Indiana University
Indianapolis, Indiana

ELSEVIER

Elsevier
3251 Riverport Lane
St. Louis, Missouri 63043

GETTING STARTED IN TEACHING FOR NURSING AND
THE HEALTH PROFESSIONS   ISBN: 978-0-323-82898-7
Copyright © 2024 by Elsevier Inc. All rights reserved.

Notice

Executive Content Strategist: Lee Henderson
Content Development Specialist: Angie Breckon
Publishing Services Manager: Deepthi Unni
Project Manager: Thoufiq Mohammed
Design Direction: Bridget Hoette

Printed in India

Last digit is the print number: 9 8 7 6 5 4 3 2 1

Working together
to grow libraries in
developing countries

www.elsevier.com • www.bookaid.org

This book is dedicated to all newly appointed nursing and health professions educators whose students will be our next generation of health care professionals. It is our hope that this book provides a blueprint for ensuring that all new faculty receive the support and mentoring they deserve as they are "getting started" in the teaching environment.

PREFACE

The idea for this book started with an awareness that many new faculty in nursing and the health professions begin their first teaching positions with little or no preparation for how to teach. They also may have limited opportunities for an orientation to their new teaching responsibilities before they find themselves facing their first class of students. With an acute shortage of educators in many of the health professions, it is not uncommon for new faculty to be hired just weeks before the semester is scheduled to begin. So, with a syllabus in hand they enter the classroom and clinical teaching environments wondering how and where to get started with developing their skills as educators. In interviews with new faculty in their first year of teaching, we confirmed that this scenario is a common one and that they frequently lacked resources to help guide them as they acclimated to their role as educators. We are hoping that this book can help fill the knowledge gap for beginning nursing and health professions educators and serve as a go-to reference to find answers to common questions new educators may have. We also believe that this book can be a valuable resource for deans, directors, and other administrators who are responsible for planning orientation programs and creating a welcoming and supportive environment for all new faculty.

Good teaching does not happen in a vacuum. It requires intentional thought and preparation on the part of the new faculty, and supportive administrators and colleagues who can provide guidance and mentoring to new faculty as they face teaching challenges for the first time. The teaching-learning environment that exists in higher education is ever changing. This is especially true in nursing and the health professions as faculty also strive to stay abreast of changes in complex health care environments. While health care disciplines have their focused areas of disciplinary expertise, the faculty who teach in the health care professions face common sets of challenges that can often be mutually addressed in interprofessional settings. It is our hope that this book, which is written from an interdisciplinary perspective, can be used to provide a foundation for teaching practices and the development and retention of new faculty in our health professions academic programs.

The reader will find that this book is arranged in five parts that focus on areas in the academic teaching-learning environment for which all new faculty will eventually need to develop competence: (1) curriculum development, (2) teaching in the classroom, (3) teaching in the clinical environment, (4) using technology to support teaching and learning, and (5) program evaluation and accreditation. The information in the chapters associated with each part is designed to help faculty with knowing how to get started in securing the resources and knowledge they need in their first year as educators. Each part of the book opens with a quick overview of the topics covered in each chapter. Appendices at the back of the book identify institution and program resources that faculty should become familiar with as they gain an understanding of their specific campus and program environments. A glossary is also included, which defines commonly used terms in education and the academic setting.

This book has many potential uses. Individual faculty can use it to help meet their own professional development needs. Administrators in nursing and health professions programs may consider providing a copy to all new faculty and using it as a guide for developing faculty orientation programs. It can also be useful as a textbook for new faculty enrolled in professional development and academic courses. It is our hope that this book will be a useful resource for all who have chosen to pursue a career as faculty in nursing and the health professions.

Judith A. Halstead
Diane M. Billings

CONTENTS

Participating in Curriculum Development

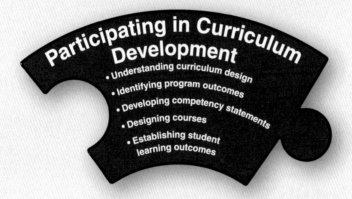

As a health professions educator you are responsible for designing and implementing a curriculum with learning experiences that enable students to develop the practice competencies necessary for safe and effective patient care. Part 1 provides you with the fundamental concepts associated with curriculum development, implementation, and evaluation. Chapter 1 introduces you to the curriculum development process, including the faculty role and responsibilities associated with curriculum development. You will have an opportunity to conduct a self-assessment related to your competencies with curriculum development and which areas you will want to develop further. Chapter 2 focuses on steps that you can take in your first year of teaching to prepare to participate in the curriculum development process. Chapter 3 addresses the key elements of the curriculum and provides you with a guide of how to develop a curriculum that is relevant and produces competent graduates. In Chapter 4 you are introduced to some common issues related to curriculum, including how faculty dynamics can affect curriculum change, how to navigate the curriculum approval process, and understanding the legal and ethical implications of curriculum development and implementation. Chapter 5 completes Part 1 with a discussion on evaluating the effectiveness of the curriculum. At the back of the book, you will find Appendix A, which contains a listing of documents to gather and review as part of your teaching responsibilities related to participating in curriculum development.

CHAPTER 1

Introduction to Curriculum Development

Congratulations on accepting a position as a faculty member in the health professions! You are choosing a career in the teaching profession at a time when the health professions are collectively experiencing many challenges in both health care and higher education. As a health professions educator, you are responsible for preparing the health professions workforce of the future and ensuring that learners acquire the competencies needed to practice in an ever-changing health care environment. This responsibility includes designing and implementing a curriculum with learning experiences that enable the learner to develop the requisite practice competencies for safe and effective patient care. Evaluating the effectiveness of the curriculum is also your responsibility. Faculty are responsible for understanding all aspects of the curriculum and being an active participant in curriculum development. As a new member of the faculty, participating in curriculum development activities may be at first intimidating. This handbook provides you with the fundamental concepts associated with curriculum development, implementation, and evaluation.

Faculty spend a considerable amount of time engaged in discussions about the program's curriculum. Examples of common curriculum questions include the following:

- Does the curriculum achieve the intended learner outcomes?
- Is the curriculum up to date and reflective of advances in your discipline and health care?
- Is there evidence that the curriculum is preparing graduates to be successful in achieving licensure or certification for the role in which they have been prepared?
- Do employers seek out the graduates of the program for hire in their agencies because of their competence?
- What areas of the curriculum could benefit from revision?

The purpose of this handbook is to provide readers with practical, how-to advice on ways to effectively participate in curriculum development, implementation, and evaluation activities that are essential responsibilities of faculty.

Faculty Role and Responsibilities in Curriculum Development

Many new educators do not have firsthand experience with curriculum development and lack formal preparation in the area. Faculty may seek formal academic preparation in curriculum development by taking coursework (academic or continuing education) to help increase knowledge of curriculum development, implementation, and evaluation. Doing so will help you gain valuable knowledge about the various curriculum elements and how they are cohesively designed to provide learners with the foundation they need to be successful in their academic studies. Besides formal coursework there are steps you can take to prepare yourself to become an informed and active participant in your program's curricular discussions and assume the faculty responsibilities associated with curriculum development within your program (Box 1.1). These steps will be covered in detail in Chapter 2.

BOX 1.1 ■ Step-by-Step: Understanding Curriculum Development in Your Institution

- Understand your institution/program's formal curriculum development process.
- Know the key players leading curriculum development in your institution and program.
- Articulate the institution/program's mission and philosophy.
- Understand how your courses fit within the curriculum.
- Read the program's curriculum policies and understand how they apply to your courses.
- Review the program's curriculum evaluation plan.

Developing the curriculum by which the knowledge, skills, and attributes (attitudes and values) of one's discipline will be conveyed to learners is the responsibility of faculty and not administration. Faculty governance bylaws of most any institution of higher education make statements upholding the role of faculty in determining the curriculum. This tenet holds true for the development of the institution's general education curriculum as well as the unique curriculum of academic disciplines. The faculty's responsibility for developing curriculum is often reinforced by accreditation bodies that set forth standards that speak to expectations of faculty being involved in institutional and program governance, especially in the area of curriculum. It is important for faculty to embrace curricular decisions and implementation and participate in curricular discussions. Box 1.2 describes faculty responsibilities associated with successful curriculum development. These responsibilities are further described in the sections that follow.

BOX 1.2 ■ Faculty Responsibilities Related to Curriculum Development

- Articulate a curriculum philosophy of teaching and learning.
- Understand the curriculum model.
- Develop skill in assessing the curriculum and evaluating its effectiveness.
- Develop policies to support curriculum implementation.
- Understand academic freedom and implications for curriculum implementation.
- Implement the curriculum as designed.
- Remain current about professional issues related to discipline, societal trends, health care, and higher education.

ARTICULATING A CURRICULUM PHILOSOPHY OF TEACHING AND LEARNING

While many formal definitions of curriculum exist, the term can be simply defined as the entirety of educational experiences that students are exposed to in their plan of study with a goal of achieving predetermined student learning outcomes. In the broadest sense, the concept of curriculum includes expected program outcomes, the courses that constitute the plan of study, learning activities delivered in a variety of settings, teaching/learning strategies used to implement the curriculum, services to support curriculum delivery, and extracurricular activities to further foster students' personal and professional development. Faculty are responsible for designing the curriculum and overseeing its implementation and evaluation.

To successfully design and consistently implement all elements of a curriculum, faculty need to be collectively guided by a philosophic framework of beliefs regarding the teaching and learning processes. The educator's views regarding the role of the teacher and the role of the learner in the teaching-learning process impacts decisions on curriculum design and implementation. Many faculty in health professions programs develop a philosophic framework that addresses faculty beliefs about core concepts related to the specific health professions discipline, health, humans, society, and the teaching-learning process. The faculty often develop a written philosophy statement to express these beliefs and guide the program. O'Riordan (2018) reported on the importance of faculty developing curriculum that is informed by their philosophic beliefs, that curriculum developed within such a context can be truly transformative. She asserted that such an approach can lead to rich discourse among faculty and provide the rationale as to which concepts should be either included or not included within the curriculum. She also stated that significant discourse lead time is needed to shape a shared faculty vision of philosophic beliefs.

New educators can review the philosophy and consider the concepts that are defined within the statement and consider how the philosophy aligns with their beliefs about practice and the teaching-learning process. Locate and review the philosophic framework that guides your program's curriculum, then consider how the framework will affect your teaching practices.

UNDERSTANDING THE CURRICULUM DESIGN

When you accepted your faculty position you were likely assigned courses that would be your responsibility to teach, either by yourself or in a team with other faculty. To effectively instruct your students it is important to understand the sequence of courses within the curriculum, the placement of your courses, and how the courses you are assigned to teach are integrated into the overall curriculum. It is important to know the courses the students have taken before they enroll in your course and understand the competencies students are expected to master while enrolled in your course to facilitate their success in subsequent coursework.

A variety of curriculum models can be used to structure health professions curricula and serve as an organizing framework to determine how students will experience the curriculum. Curricula can be organized by concepts, competencies, "blocks" of content, or by a combination of these models. Another way the curriculum can be described is by the order in which content is introduced, such as flowing from simple to complex patient care situations or from wellness to illness concepts. The curriculum model that faculty choose as an organizing framework determines where content is placed, what learning activities are implemented, and when and how students' achievement of the expected student learning outcomes will be evaluated. It is each faculty member's responsibility to understand the curriculum model used to guide the development and implementation of the curriculum.

DEVELOPING SKILL IN ASSESSING AND EVALUATING THE CURRICULUM

Another key faculty responsibility is to regularly assess the curriculum and evaluate its effectiveness in preparing students for the health care role they will assume upon program completion. Such assessment and evaluation strategies are implemented at the individual course level and the aggregate program outcome level. Faculty must be familiar with the curriculum evaluation plan that has been developed for your program. The evaluation plan can frequently be found outlined in the program's systematic evaluation plan (SEP). All faculty should be familiar with the program's SEP. The SEP provides you with a blueprint for all the program's evaluation strategies and identifies evaluation activities that faculty are expected to carry out for their courses. For example, you can anticipate gathering feedback from students through the course evaluation process for each course you teach. You may also seek peer review of your teaching practices and course materials. Curriculum evaluation is discussed in further detail in Chapter 5.

DEVELOPING POLICIES TO SUPPORT CURRICULUM IMPLEMENTATION

For the curriculum to be effective in achieving desired program outcomes it must be implemented in a consistent and equitable manner for all learners. To achieve this consistency the implementation of the curriculum is guided by policies as determined by the institution and program, as well as faculty. Faculty are responsible for knowing where to access these policies, understanding them and their implications for the courses they teach, following them as written, and articulating them to students. It is also faculty's responsibility to participate in the regular review and revision of the curriculum policies.

Curriculum policies can encompass any number of issues and exist at the institutional and program levels. For example, institutional level policies can dictate the number of credit hours required to graduate with a specific academic degree (associate, bachelor, etc.), number of credit hours that can be transferred in from another institution, the university/college grading scale, and number of general education credits required of each undergraduate. Institutional policies can also provide guidelines for how to manage cases of academic dishonesty or incivility in the classroom. At the program level, policies often exist to dictate course credit hour allocations for classroom and clinical instruction, clock hour to credit hour ratios, specific grading scales for the academic discipline, attendance policies, circumstances when a student may be dismissed from a program due to course failure, how a student may file a grievance in response to a grade received, and the grade point average a student must maintain to progress in the curriculum. These are just a few examples of the types of curriculum policies that may exist in the institution and program to illustrate the wide breadth of topics covered. Faculty must understand the curriculum policies that guide their actions. You will want to closely review the policies of your program and seek clarification as needed from your peers, mentor, or supervisor.

Faculty are responsible for understanding and following all established policies. Failure to follow policy on the part of faculty that leads to an adverse action for the student (e.g., course failure) can provide the student with a legal basis upon which to file a grievance alleging capricious and arbitrary action by the faculty member. Do not hesitate to ask questions about policy statements and their implications. Curriculum policies can be difficult to understand, especially for someone new to teaching within the program. It is wise to ask for clarification of policies that are not clear. You will notice that faculty spend a lot of time reviewing, discussing, and revising policies related to the curriculum. You can prepare to participate in these discussions by reading the policies and noting the areas where you have questions or suggestions for achieving greater clarity.

UNDERSTANDING ACADEMIC FREEDOM AND IMPLICATIONS FOR CURRICULUM IMPLEMENTATION

In your institution and program you will likely hear references to the faculty's right to academic freedom. Academic freedom is an important concept that emerged in 1940 from a statement developed by the American Association of University Professors (AAUP) entitled "Statement of Principles on Academic Freedom and Tenure" (AAUP, 1940). The 1940 statement was a restatement of academic freedom ideals that first originated in 1915. The 1940 statement itself has been updated with additional interpretative comments over the years, but the basic tenets remain unchanged. Academic freedom is considered essential to protecting the research and teaching enterprises of faculty. The AAUP principles state that professors have the full freedom to conduct and publish research to meet their academic obligations without interference or retaliation from their institution, even if the findings may be viewed as controversial by some. They also have the full freedom to discuss issues related to their academic disciplines in the classroom if they do not introduce controversial topics that lack relevance to their subject matter. Academic freedom does not protect professional incompetence or the conduct of research that does not abide by institutional regulations or ethical guidelines.

A third principle is that as private citizens professors can freely express their opinions on issues without institutional censor but must avoid asserting their own opinions while appearing to speak on behalf of their institution in their professorial role. These basic rights also carry with them the responsibility to conduct oneself in a manner that is always civil and respectful of others.

Academic freedom, however, does not mean that faculty have the right to alter the program's curriculum or change the content of their assigned courses without the input and feedback of their faculty colleagues. To maintain the integrity of the curriculum it is important for faculty to realize they must teach the courses as designed and use the appropriate approval process when recommending any substantive course changes. The concept of what constitutes substantive change is discussed next.

IMPLEMENTING THE CURRICULUM AS DESIGNED

While faculty have the right to determine the curriculum of their disciplines, the principles of academic freedom do not extend them the freedom to unilaterally alter the curriculum to suit their own preferences. When joining a faculty you become a member of a collective decision-making body; as such, are expected to implement the curriculum as it has been designed by the total faculty. For example, you may not alter the course description, course objective or outcomes, assigned content, allotted credit hours, prerequisites, and corequisites without going through the appropriate approval processes. Any of those changes would be considered substantive. Such decisions require the input and approval of the total faculty. Your responsibility will be to implement the curriculum as it has been designed and to be an informed participant in any curriculum discussions.

STAYING CURRENT IN YOUR KNOWLEDGE

As a faculty member in health professions education you have the multifaceted responsibility to stay current in the professional issues and societal trends that affect your discipline, health care, and higher education. You also have the responsibility to remain competent in your clinical practice. Your ability to develop and implement a relevant curriculum that will provide your students with the requisite knowledge and skills for competent practice is dependent upon remaining up to date and knowledgeable of the forces that are affecting your practice discipline and your role as a teacher. Van Schaik (2021) supported this need when he stated that many medical school faculty are being asked to undertake significant curriculum reform efforts to integrate concepts into the curriculum that they themselves have not had experience with. This leaves faculty unprepared to implement new curricular revisions without significant support. As examples of such concepts, he cited interprofessional education, improving health care systems, and diversity, equity, and inclusion. He stated

---

BOX 1.3 ■ Strategies for Staying Current

- Join professional organizations that support the teaching and practice of your discipline.
- Develop a list of relevant professional journals, newsletters, and websites to regularly read.
- Attend webinars and professional conferences for continuing education.
- Maintain your clinical practice through part-time or joint clinical appointments.
- Attend faculty development activities offered by your institution and program.
- Develop a network of faculty colleagues outside of your institution.
- Create a plan to achieve and maintain relevant certifications.

---

that faculty need strong programs of continuing education to remain current in their knowledge about emerging trends and adequately prepared to participate in curriculum development efforts. While van Schaik's comments were directed toward medical faculty, a similar case can be made for all health professions faculty. Inevitably, society and health care needs will eclipse what educators have had experience with in their own education, meaning that a commitment to continuing development is essential throughout the length of their academic career.

As you enter the academic environment and are no longer immersed in clinical practice full time, it can become a challenge to stay up to date with emerging health care trends. At the same time, you are now working in the higher education environment, which has its own set of unfamiliar issues you are discovering. As a faculty, you will want to proactively consider strategies to stay current in the faculty role while maintaining your competence in clinical practice. Box 1.3 includes a list of suggested strategies that may be helpful to developing a plan for remaining current in one's clinical practice while teaching.

Educator Competencies Related to Curriculum Development

Curriculum development in the health professions is a complex activity requiring the contributions of many to produce and maintain a relevant curriculum. Some faculty may lead the design process. Others help develop effective evaluation strategies to determine if the curriculum is working as it is intended. All faculty implement the curriculum as planned at the course level. Novice educators also provide ongoing feedback and reviews of courses to contribute to the curriculum development process. As someone who is new to the process, novice faculty may provide valuable insight as to how the curriculum meets current clinical practice standards and to underscore the clarity, or lack of clarity, of academic policies.

There are a core set of competencies associated with curriculum development. The National League for Nursing (NLN) established core competencies for nurse educators in 2005 (most recent revision in 2020 by Christensen & Simmons), including competencies that addressed curriculum development. While these core competencies were developed for nurse educators, the competencies themselves were drawn from evidence-based literature contained in databases from the psychology, sociology, allied health, medicine, social work, and nursing professions (Christensen & Halstead, 2019). Thus the competencies have relevance for other health professions educators.

From the comprehensive set of NLN core competencies (Christensen & Simmons, 2020) some basic curriculum competencies can be derived for new educators to focus on acquiring during their first 1 to 2 years of teaching. Those competencies can be organized into four overarching themes: (1) competencies related to the context of the institution/program's mission and professional discipline, (2) competencies related to having knowledge of the various elements that make up the curriculum, (3) competencies related to curriculum evaluation, and (4) competencies related to stakeholder collaboration (Box 1.4). This handbook introduces readers to the competencies associated with each of these themes. Do not be discouraged if it takes time to feel comfortable doing "curriculum work." Intentionally seek out opportunities to develop and increase your understanding of these core curriculum competencies, and your proficiency in curriculum development will continue to grow.

BOX 1.4 ■ Expected Novice Educator Competencies Related to Curriculum Development

Competencies Related to Context of Mission and Discipline

- Understands how the curriculum supports the stated mission of the institution and program, and practice role for which the learner is being prepared
- Develops and revises curriculum based on current knowledge regarding health care trends, discipline-specific issues, community and societal needs, and learner needs
- Demonstrates an awareness of the impact of cultural inclusivity on curriculum development

Competencies Related to Knowledge of Curriculum Elements

- Demonstrates knowledge of curriculum theory, educational theories, and principles to form the foundation of curriculum design
- Possesses knowledge of how to identify and write curricular elements: program outcomes, competencies, course syllabi, learning outcomes, and learning activities

Competencies Related to Curriculum Evaluation

- Uses assessment and evaluation strategies to determine curriculum effectiveness in achieving expected program outcomes
- Participates in program evaluation efforts
- Participates in fostering a culture of continuous quality improvement to maintain relevance and effectiveness of curriculum

Competencies Related to Stakeholder Collaboration

- Demonstrates an awareness of the change process as applied to curriculum revision
- Works collaboratively with all stakeholders to participate in curriculum development and revision activities
- Forms partnerships with external stakeholders to implement all aspects of the curriculum

The first competency area is related to the institution/program's mission and your professional discipline. For example, how does the curriculum support the stated mission of the institution and program? How is the curriculum designed to support a learner in achieving outcomes in preparation to practice as a physical therapist, nurse, dental hygienist, or other field? Faculty need to learn how to develop and revise curriculum that is based on current knowledge regarding health care trends, discipline-specific professional issues, community and societal needs, and learner needs. This requires faculty remain familiar with how your discipline is evolving in its practice expectations so that the curriculum faculty design remains forward looking and does not become outdated. In addition, faculty want to demonstrate an awareness of the importance of developing a curriculum that is culturally inclusive, recognizing the rich diversity of learners and addressing the unique learning needs of all.

The second competency area is related to expanding knowledge of the various elements that make up the curriculum and how to develop them. For example, faculty need to understand the role of program outcomes, leveled competencies, course syllabi, learning outcomes at the course level, and learning activities. You will also want to familiarize yourself with the curriculum, educational theories, and learning principles that form the foundation of curriculum design. These theories guide the decisions that faculty make regarding how to construct the curriculum.

The third competency area that is essential to understanding curriculum development is learning how to evaluate the effectiveness of the curriculum. To maintain a relevant curriculum, it is important for faculty to foster a culture of continuous quality improvement within the program and engage in evaluation activities that allow faculty to measure curricular outcomes and revise the curriculum as needed. You will be expected to participate in program evaluation activities with your initial responsibilities associated with evaluating the courses you are assigned to teach. To engage in course evaluation activities, faculty must be competent in using assessment and evaluation strategies to determine if their course is successful in helping learners achieve expected program outcomes.

The fourth competency area for educators to develop is how to effectively collaborate with the various stakeholders who are vested in the success of the program. For example, stakeholders may include students, faculty peers, clinical practice partners, community leaders, and professional organizations. As faculty debate the continued relevance of the program's curriculum and the need for revision they will want to seek the input of these stakeholders. Faculty collaborate with stakeholders as they engage in curriculum revision activities, so developing teamwork and collaborative skills is essential for engaging in curriculum work. Faculty often form partnerships with external stakeholders to implement the curriculum as designed, especially in the clinical teaching areas. Finally, since curriculum is dynamic and always in need of regularly scheduled review, faculty need to become familiar with the change process as it is applied to curriculum revision.

TABLE 1.1 ■ **Self-Assessment of Competencies Related to Curriculum Development**

Consider to what extent you feel comfortable performing the following competencies, then check the appropriate box. After you complete the checklist, develop a plan to gain skill in the competencies in which you have less experience. Share your plan with your mentor for additional feedback.

Educator Competency	I Have No Experience	I Have Some Experience	I Have Much Experience
Understands how the curriculum supports the stated mission of the institution and program, and the practice role for which the learner is being prepared			
Develops and revises curriculum based on current knowledge regarding health care trends, discipline-specific issues, community and societal needs, and learner needs			
Demonstrates an awareness of the impact of cultural inclusivity on curriculum development			
Demonstrates knowledge of curriculum theory, educational theories, and principles to form the foundation of curriculum design			
Possesses knowledge of how to identify and write curricular elements: program outcomes, competencies, course syllabi, learning outcomes, and learning activities			
Uses assessment and evaluation strategies to determine curriculum effectiveness in achieving expected program outcomes			
Participates in program evaluation efforts			
Participates in fostering a culture of continuous quality improvement to maintain relevance and effectiveness of curriculum			
Demonstrates an awareness of the change process as applied to curriculum revision			
Works collaboratively with all stakeholders to participate in curriculum development and revision activities			
Forms partnerships with external stakeholders to implement all aspects of the curriculum			

To increase one's skill with curriculum work, you will find it helpful to conduct a self-assessment of your competence in curriculum development. Table 1.1 provides a listing of curriculum competencies for novice educators. Take the time to evaluate your experience level with each competency, review your self-assessment, and create a plan to increase your competence in the various areas. It may be helpful to consult with a mentor or your supervisor to better understand the areas in need of improvement and prioritize the self-improvement activities that will be most beneficial. With focused effort on improving your skill set, you will find you enjoy working with students and colleagues to design and implement an effective curriculum.

Chapter Summary

This chapter introduced the competencies related to curriculum development and how to prepare yourself to participate in curriculum discussions. The following are key points to consider as you prepare to become a participant in your program's curriculum development work:

- Understanding the curriculum development process in place in your institution and program is an important first step to participating in curriculum work. Set aside time to gather the information listed in Box 1.1, consider how it applies to your assigned courses, and meet with your mentor to discuss any questions you may have.

- Developing curriculum is a faculty responsibility. As a faculty member you will be expected to regularly participate in the ongoing curriculum development activities that take place in your program. These activities may occur at either the course level or the program level. Box 1.2 identifies the faculty responsibilities associated with curriculum development that are essential to fulfilling the faculty role.

- Developing and maintaining a relevant curriculum requires faculty to stay current in their knowledge of professional issues occurring in their discipline, health care trends, societal needs, and higher education needs. Health professions faculty also need to maintain the clinical skills needed to be effective role models for students. Review the strategies suggested for staying current (see Box 1.3) and select two to three strategies to get started with a plan for staying up to date in your teaching role.

- Engaging in curriculum evaluation activities allows you to measure the effectiveness of the curriculum in achieving expected student learning outcomes. Faculty will be expected to evaluate the effectiveness of the courses they are assigned to teach. To engage in course evaluation activities you will want to become competent in using assessment and evaluation strategies. Seek out opportunities to increase your knowledge of evaluation strategies appropriate for the courses you are teaching.

- Becoming comfortable with the change process as applied to curriculum development is a valuable skill to develop as a faculty member. Do a literature search and seek out articles on how to successfully navigate change and remain a productive contributor to your program's curriculum development and revision activities.

- Staying current in your discipline knowledge is a critical step in maintaining your confidence as a teacher. Consider ways that you can remain knowledgeable and current about your discipline, societal needs, health care, and educational trends. Outline a plan to follow that will keep you informed so that you in turn can keep the curriculum and your courses up to date.

- Understanding the term academic freedom and how it impacts your teaching role is important. Review your institutional faculty handbook and read any sections related to academic freedom. How is it defined by your institution? How does that definition differentiate academic freedom from your responsibilities pertaining to curriculum development?

References

American Association of University Professors. (1940). *Statement of principles on academic freedom and tenure*. https://www.aaup.org/report/1940-statement-principles-academic-freedom-and-tenure

Christensen, L., & Halstead, J. (2019). The influence of the core competencies for nurse educators: 2005-2015. In J. Halstead (Ed.), *NLN core competencies for nurse educators: A decade of influence.* National League for Nursing.

Christensen, L., & Simmons, L. (2020). *The scope of practice for academic nurse educators and academic clinical nurse educators* (3rd ed.). National League for Nursing.

O'Riordan, F. (2018). Curriculum development discourse and practice. In G. Craddock (Ed.), *Transforming our world through design, diversity and education.* Open Access/IOS Press.

van Schaik, S. M. (2021). Accessible and adaptable faculty development to support curriculum reform in medical education. *Academic Medicine, 96*(4), 495–500. https://doi.org/10.1097/ACM.0000000000003804

CHAPTER 2

Getting Started With Curriculum Development

Curriculum development is a dynamic, ongoing process that faculty engage in regularly as part of their faculty responsibilities. As a new faculty member you will be expected to participate in curricular discussions and understand how the discussions and resulting decisions affect the courses you are assigned to teach. If you have not had formal academic preparation in curriculum development, then you may wish to consider taking coursework (academic or continuing education) to increase your knowledge of curriculum development, implementation, and evaluation. However, there are other steps that you can take to increase your knowledge of the curriculum development process at your institution and prepare to be an active and informed participant in curriculum discussions.

This chapter addresses steps you can take in your first year of teaching to prepare to participate in the curriculum development process. These initial steps include (1) understanding your institution/program's formal curriculum development process, (2) knowing the key players leading curriculum development in your institution/program, (3) articulating the institution/program's mission and philosophy, (4) understanding how your courses fit within the curriculum, (5) reading the program's curriculum policies and applying them to your courses, and (6) reviewing the program's curriculum evaluation plan. Appendix A contains a listing of documents to gather and review as part of your teaching responsibilities related to participating in curriculum development.

Understanding Your Institution/Program's Curriculum Development Process

Internal and external institutional stakeholders have a role in determining academic degree curricula. All higher education institutions and programs have specific policies and committees in place to govern the curriculum development process. In the case of public institutions of higher education, state legislatures and higher education commissions may also determine the total number of credit hours that can be awarded in undergraduate academic degrees and hold approval rights over the type of degrees offered by the institution. For programs in which graduates are required to sit for professional licensure or certification to practice in their chosen discipline, regulatory boards (e.g., boards of nursing, occupational therapy) may also prescribe curriculum standards. Accrediting agencies can also influence curriculum at both the institutional and program levels.

Within the institution the faculty hold primary responsibility for the curriculum and determine the plan of study, allocate credit hours, and set course requirements for any given degree (American Association of University Professors, 1966/1990). Understanding the role of these various stakeholders in the curriculum development and approval process is essential; the number of stakeholders involved in approving curricula can be significant with predetermined timelines for review of the proposed curricula. This is one reason that seeking curriculum approval for new programs or courses is often a lengthy process within an institution. As a new faculty it is important to appreciate the fact that curriculum development is a collaborative process requiring faculty to work across several committees and approval bodies. While faculty hold responsibility for curriculum development, it is a collective responsibility and rarely something that a single faculty member can accomplish without the input and eventual approval of other stakeholders.

The curriculum plan of study for any undergraduate degree program consists of two categories: the general education curriculum and the discipline-specific curriculum. The general education requirements of an institution are set by the faculty of the institution, typically by an institution-level general education curriculum committee that consists of representatives from all the major academic divisions within the institution. In public institutions of higher education, state government may also influence general education credit hours and the transfer of credits across public institutions. The general education requirements adopted by the institution must be met by all undergraduate students regardless of academic major to earn the degree from the institution.

When developing a plan of study for specific degrees faculty must incorporate the general education courses into the overall curriculum. If the institution modifies the required general education curriculum, faculty ensure the academic majors comply with the changes. While graduate degree programs do not have general education requirements, most institutions that offer graduate degrees also have a graduate curriculum committee at the institutional level that sets academic policies for all academic graduate programs. In addition to the general education courses required by the institution, health professions programs also require courses in the basic sciences and humanities, which will need to be factored into the plan of study.

The faculty of an academic program hold the responsibility for designing the discipline knowledge-specific part of the curriculum that students need to complete to earn the degree. Most academic programs have a curriculum committee at the program level that approves curriculum changes related to discipline-specific courses. Depending on the governing structure within which your program is situated, there may also be curriculum committees at the department or school levels. In the cases of small programs that have few faculty, all the faculty may serve as a "committee of the whole" to develop the curriculum.

As a new faculty you will be asked to participate in the development of the discipline-specific curriculum.

Knowing the Key Players in Curriculum Development in Institution and Program

Once you understand the curriculum development and approval processes that are in place in your institution and program, you will want to identify the key players and the roles they play in these processes. This can vary significantly based on the size of the institution and program.

The membership of institutional curriculum committees is usually made up of representation as determined by the institution's governance structure and how academic programs are organized within the institution. Representatives on curriculum committees at the institutional level are either elected by their colleagues or appointed by the administration of each academic department. The academic department's representative to the institution curriculum committee provides regular updates about the committee's actions and seeks input from faculty about issues that have been brought before the committee. The institutional representative can be a source of information for you regarding the process associated with obtaining course approvals within the institution.

At the program level there may be several faculty who play formal roles in curriculum development and implementation. If your program has a curriculum committee, you should familiarize yourself with who is responsible for chairing and serving on the committee, and how the committee's membership is structured. If your program has small enough numbers of faculty who are all expected to serve on the curriculum committee, you will automatically be involved in curriculum discussions and decisions, even as a new faculty. Other programs elect faculty representatives to serve on the curriculum committee. These representatives may be elected as course representatives, level or year representatives, or department representatives. Program level curriculum committees typically have the responsibility for developing curriculum policies, approving the curricular plan of study for degrees and courses, as well as changes to the existing curriculum. The curriculum committee may also be charged with overseeing evaluation of the curriculum. Following approval by the committee, any curriculum proposals or policy recommendations are forwarded on to the faculty committee for overall approval by the faculty.

If you teach in a large program in which there are multiple faculty assigned to teach various sections of the same course, you may also have an appointed course leader who is responsible for coordinating the teaching of the course. The course leader brings the course faculty together to discuss course issues and to ensure consistency in learning experiences across the courses. If you have a course leader assigned to the courses you teach, that individual will be the one you go to when you have questions about the curriculum and your course or student issues that may arise as you teach the course.

Articulating the Mission and Philosophy of the Institution and Program

In higher education there are many factors that influence curriculum development at institution and academic program levels. However, one of the most influential factors that provides a foundation upon which the curriculum will be built is the stated mission and philosophy of the institution. The mission statement provides direction for faculty, staff, and administrators as they make decisions about academic program offerings and the teaching-learning environment that is created for students.

The mission of a higher education institution is a public statement of the institution's purpose for existing (Valiga, 2020). It addresses the goals the institution intends to achieve, how it serves its constituency, and the values it espouses as related to the teaching/learning enterprise. Mission statements vary depending on the type of institution. For example, higher education institutions may be research intensive providing doctoral degrees and located in academic health centers. They may be 4-year liberal arts colleges or community colleges primarily offering associate degrees.

How institutions are funded can also differentiate the mission of the institution as they can be public institutions that receive state funding and are expected to primarily serve the state's citizens, or private institutions deriving their funding from nongovernmental sources. The institutions may be nonprofit or for-profit. Some institutions are specialized, offering a singular education focus (e.g., law, engineering, health care). Other institutions primarily serve specific populations such as faith-based institutions, historically Black colleges and universities, and tribal universities and colleges. The type and nature of the institution will influence the mission statement. The curriculum will be influenced by the mission of the institution. For example, a research-intensive institution may demonstrate a commitment to providing research opportunities to all students. A faith-based institution may require coursework that reflects faith-based values. An institution that has close community-based ties may emphasize service-learning experiences for students.

The mission of the institution influences the program's stated mission, as it is expected that academic programs align their mission with their institution's mission. This will inevitably affect the curriculum design of the academic programs. In the health care profession disciplines, faculty design curriculum that integrates institutional and program mission values into mission-driven, value-based learning outcomes that apply to health care practice.

Your program may have a stated philosophic statement that outlines the values and beliefs that the program faculty hold and use to guide curriculum development, implementation, and program decision making. Philosophic statements draw upon the institution's mission and values as well as the professional values of the respective discipline. While mission statements represent the purposes of the institution and program, philosophic statements express the beliefs and values that guide faculty as they strive to achieve the purposes of the institution and program. There are several core concepts that

---

> **BOX 2.1** ■ **Examples of Core Concepts in Philosophical Statements**
>
> - Health and well-being
> - Discipline-specific professional values
> - Societal and environmental contexts
> - Beliefs and values about human beings
> - Education
> - Teaching and learning
>
> _____
>
> Adapted from Valiga, T. (2020). Philosophical foundations of the curriculum. In D. Billings & J. Halstead (Eds.), *Teaching in nursing: A guide for faculty* (6th ed., pp. 135–146). Elsevier.

---

are commonly found in philosophic statements (Valiga, 2020). Box 2.1 provides a list of concept examples. The philosophic statement elaborates on the beliefs that faculty hold for each of these concepts.

It is important for all faculty to understand the stated mission of your institution and program. Ideally you will have reviewed the mission statements prior to accepting your faculty position as doing so helps ensure that it fits with the mission and your own personal philosophy regarding education, teaching, and learning in a health professions discipline. If you have not previously had the chance to review the mission statements of your institution and program, take the time now. Look at the example of concepts in Box 2.1, then critically read your mission statements to identify key concepts that are defined in those statements and consider how those concepts can be applied to your practice as a health profession educator.

Understanding How Your Courses Fit Within the Curriculum

The various courses that make up the program's curriculum are interrelated and serve as progressive building blocks for student learning. For a curriculum to remain coherent and cohesive for the learners, faculty need to understand how the courses they teach facilitate the achievement of student learning outcomes across the curriculum. While faculty are assigned the responsibility to teach certain courses, it is important for the faculty to realize their courses are an integral part of the bigger curriculum design; as such, they are not free to substantively alter courses without going through the curriculum approval process.

Box 2.2 provides an overview of information that will help you orient yourself to the placement of your course within the curriculum. You can seek this information by reviewing curriculum sequencing plans and course syllabi, reviewing policies related to the curriculum, and making a list of questions to ask your leadership, mentors, and colleagues. Reviewing this information is one of the first activities you should engage in when you receive your teaching assignment and before you enter the classroom and meet your students on the first day of class. Having this knowledge will prepare you to understand what the students have already learned and what outcomes they will need to demonstrate to successfully complete your courses and progress in the curriculum.

BOX 2.2 ■ Understanding Your Course's Placement Within the Curriculum

- Review the general education course requirements for your program's curriculum. Note the total credit hours assigned to general education courses and the placement of the general education courses throughout the curriculum sequencing plan.
  - Which general education courses will the students have taken before they enroll in your course?
  - What knowledge can you anticipate students will bring with them from their general education courses to apply to their learning in your course?
- Note the course sequencing plan and total credit hours assigned to the discipline-related courses.
  - Where in the sequence plan is your course situated?
  - What foundational discipline knowledge have students acquired prior to enrolling in your course?
  - What knowledge, skill, and values do you need to introduce your learners to, to facilitate their success in courses they will take following your course?
- Determine if your course has any prerequisite courses or corequisite courses that you will want to reference in your course.
- Validate the total number of credit hours for your course and how those credit hours translate in weekly contact (clock) hours.
  - Didactic courses typically have a 1:1 ratio of credit/contact hours, thus 3 credit hours of coursework translates into 3 hours of classroom contact.
  - If you are teaching a clinical course, clarify the credit hour to contact hour ratio established for your program. For example, if the ratio is a 1:3 ratio of credit/contact hours, and your clinical course is a 3-credit hour course, that translates into 9 contact hours/ weekly throughout the semester.
  - If your course may also be a combination of didactic and clinical hours, you would need to allocate weekly contact hours accordingly.

Applying Curriculum Policies to Your Courses

Reading the policies that guide the development and implementation of curriculum for your program is another key activity for you as you prepare to teach your courses. These policies outline the procedures to follow as you interact with students, administer tests, and assign grades. They also can provide guidance about how to propose course revisions. Student handbooks are another source of policy that you will need to be familiar with, as you will be responsible for holding students accountable for following all student policies that relate to implementation of the curriculum.

Each program has its own unique set of curriculum and student policies. Box 2.3 provides a list of some common curriculum and student program elements that are guided by policy. Many programs maintain an online database of policy handbooks for ease of access by faculty and students. If not in electronic form, they are likely available in hard copy. Confirm your access to these policies. As you review the list in Box 2.3, find the corresponding policy for your program. Ask your administrator, mentor, or colleagues if there are additional policies for which you need to be familiar.

BOX 2.3 ■ Examples of Policies Impacting Curriculum Development and Implementation

- Revision of course title, course description, course outcomes, and course credit hours
- Credit hour/clock hour ratios for didactic and clinical courses
- Institution and program grading scales
- Faculty office hours schedules
- Required course evaluation methods at institution and program levels
- Selection of required textbooks in discipline-specific courses
- Test administration and review procedures
- Classroom/clinical attendance and tardiness
- Student attire in classroom and clinical settings
- Implementation of Americans with Disabilities Act (ADA) in classroom and clinical settings
- Student academic integrity
- Incivility in the classroom and clinical setting
- Student grievances
- Student remediation
- Academic progression in the program

Reviewing Your Program's Curriculum Evaluation Plan

For your program's curriculum to remain current and integrated as a whole, faculty must commit to regular review and evaluation of the curriculum's integrity and effectiveness. Most programs have systematic program evaluation plans that include the timelines for regular evaluation of the curriculum. Faculty are responsible for completing the evaluation plan components that apply to their courses. Many programs have annual faculty meetings where they discuss the curriculum evaluation data and recommend curriculum revisions to address any areas of concern.

Box 2.4 identifies the most common areas of curriculum evaluation. A variety of evaluation methods are typically used to gather data about curriculum effectiveness, such as quantitative methods (e.g., surveys, Likert scales) and

---

BOX 2.4 ■ Curriculum Evaluation Elements

- End-of-program curriculum outcomes
- Curriculum link to institution/program mission and philosophy
- Integration of major curricular concepts, professional standards
- Curriculum framework design
- Course, level, and program outcomes
- Variety and effectiveness of teaching and learning strategies
- Achievement of student learning outcomes (individual and aggregate)
- Relevance of general education courses to the major discipline
- Evaluation of teaching effectiveness
- Student and peer evaluation of teaching strategies
- Adequacy of learning resources
- Classroom and clinical assessment of student learning
- Classroom and clinical evaluation strategies
- Effective use of technology by faculty and students

qualitative methods (e.g., focus groups, exit interviews). Ideally, the program's systematic evaluation plan outlines established timelines and data collection strategies, identifies those responsible for gathering and analyzing data, and disseminates findings to the faculty to aid in decision making. All faculty participate in these evaluation efforts. Seek out your program's systematic evaluation plan and review the portion of the plan that is related to curriculum. Chapter 5 discusses curriculum evaluation in greater detail.

BOX 2.5 ■ Preparing Yourself to Participate in Curriculum Development

- Thoughtfully consider and write down your beliefs about the teaching-learning process.
  - Do your personal beliefs align with the philosophic beliefs of your program?
  - How do you see these beliefs informing your decisions about the curriculum?
- Familiarize yourself with the curriculum design of your program.
  - How many credit hours do the students take? In what order are the courses sequenced?
  - How do the courses you are assigned to teach integrate into this design? Understand the curriculum of the program you are teaching in and how your course is integrated into and supports the implementation of the curriculum.
- Read the course syllabi for the courses you have been assigned to teach.
  - Note the course objectives, learning activities, and evaluation strategies.
  - Note if your course is a prerequisite for other courses in the curriculum; if so, familiarize yourself with the syllabi of those courses as well.
  - Write down any questions you have so that you can raise them with the appropriate individuals.
- Do a literature search on assessing student learning and how to evaluate course effectiveness.
  - Select some articles to read to build your knowledge base related to assessment and evaluation, especially at the course level.
- Locate and read the curriculum policies for your program.
  - How do these policies apply to the courses you have been assigned to teach?
  - How do these policies impact the students that you teach?
  - What is your role in implementing the policies?

Chapter Summary

This chapter introduced steps you can take in your first year of teaching to prepare yourself for participating in the curriculum development process. Key points to consider as you prepare yourself to be a participant in the curriculum discussions taking place in your program include the following:

- Familiarizing yourself with the curriculum development and approval processes in place in your institution and program and determining your role in those processes is the first step toward becoming a knowledgeable participant in curriculum development.
- Identifying the key players in the curriculum development and evaluation process and seeking out their guidance to increase your understanding of your faculty responsibilities related to curriculum development is also key.
- Understanding how the courses you teach contribute to the curriculum's integrity helps you appreciate that how you teach and evaluate your courses may impact the student learning outcomes of other courses.
- Reviewing and thoughtfully considering the questions in Box 2.5 will serve as a useful primer to preparing yourself to effectively teach your assigned courses.

References

American Association of University Professors. (1966/1990). *Statement of government of colleges and universities.* https://www.aaup.org/report/statement-government-colleges-and-universities

Valiga, T. (2020). Philosophical foundations of the curriculum. In D. Billings & J. Halstead (Eds.), *Teaching in nursing: A guide for faculty* (6th ed., pp. 135–146). Elsevier.

CHAPTER 3

Key Components of Curriculum Development

As the curriculum is the responsibility of the faculty, it is important for you to understand how the curriculum development process works and the various elements of the curriculum. Ideally faculty work collaboratively to produce a logically sequenced curriculum that provides student learning experiences that are thoughtfully designed to progressively lead learners toward the achievement of preestablished program outcomes. In all health professions disciplines, the goal of the curriculum is to produce safe, competent practitioners who are prepared to deliver patient care in various health care settings. There are many variables that can affect the curriculum development process.

The purpose of this chapter is to introduce readers to the key elements that make up the so-called curriculum and provide a step-by-step guide that can be used to help faculty craft a curriculum that is relevant and successful in producing competent graduates. Let's start the discussion with an overview of the professional issues currently affecting curriculum development in health professions programs.

Professional Issues Affecting Curriculum Development in Health Professions Programs

Professional issues internal and external to a specific health profession discipline can influence curriculum development. The education of health professionals has been a source of debate within the health professions, resulting in some calls to action. For example, the Institute of Medicine (IOM), which is now the National Academy of Medicine (NAM), published a report in 2001 called *Crossing the Quality Chasm*. In this publication the IOM called for changes in health care delivery that would improve quality of care, including a vision for 21st-century education for health care professionals. The report described the relationship between education and the quality of patient care delivered by practitioners, resulting in a call to identify how health care professionals can most effectively learn the competencies necessary for safe, competent practice (IOM, 2001).

The *Quality Chasm* was followed by the IOM's 2003 report, *Health Professions Education: A Bridge to Quality.* In this writing, which was generated by experts from medicine, nursing, allied health, and pharmacy, the IOM stated that health professions education lacked an evidence base and that teaching in the health professions was guided by personal beliefs and opinions and dominated by intuition and tradition instead of scholarly inquiry. The report asserted that there was a need for the health professions to focus on allocating resources to develop an evidence base about what should be emphasized in health professions education and what should be eliminated. The IOM (2003) identified five core competencies for all health care professionals that health professions programs should incorporate into their program curricula: (1) patient-centered care, (2) interdisciplinary work, (3) evidence-based practice, (4) quality improvement, and (5) informatics. While these two influential IOM reports are now 2 decades old, the identification of the five core competencies had a profound impact on curriculum development in health professions and remain seminal works in health professions education. More recently IOM produced reports on the future of nursing (IOM, 2010; NAM, 2021) that have influenced education and curriculum development in the profession.

These are just a few examples of how forces external to your specific discipline can influence the professional discussions that occur within the discipline and subsequently the program's curriculum development efforts. Other entities that can impact curriculum include the discipline's licensing board, professional organizations, and accrediting agencies. Professional standards and guidelines, such as the core competencies for the Interprofessional Education Collaborative (IPEC, 2016), also influence how curriculum is designed. Faculty regularly engage in periodic environmental scans of relevant organizations, regulatory bodies, and other entities to remain aware of emerging reports that have the potential to impact a program's curriculum.

Examples of other professional issues that can impact curriculum development efforts include workforce shortages and faculty shortages and calls for innovative approaches to curriculum implementation to continue educating the number of needed graduates. Changing student demographics and learning needs, as well as the emphasis on student-centered, active learning strategies can influence curriculum development. The constantly changing health care environment and increasing integration of technology in both patient care settings and educational settings are further examples of issues that influence how faculty develop and implement curriculum. Selecting the appropriate pedagogic strategies for teaching the curriculum and designing relevant learning assignments are key components to the curriculum and directly influence how faculty teach their courses.

This preliminary discussion of professional issues illustrates the importance of staying abreast of the emerging trends and issues impacting one's discipline to fully participate in curriculum development. For curriculum development efforts to be relevant, faculty must be fully engaged and understand current professional issues.

The Purpose of Curriculum

The purpose of the curriculum is to facilitate the learner in achieving identified goals and outcomes. As such, the curriculum consists of selected concepts and learning experiences that have been sequenced in a series of courses to form a program of study leading to the achievement of end-of-program outcomes. It is the responsibility of the faculty to determine the essential concepts and learning experiences necessary to achieve the identified outcomes, and to select settings (context) in which the students' learning will take place. In addition, the faculty must make these decisions with an understanding of the resources that will be required to fully implement the curriculum as designed.

You can envision the curriculum to be an educational roadmap (Sullivan, 2020) with a sequence of learning experiences that lead to the final destination of graduation when the desired educational outcomes have been achieved. The curriculum is organized within a framework that consists of several elements designed to facilitate learner acquisition of the knowledge, skills, and attributes required to graduate from the program.

DEVELOPING THE CURRICULUM FRAMEWORK

A curriculum framework provides how the curriculum is conceptualized. A well-designed framework logically organizes the teaching and learning of the requisite knowledge, skills, and attributes of a competent health care professional into a coherent, meaningful structure. Faculty use the framework as a guide to help in the design, implementation, and evaluation of student learning experiences. To maintain curricular integrity, faculty must work collectively to implement the curriculum. The use of a curriculum framework provides direction to the faculty so that all teaching efforts are focused on achieving the same outcomes, thus preserving the integrity of the curriculum.

Box 3.1 lists the elements that comprise the curriculum framework. This chapter discusses each of these interrelated elements, providing a step-by-step guide as to how faculty can most effectively develop these individual components into an integrated, systematically organized and coherent curriculum. While there are various methods by which to design a curriculum, the most logical starting point is to begin with where you want your graduates to end up (i.e., with the achievement of the program outcomes). To continue the curriculum roadmap analogy, faculty must recognize the destination before they can map out how to facilitate students reaching that destination. Program outcomes represent the destination of your program's curriculum. Program outcomes must be consistent with the program's

---

BOX 3.1 ■ Curriculum Framework Elements

- Mission Statement
- Philosophy Statement
- Conceptual (Organizing) Framework
- End-of-Program Outcomes
- Competencies
- Course Outcomes (Objectives)
- Learning Experiences
- Evaluation

mission and the faculty's philosophy statements and any conceptual (organizing) framework that may exist.

Mission and Philosophy Statements

The program's mission and philosophy statements (see Chapter 2) provide the foundation for the program's curriculum. The mission statement describes the purpose of the program and what it hopes to accomplish through its activities. The mission of the program also informs the faculty regarding the essential values and concepts that will be emphasized in the curriculum.

For example, consider the mission statement in Box 3.2 from a college of nursing and health professions. As you read the mission statement, make

---

BOX 3.2 ■ Examples of Program Mission and Vision Statements

Mission and Vision Statements

Mission

Deeply committed to health equity in Philadelphia and around the world, CNHP rigorously prepares nurses and health professionals for successful careers through experiential learning and interprofessional research that advance person and family-centered care in all settings and across the life course. Specifically, CNHP works towards greater health equity in Philadelphia and around the world by:

- Preparing nurses and health professionals to deliver interprofessional care and address the social and structural determinants that prevent many people, and particularly Black and Brown individuals and families, from attaining their full health potential
- Conducting needed, cross-cutting research on the core problems facing health care and health care systems with particular focus on health equity
- Providing high quality health services in the community that addresses social and structural determinants of health

Vision

Leading in interprofessional nursing and health profession education, research and clinical practice to assure health and wellness for everyone, everywhere
©Drexel University College of Nursing and Health Professions.

Vision Statement

The vision of Texas State University's College of Health Professions is to be recognized for educating healthcare professionals who can recognize, respond, and mitigate current and future healthcare challenges and disparities in our diverse society.

Mission Statement

The College of Health Professions educates and prepares healthcare professionals with innovative teaching, evidence based practice and principles, and a commitment to life-long learning in a student-centered environment. The College excels in teaching, clinical practice, scholarship, and service while responding to the diverse healthcare needs of the State of Texas, the nation, and the global community. The College unites faculty, students, communities, and consumers in coalitions to expand the body of knowledge in healthcare practice and management.

From Texas State University's College of Health Professions website. College of Health Professions Vision and Mission © 2017 Accessed July 28, 2022. https://www.health.txstate.edu/About/Vision-and-Mission.html

---

BOX 3.2 ■ Examples of Program Mission and Vision Statements (Continued)

Our Mission Statement

We continue the teaching and healing ministry of Jesus Christ by creating experiences that challenge our students to be competent and compassionate professionals serving local and global communities.

Our Vision Statement

We will create a learning environment that inspires our students to lead, to heal, to serve, bringing wholeness to the world.

Our Values Statement

We foster transformational experiences that inspire compassion, integrity, and excellence, which promote a culture of service.

From Loma Linda University website. School of Allied Health Professions Missions, Vision, and Values © 2022 Accessed June 28, 2022. Alliedhealthllu.edu/about/school-allied-health-professions-mission-vision-and-values

---

note of the context, concepts, and values identified in the statement. Based on this mission statement you may expect faculty to design a curriculum that emphasizes competence and compassion in the patient care delivered by graduates of the school's programs. Building curricula that is evidence based and effectively integrates technology is another guiding mission tenet. You would also expect to find concepts related to community-based practice, health care disparities, and improving health care outcomes integrated throughout the curriculum, supported by community-based clinical learning experiences.

Mission statements have implications for faculty as well. Based on this mission statement, faculty would be expected to design creative, innovative teaching strategies and to be engaged in interprofessional research. Take this opportunity to review your program's mission statement and identify the values, beliefs, and concepts that are embedded within the statement. Consider how the statement informs the curriculum development efforts of your program.

Philosophy statements (see Chapter 2) profess the beliefs and values related to core concepts that guide faculty in their teaching role. Not all programs have written philosophic statements. In some programs, faculty may have developed a vision statement and/or core values to guide their teaching. A vision statement differs from a mission statement or philosophy statement, in that the program's vision is aspirational and describes what the program wants to achieve (Valiga, 2020). To prepare for your teaching role, seek out the guiding beliefs and values that shape the program's curriculum by reviewing your program's vision, philosophy, and/or core values and considering how they will influence your teaching.

Conceptual (organizing) Frameworks

In addition to written philosophy statements, some health professions programs develop a conceptual framework, also known as an organizing framework, that builds on the core concepts identified in the philosophy statement by defining, organizing, and expanding on major curriculum concepts, as well as explaining the linkages between the concepts. The intent of the conceptual framework is to organize the curriculum for both faculty and students, moving the concepts from abstract representations to operational definitions upon which knowledge can be built.

Conceptual frameworks can be organized not only by concepts but also by the context for understanding and applying the concepts. Some curricula are organized to move from wellness to illness, simple to complex, or from health promotion and illness/disease prevention to acute care and chronic care of disease/illness. Environmental settings such as acute care, long-term care, rehabilitation, community health, and home care may also be organizing constructs within a curriculum. In some health care professions, conceptual frameworks can be organized using concepts from a singular theorist. More often the conceptual framework is eclectic, drawing its concepts from multiple theories.

There are several ways to approach the creation of a program's conceptual framework. Professional organizations for the health care disciplines may provide a conceptual framework for faculty to use as a guide, or faculty may develop their own. The overriding principle is that the conceptual framework must have meaning for the faculty and students and be aligned with the program's mission and the faculty's philosophy of teaching and learning related to the practice of their given discipline.

Essentially frameworks guide the faculty in making decisions on what to include in the curriculum and what not to include. Organizing concepts are defined for both the faculty and the students, and linkages among the concepts are explicated to guide the practice of the discipline (Sullivan, 2020). The framework is best focused on main concepts for clarity and ease of implementation. You will want to explore whether your program's curriculum is guided by a conceptual/organizing framework. If it is, review the concepts and how they are defined, then relate them to the courses you are assigned to teach.

Identifying Curriculum Outcomes for the Program

Curriculum program outcomes, also known as end-of-program outcomes, can be defined as statements that broadly represent what the graduates of your program have been prepared to do as they successfully complete the program's curriculum and assume their practice roles. The outcomes are the endpoint of the students' journey through the curriculum, and their achievement of the end-of-program outcomes indicates that they possess the practice competencies (knowledge, skills, and attributes) required of the role for which they have been prepared. Frequently health professions programs publicly disseminate their program's curriculum outcomes through websites, catalogues, or brochures and other printed materials so that stakeholders are informed as to what graduates of the program will be prepared to do when they complete the program.

In addition, the end-of-program outcomes are used to measure the effectiveness of the curriculum in achieving desired outcomes. Program stakeholders, such as employers and alumni, are often asked to measure how well graduates of the program are prepared to perform in clinical settings. Program evaluation seeks to measure if graduates demonstrate the end-of-program outcomes in their practice, typically measured 6 to 12 months postgraduation.

Every course in the curriculum is developed by the faculty to collectively lead to the achievement of the program's curriculum outcomes. Every learning experience is designed to facilitate learners' acquisition of required practice competencies. Therefore the end-of-program curriculum outcomes must be carefully crafted by faculty to reflect the desired knowledge, skills, and attributes each graduate will possess when they successfully complete the program.

Following the development of the mission and philosophy statements, and the conceptual/organizing framework, the next step in the curriculum development process is for faculty to determine the end-of-program curriculum outcomes. Without knowing what the expected end-of-program outcomes are, it is not possible to design a cohesive curriculum that will consistently produce the desired learning outcomes for all students. Having clearly written, clinically relevant program outcomes is critical to the curriculum development process, as the program outcome statements will guide faculty as they develop competency statements and design courses that will help students achieve the program outcomes. Let's talk about the process used to determine these important end-of-program outcomes.

DETERMINING END-OF-PROGRAM CURRICULUM OUTCOMES

As presented in this chapter, curriculum development is a process that begins with the establishment of the program's mission, philosophy, and conceptual framework, and then proceeds with faculty developing end-of-program expected outcomes, competency statements, and courses. At the course level faculty must also design learning experiences and determine how student achievement will be evaluated. Fig. 3.1 depicts an overview of this process beginning with the development of end-of-program outcomes and the order in which the process flows. Before beginning the development of end-of-program outcomes, the faculty should consider the flow of the process and how the end-of-program outcomes will guide development of the remaining curriculum.

First and foremost, to determine end-of-program outcomes the faculty need to answer the question, "What is the graduate of our program being prepared to do?" Yes, they are being prepared to be health care professionals in a specific health care discipline, but what unique set of behaviors will epitomize their practice? When viewed collectively, the end-of-program outcome statements identified by the faculty communicate to the public what can be expected from the program's graduates when they are employed in real-world practice settings.

The next question the faculty need to ask is, "What competencies must the student develop to achieve the desired program outcomes?" Competencies represent the knowledge, skills, and attributes (beliefs, values) that students need to acquire and demonstrate to successfully achieve the program outcomes. What

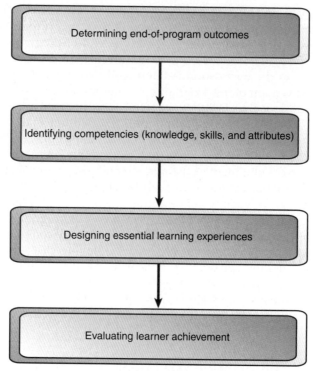

Fig. 3.1   Steps to the Curriculum Development Process

knowledge must the curriculum be designed to convey to students, so they emerge from the program as safe, competent practitioners? What skills do students need to demonstrate as they progress through the program? What professional attributes does the curriculum need to emphasize to support the formation of the students' professional values and identity as health care professionals in their chosen discipline? While the program outcomes are written to represent the expected destination, or end goal, of the curriculum, the competencies represent the path or road that will lead the students to reach that goal. Progressively and successfully demonstrating the identified competencies as integrated throughout the curriculum should lead students to achieving the expected program outcomes. Developing curriculum is a reiterative process, and outcome statements are closely aligned to the competencies that students will need to acquire.

Finally, after identifying the curriculum outcomes and accompanying competencies, faculty need to consider how to foster the students' ability to achieve the desired outcomes. What course-level learning experiences are essential to helping students acquire the identified outcomes and competencies? What methods will be used to evaluate students' individual and aggregate achievement of the competencies and program outcomes?

Determining end-of-program outcomes for the curriculum can be a challenging exercise for faculty, one that requires a fair amount of dialogue among

> **BOX 3.3 ■ Determining End-of-Program Outcomes: Questions for Faculty to Consider**
>
> - How does the program's philosophy and/or conceptual framework provide a context for the end-of-program outcomes?
> - What qualities and characteristics do faculty want graduates to demonstrate upon graduation?
> - What outcomes are consistent with practice needs in today's health care environment?
> - Why is the outcome important or critical to practice?

the faculty before the final set of outcomes is produced. But there are steps that faculty can take collectively to make the process an engaging one. Box 3.3 identifies some questions that faculty can consider to launch these discussions. One of the most productive ways to focus on these questions and begin the dialogue is to schedule a day or two in a comfortable setting, in which faculty are encouraged to set aside their usual teaching responsibilities and solely concentrate on the task of determining end-of-program outcomes that represent the qualities and characteristics that faculty want graduates to display in their practice.

Prior to the scheduled retreat days, faculty should participate in anticipatory activities to prepare them for the discussion. Reviewing the discipline's professional standards, guidelines, scope of practice regulations, national accreditation guidelines, seminal reports affecting health care and your discipline, and other influential literature informs faculty to align decisions with contemporary practice, and discipline-specific issues and trends, leading to evidence-based curriculum decisions. Grounding the discussions in the literature ensures that the program's outcomes are consistent with practice needs for today's complex health care environment and appropriate for the role for which graduates are being prepared. Faculty can also interview clinical practice partners, advisory committee members, and other stakeholders to get input on what behaviors and characteristics are expected in the practice setting for the delivery of competent care.

There are two caveats that faculty should keep in mind as they determine their program outcomes. First, as they begin to identify the end-of-program outcomes, faculty may question how many outcomes are needed. Secondly, faculty may question how often end-of-program outcomes should be reviewed and revised.

While there is no magic number to answer the question of how many outcomes a program should expect to have for its graduates, it may be tempting to create a comprehensive list. However, keep in mind that program outcomes represent the overall behaviors or characteristics that are important or critical to your graduates' practice; as such, they should be written at a macro level broad enough to encompass the many competencies the graduate will need to demonstrate while progressing throughout the program. Most programs can accomplish this with eight to ten well-written end-of-program outcomes. In addition, the outcomes should be written to withstand scrutiny over time, as it would become cumbersome to subject them to frequent revision. Making

---

BOX 3.4 ■ Example of End-of-Program Curriculum Outcomes

As a graduate of the BSN program, you will:

- Demonstrate intellectual engagement and use evidence as a basis for clinical reasoning and decision-making.
- Provide culturally sensitive, holistic, individual, family, community, and population-centered nursing care.
- Coordinate care and facilitate access to resources across the continuum of healthcare environments to meet the evolving needs of individuals, families, communities, and populations.
- Understand and consider the impact of healthcare policy, finance, and regulatory environments on care deliver.
- Practice in diverse healthcare environments with competence and professionalism.
- Embody the professional identity of the nurse who translates the inherent values of the nursing profession into the ethical and legal practice of nursing.
- Communicate effectively and collaborate with interprofessional team members, patients, and their support systems for improved health outcomes.
- Lead and manage while applying principles of systems, organizational processes, and balancing resources to promote quality care and patient safety.
- Embrace and employ innovations in information management and technology in the delivery of quality patient care.

(**Copyright** Indiana University School of Nursing, Indianapolis, IN)

---

significant changes in the program outcomes will necessitate other changes throughout the curriculum.

Box 3.4 provides an example of end-of-program outcomes for a baccalaureate nursing program. As written, these program outcomes will remain relevant for some time, as the expected behaviors referenced in the outcome statement will likely not change. Faculty expect their graduates to be safe practitioners, effective communicators, and to practice within a legal and ethical framework as outcomes of the program. However, the competencies may need revision and the nature of student learning experiences changed so that students continue to acquire the requisite knowledge, skills, and attributes for practice.

WRITING OUTCOME STATEMENTS

Once faculty have determined what the graduates of the program are being prepared to do, the next step is to write outcome statements that reflect those expected behaviors. The outcome statement should emphasize two elements: the expected graduate outcome and what will be accomplished when the outcome is met.

For example, let's say that your program faculty decided that one of your program's outcomes is to produce a graduate who is an effective communicator. Being an effective communicator is an essential skill for any health care professional, regardless of discipline, so it is common to see communication referenced as a program outcome. In writing the actual outcome statement, faculty address the question as to why graduates should be effective communicators. For what reason should graduates be effective communicators? The exemplar outcome statement found in Box 3.4 states the program has an expected outcome statement that asserts program graduates will be able to demonstrate they "communicate effectively and collaborate with interprofessional team members, patients, and their support systems for improved health outcomes" (Indiana University School of Nursing, 2021). The expected behavior is for the graduate to be an effective communicator in interprofessional clinical situations and to do so in a collaborative manner with other team members, patients, and their significant others. For what reason should graduates be effective communicators? The answer is "to improve the health outcomes of patients."

When program outcomes are written with an emphasis on the desired graduate behaviors or characteristics coupled with the reason for the individual to demonstrate these attributes in their practice, the outcome becomes a meaningful guide to the competencies that students need to develop to achieve these outcomes. With this understanding, faculty can design student learning experiences that will facilitate acquisition of the competencies and achievement of the expected program outcomes.

Box 3.5 identifies statements for faculty to thoughtfully consider to ensure they are crafting practice-relevant outcome statements for their program's graduates. The outcome statements should collectively express the faculty's informed and evidence-based beliefs about contemporary health care practice in their respective disciplines. Additionally, faculty will want to consider what students will need to do to achieve the expected outcomes. Does the outcome statement communicate expectations? Is it possible to identify the competencies that students need to acquire to achieve the outcome? Answering these questions helps faculty determine the competencies that students need to demonstrate by the end of the program and identify the learning experiences that need to be incorporated into the curriculum. Are the outcome statements measurable? Outcome statements need to be measurable so that faculty can assess and evaluate student achievement of the outcomes.

Given these questions, let's examine once again the outcome statement cited earlier that is related to being an effective communicator. The statement

---

BOX 3.5 ■ Getting Started: Writing End-of-Program Outcome Statements

When writing end-of-program outcome statements, the faculty should ensure that the statements:

- Reflect discipline and faculty beliefs and expectations for contemporary practice
- Describe the characteristics or behaviors that graduates should possess upon program completion
- Emphasize the desired impact of the outcome's identified behavior or characteristic of the graduate on practice of the profession
- Are measurable to determine successful outcome achievement
- Provide direction as to the competencies (K, S, A) students will need to acquire to achieve the outcome

indicates that graduates will be effective communicators who are collaborators in interprofessional teams. To determine what the students need to do to achieve this outcome by the end of the program, faculty must define the major concepts that are referenced in the statement. In this case, the concepts include communication, collaboration, and interprofessional teamwork. Ideally, if the program has a conceptual/organizing framework for the curriculum, the framework defines the major concepts in the curriculum and describes how the concepts are linked and interrelated. Understanding these conceptual links can guide faculty in their curriculum development activities.

Based on the concept's definitions, faculty proceed to the next step of determining what competencies the students need to acquire to achieve the expected outcomes. To measure and evaluate achievement related to outcome statements and the associated competencies, students need to have learning experiences integrated throughout the curriculum that provide opportunities to progressively develop and demonstrate they have acquired the necessary competencies. In this example, students will need to demonstrate their communication and collaboration skills, function in an interprofessional team, and interact with health care professionals, patients, and their significant others.

Developing Competency Statements Related to Program Outcomes

Once program outcomes have been determined, the faculty are ready to identify the competencies that students will need to acquire to achieve the outcomes. Competencies are written as behavioral statements that are student focused, leveled across the curriculum to the appropriate stage of student learning, and situated within the context or environment in which the student needs to demonstrate the competency. While the program outcomes represent the desired destination of the curriculum, competencies represent the mileage markers leveled across the curriculum. Achieving each competency level allows the student to progress along the curriculum pathway to achieve the program outcomes and graduate from the program.

Competency statements are written in measurable terms and are used to assess and evaluate student learning throughout the curriculum. Students who can demonstrate the competencies as expected continue to progress through the curriculum; however, if at some point in the curriculum students cannot demonstrate the expected competencies at the required level, then this will indicate the need for remediation or possible failure.

Competency behaviors encompass the three foundational domains of learning that students must develop to function as a competent professional in their chosen health care discipline. Students must acquire the knowledge of their discipline, demonstrate the skills required for safe practice, and incorporate the desired professional attributes (attitudes or values) into their practice. When writing the competency statements associated with each program outcome, faculty must address the essential knowledge, skills attributes, and attributes required to achieve the program outcomes. Overlooking any one of the domains when identifying the competencies can impact student learning and cause students to struggle in meeting the outcomes required to perform as competent health care professionals.

LEVELING COMPETENCY STATEMENTS

We often refer to the leveling of competencies across the curriculum. Leveling, applied to competencies, refers to the levels of knowledge, skills, and attributes related to a concept that are expected to be demonstrated by the students at different points in the curriculum. The learning outcomes that faculty expect of students vary depending on placement of the learning experience within the curriculum and level of competency that needs to be demonstrated. Competencies can be leveled by year, semester, and from course to course to ensure faculty expectations of student performance progress across the curriculum leading to achievement of end-of-program outcomes. The design and sequencing of the curriculum's courses is often how leveling of the competencies is achieved.

Once again, let's consider the program outcome related to being an effective communicator. The communication competencies expected of students who are in their first semester of study are less complex than what faculty will expect students to demonstrate in their final semester prior to graduation. The competency statements are scaffolded across the curriculum to reflect increasing difficulty and the students' progression in acquiring the knowledge, skills, and attributes related to being an effective communicator.

Additionally, competencies are frequently written to indicate the context within which each competency behavior will be demonstrated. For example, in the early stages of the curriculum, students may be expected to demonstrate competency in their care of one or two patients in an acute care setting under the direct supervision of their clinical instructor. In the later stages of the program, students may be expected to demonstrate competency in independently caring for multiple patients in more complex settings.

Written competency statements provide guidance as to the type of learning environment faculty must design to support students acquiring the expected level of knowledge, skills, and attributes. Competency statements also help faculty to select relevant evaluation measures to evaluate student learning associated with each competency.

Writing leveling competency statements and progressively leveling them is a time-consuming process that involves the entire faculty. It is important that all faculty are fully aware of what is expected of students at each level of the curriculum, so that appropriate learning experiences can be designed to support student attainment of the competencies and progression through the curriculum. If competencies are not progressively leveled, the students' ability to achieve the desired performance level by the end of the program may be hampered.

In many cases, health professional students must pass a licensure examination at the end of their program to demonstrate their competence and safety to practice. Programs that experience significant licensure examination failure by their graduates may not have leveled curriculum competencies or designed learning experiences that allow students to progressively demonstrate competence at the levels required to achieve professional licensure. We will come back to the concept of leveling competencies as we continue our discussion of how to write competency statements.

WRITING COMPETENCY STATEMENTS: LINKING COMPETENCIES TO OUTCOMES

To begin the process of writing competency statements, the faculty must carefully consider the program outcomes and identify the major concepts associated with each one. Each program outcome will undoubtedly have several competencies linked to it that students need to acquire to demonstrate the outcome by the end of the program. Box 3.6 outlines a process and sequence of activities that faculty may consider when writing the program's competency statements. While the activities are written linearly, in actual practice they may unfold in a more reiterative fashion through multiple faculty discussions. At the completion of this process, faculty should have a set of competencies identified for each program outcome that are ready to be integrated throughout the curriculum.

BOX 3.6 ■ Getting Started: Writing and Implementing Competency Statements

- Consider each end-of-program outcome and identify the *major* concepts addressed in each outcome statement.
- Ensure each major concept identified is clearly defined by the faculty to promote consistency in application across the curriculum, noting the definition in a curriculum glossary.
- For each defined concept identify the knowledge, skills, and attributes students will need to acquire to competently apply the concept to their practice as health care professionals by program completion.
- Begin the leveling process by identifying the behaviors or characteristics faculty expect students *to do or exhibit* using the knowledge, skills, and attributes associated with a concept, citing at what point in the curriculum and in what context students will be expected to demonstrate a defined level of competency (end of a year, end of a semester, end of a course, etc.).
- Design and scaffold learning experiences across the curriculum that support student demonstration of the competency, assigning the learning experiences to the appropriate course(s); not all competencies need to be addressed in all courses.
- Determine how the competency will be assessed and evaluated, selecting evaluation strategies that are appropriate to the learning experience and desired student learning.

Continuing with the previous example of a program outcome in which graduates will be effective communicators who are collaborators with interprofessional teams and patients to improve health care outcomes, let's begin to link the outcome to possible competency statements. As identified previously, major concepts associated with this outcome include communication, collaboration, and interprofessional teamwork. To develop competency statements linked to this program outcome, faculty need to identify the essential knowledge, skills, and attributes related to the major concepts of communication, collaboration, and interprofessional teamwork. As an example, Table 3.1 briefly outlines the possible types of knowledge, skills, and attributes students may need to develop their competence

TABLE 3.1 ■ Examples of Knowledge, Skills, and Attributes Related to Effective Communication

	Concept: Communication	Concept: Collaboration	Concept: Interpersonal Teamwork
Knowledge	- Communication process - Verbal communication - Nonverbal communication - Technology communication - Cultural implications - Patient education	- Definition of collaboration - Collaborative skills applied to health care - Negotiation - Conflict resolution	- Definition of interprofessional practice - Understand roles of health care professionals - Effective team-based care practices
Skills	- Therapeutic communication skills in the clinical setting - Listening skills - Interview/health assessment skills - Documenting patient care	- Clarity of written and oral communication with other providers and patients - Collaborative care strategies (rounds, huddles, etc.)	- Interact with other health care professionals to plan/implement/evaluate patient care
Attributes	- Empathy - Nonjudgmental - Respect - Confidentiality	- Mutual respect and trust - Value opinions of others	- Responsibility and accountability for own role in team - Respectful communication with team members

as effective communicators with collaborative skills on interprofessional teams. As you review the information in Table 3.1, can you think of additional content to add? As you review this example, consider how these concepts can be integrated into courses and leveled across the curriculum into competency statements.

The next step to consider is the context of the learning experiences that require students to demonstrate their competency as communicators. Health care professions are practice disciplines. Students need to demonstrate that they are effective communicators not only in the classroom but also in the clinical setting where they care for patients and interact in interprofessional health care teams. Box 3.7 provides an example of competency statements

BOX 3.7 ■ Examples of Course-Level Competency Statements Related to Communication in the Clinical Setting

- Functions proficiently within inter/intra professional teams to achieve quality patient care.
- Formulates individualized teaching plans for patients with complex alternations in health in collaboration with patients, families, and the inter/intra professional team.
- Demonstrates proficient use of technology and incorporation of evidence-based practices to support safe, effective, quality patient care.

From Ivy Tech Community College, Associate Degree Nursing Program, Indianapolis, IN, used with permission.

written for a clinical course that are related to effective communication in patient care situations.

It is clear from this one brief example that developing competency statements associated to each program outcome can become an expansive activity. For this reason, it is important for faculty to identify the critical, essential concepts and competencies required for safe practice and to resist the temptation to create exhaustive listings. Many health care professions have published standards and essential competencies for their discipline that faculty can use as guides for identifying major concepts and competencies for their curriculum. Accreditation standards and regulatory licensing bodies also provide invaluable guidance. Take the time to familiarize yourself with the professional standards and guidelines related to your discipline before participating in any curriculum development activities.

Course Design and Writing Course Outcomes

Following the development of program outcomes and competencies, the next step in the curriculum development process is to identify the courses that make up the curriculum and are used to integrate (or thread) the competencies across the curriculum, providing students with learning experiences needed to support the acquisition of the program's outcomes and competencies. The courses are organizing units of the curriculum, providing structure through which the curriculum will be implemented. Each course is designed to address one or more program outcomes and the related competencies. All required courses should have relevance to the program's end-of-program outcomes and competencies.

Course design begins with the faculty considering the relevance of each required course and how each course helps students develop the required knowledge, skills, and attributes of the profession and at what level. The sequencing of courses within the curriculum, prerequisite coursework, and the need for concurrent courses are factors for which faculty need to make decisions. Faculty determine the course title, description, and number of credit hours and develop the course outcomes (objectives). These course elements must be approved by the faculty following the institution's and program's curriculum approval processes.

The course description is typically written to briefly outline the main purpose or goal of the course, the major concepts to be taught, a broad overview of student learning experiences, and the context within which learning will occur. When reading the course description, it should be evident which program outcome(s) and competencies are to be addressed in the course.

The course outcomes (objectives) flow from the course description and are written to describe what students need to know and do, and the professional attributes they must exhibit, by the completion of the course. The course outcomes are aligned with the program's competency statements and used by faculty to guide the development of the course's learning experiences and evaluation strategies. Just like the course description, course outcomes are defined by the faculty and require faculty approval. Typically, you cannot alter or

---

BOX 3.8 ■ Teaching Leadership Concepts: Course Description, Related Competencies, and Course Outcomes

Course Description

Focuses on principles of leadership and management as they are practiced in nursing. Concepts of organizational behavior, transformational and transactional leadership are emphasized along with client advocacy, change agency, power, and politics.

Competencies

- Practices as a member of a multidisciplinary team at a level consistent with beginning professional practice
- Demonstrates competence in leadership and management skills at a level consistent with beginning professional practice
- Practices within the moral, ethical, and legal framework of the nursing profession

Course Outcomes

Upon completion of this course, the student will be able to:

- Compare and contrast communication strategies used to ensure attainment of quality outcomes, manage conflict, implement change, and enhance accountability within healthcare institutions.
- Identify skills needed to develop and build teams including negotiation, and conflict management.
- Analyze the relationships among power, influence, and problem solving in effecting change within health care organizations.
- Understand the nurse's responsibility to balance human, fiscal, and material resources to achieve quality health care outcomes.
- Explore principles related to case management and managed care.
- Articulate personal beliefs and values and their impact on leadership styles.
- Analyze current best practices related to leadership on a personal, local, regional, national, and global level.
- Analyze dilemmas in nursing leadership using ethical and legal standards of the profession.

From University of Evansville, used with permission.

---

revise course outcomes of your course without following your program's curriculum approval process.

Box 3.8 provides an example of a brief course description that is focused on leadership concepts, related program competency statements, and the accompanying course outcomes. Note how the course outcomes are related to the competency statements. As you read the course outcomes, identify the knowledge, skills, and attributes (values) that the students are expected to demonstrate to complete the course successfully. Note that each course outcome statement starts out with an action verb that provides students with direction as to what level of behavior they are expected to demonstrate their mastery of the course content.

When writing course outcomes it is important for faculty to carefully consider the action verb that is used to structure the outcome statement, as it should correlate to the level of competency the student needs to demonstrate to successfully complete the course. The level of verb chosen sets the expectation for the desired student learning outcomes. It also directs the nature of the

---

BOX 3.9 ■ Learning Domains: Cognitive, Psychomotor, and Affective Domains

Cognitive Domain (Bloom et al., 1956; Anderson & Krathwohl, 2001)
- Remembering: define, identify, recall, recognize
- Understanding: classify, compare, contrast, comprehend
- Applying: apply, demonstrate, develop, modify
- Analyzing: contrast, relate, analyze, differentiate
- Evaluating: evaluate, interpret, critique, appraise
- Creating: create, design, generate, revise

Psychomotor Domain (Dave, 1975)
- Imitation: replicate, repeat, participate
- Manipulation: demonstrate, show, acquire
- Precision: organize, achieve, perform
- Articulation: construct, design, adapt, modify
- Naturalization: create, initiate, compose, adapt

Affective Domain (Krathwohl et al., 1964)
- Receiving: use, select, identify
- Responding: question, discuss, participate, report
- Valuing: demonstrate, justify, propose
- Organizing: compare, defend, synthesize, integrate
- Internalizing values: display, discriminate, practice, act

Adapted from Hoque, M. E. (2016). Three domains of learning: Cognitive, affective, and psychomotor. *The Journal of EFL Education and Research (JEFLER)*, 2(2). www.edrc-jefler.org

---

learning experiences and student evaluation. Bloom's taxonomy (1956), revised by Anderson and Krathwohl in 2001, has long been used by educators to frame the cognitive domain level at which students need to demonstrate a given concept. Krathwohl et al. (1964) later developed the affective learning domain, followed by the psychomotor learning domain developed by Dave (1975), among others. Box 3.9 identifies the categories associated with each learning domain by order of increasing complexity. Included are some examples of action verbs that can be applied to each level. To help you develop relevant course outcomes, take the time to search the literature and read more about the use of Bloom's taxonomy and learning domains; you will easily find extensive listings of action verbs correlated to each domain level.

Designing Learning Experiences to Meet Course Outcomes

After writing course outcomes, faculty design learning experiences for students and identify strategies to evaluate their learning. Given the course outcomes listed in Box 3.8, what learning experiences would you expect to design if you were assigned to teach this course? What evaluation strategies could you use to measure student performance?

To apply the concepts of curriculum design to your own courses, consider the courses that you have been assigned to teach. Can you relate the course outcomes to your program's outcomes and competency statements? Are the action verbs that are used to anchor each course outcome written at an appropriate level? Can you use the course outcomes to envision the learning experiences your students will need to have to achieve the course outcomes?

The course outcomes provide an outline of the concepts that you will need to cover in the course and indicate the learning experiences that you will need to create. Courses are the organizing structures of the curriculum and are sequenced to facilitate student progression through the curriculum. Failure to implement your courses in accordance with the approved course outcomes can impact the integrity of the curriculum, potentially creating redundancy and/or gaps in student learning. Course outcomes also communicate expectations to students regarding content they can anticipate learning in the course. It is important for you to carefully consider course outcomes and use them as a guide to design learning assignments. If you have any questions about how to interpret your course's outcome statements, seek out your mentor or supervisor, curriculum coordinator, or a colleague for guidance.

While courses represent the organizing structure of the curriculum, faculty also create an organizing structure within their course for teaching and learning experiences. There are several ways you can approach the organization of your course. Common organizational structures at the course level include units of study and learning modules. Lesson plans are the most basic organizational structure within a unit of study or module where student assignments and learning experiences are explicated. How you choose to organize your course is dependent on the course concepts and content, the complexity and length of the course, and any expectations for organizational consistency across courses that may have been established by the program.

If the course covers multiple concepts, you may wish to develop units of study as one level of organizing structure, with learning modules imbedded within each unit. If the course is focused on one major concept, it may be sufficient to organize content solely by learning modules. Whichever approach is chosen, the important principle is that faculty are consistent across the course and provide clear expectations for students. The length of time it takes to cover the units, modules, and lesson plans varies depending on the scope and depth of the material being covered.

Box 3.10 is an example of a course that has units of study, modules, and lesson plans. The unit of study described in this example is focused on the assessment of a patient's vital signs. The unit of study has an overall set of outcomes identified for the unit. To achieve these outcomes, the unit has been divided into four learning modules with each one dedicated to one type of vital sign assessment.

In this example, module 1 focuses on the assessment of body temperature, and the lesson plan learning outcomes have been developed for the module. The outcomes identified within the lesson plan are used to guide the learning assignments and the knowledge, skills, and attributes the students will be expected to demonstrate. From this example you can determine what learning resources will need to be made available to the students to achieve the lesson

---

BOX 3.10 ■ Units, Modules, and Lesson Plans

Unit of Study—Assessing Vital Signs in the Adult Patient

At the completion of this unit of study the student will be able to:

1. Explain the physiologic and pathophysiologic processes that can affect an adult patient's temperature, blood pressure, pulse, and respiration.
2. Discuss the safety protocols associated with assessing the vital signs of an adult patient.
3. Demonstrate competence in safely assessing and documenting an adult patient's temperature, blood pressure, pulse, and respiration.

   Module 1: Assessing the Patient's Temperature
   Module 2: Assessing the Patient's Blood Pressure
   Module 3: Assessing the Patient's Pulse
   Module 4: Assessing the Patient's Respirations

Lesson Plan for Module 1: Assessing the Adult Patient's Temperature

At the completion of this lesson plan, the student will be able to:

1. Explain the physiology associated with the regulation of body temperature.
2. Understand conditions that can affect body temperature.
3. Identify the sites appropriate for taking the temperature of an adult patient.
4. Identify the different types of thermometers used to measure temperature.
5. Explain the safety guidelines associated with taking oral, rectal, axillary, and tympanic temperatures.
6. Demonstrate the technique for safely taking an oral, rectal, and axillary temperature in a simulated laboratory setting.
7. Demonstrate the assessment of an oral temperature on an adult patient in the clinical setting using appropriate guidelines.
8. Document with accuracy the measured temperature in the patient's electronic medical record.

---

plan outcomes. You can also determine how the students will be evaluated in their achievement of the outcomes. Based on the module outcomes, you can anticipate evaluating students using written examinations, simulated learning checkoffs, and clinical patient learning experiences.

Using the approach outlined here, you can design the learning experiences for your course in an organized manner that facilitates student learning. There are resources available to help you design course learning experiences, such as textbooks, internet, professional standards and guidelines, and published instructional resources. One's expertise as a practitioner may inform the learning experiences to develop students' competence as health care professionals.

Additionally, you will want to consider how each learning experience addresses the students' learning needs and how to actively engage students in learning. This is a critical step in course design and provides faculty with an opportunity to be creative and innovative in their teaching. Box 3.11 provides guidelines to use when designing student-centered learning experiences.

For additional information on teaching-learning strategies and evaluation of student learning, see Parts 2 and 3.

BOX 3.11 ■ **Getting Started: Designing Student-Centered Learning Assignments for Your Course**

- Focus on student learning: What do students need to know, do, and value?
- Shift from faculty-driven learning environments to student-driven learning environment based on learning needs.
- Assess student learning needs: What are their goals for the course? What do they see as their strengths? Where would they like to improve their performance?
- Promote student engagement with the content: Ask how they see the course's content and learning experiences having relevance to their practice as a health care professional.
- Use active learning strategies that encourage collaboration, peer interaction.
- Give learners a voice in the selection of learning strategies: Ask your students how they want to learn.
- Foster co-creation of learning experiences and development of a learning community.

PREPARING THE COURSE SYLLABUS

The course syllabus is your contract with your students, setting forth the course requirements that students must meet to successfully complete the course, and is your first opportunity to communicate with the students enrolled in your course. The course syllabus identifies the course outcomes (objectives) and competencies that students will need to achieve to pass the course, and thus is an integral representation of the curriculum as it is intended to be taught.

It is important that the syllabus be accurate and made available to the students on the first day of class. Plan on setting aside some time during the first day of class to review the syllabus with students, allowing them time to have their questions about the course answered. This is the opportunity for students to review course requirements and make a final decision about whether to remain enrolled in the course. When students review the course expectations as distributed in the syllabus and remain enrolled in the course, they are accepting the responsibility and accountability to meet the course expectations to the best of their ability. However, if certain students do not believe they can meet the requirements of the course, then they may choose to withdraw at that time. You will want to ensure that your syllabus includes all the required elements before disseminating it to students. Once the syllabus is shared with students and the course has started, it is not acceptable to make changes in the course expectations. Although you may have a statement on your syllabus stating that you reserve the right to make changes, it is still not a recommended practice, and changes should be avoided unless necessary due to unforeseen circumstances.

Institutions usually have an approved syllabus template that identifies the minimal elements that are required to be included on all syllabi regardless of the program. Programs may also have additional syllabi requirements. The first step before preparing your syllabus is to familiarize yourself with any institutional and program requirements that may exist for an official course syllabus. Box 3.12 lists essential elements for a syllabus that effectively communicates course expectations to students who enroll in the course.

BOX 3.12 ■ Getting Started: Essential Elements for Your Course Syllabus

- Course title
- Allotted credit hours
- Course prerequisites and/or corequisites
- Course description
- Course outcomes/objectives
- Required textbooks/learning resources
- Optional resources
- Topical outline
- Evaluation methodologies for course (tests, written papers, special projects, class participation, etc.) with brief descriptions, due dates, and assigned percentage of total course grade
- Description of what constitutes a passing course grade
- Grading scale
- Policy statements (attendance, academic honor code, examination administration, ADA, late assignments, etc.)

Certain elements of the syllabus will be preset by institutional and program policy: Course title, credit hours, course description, and course outcomes/objectives may require institutional or program approval, and faculty need to use them as they have been written and approved. For the remainder of the syllabus, you may have more freedom to create it in a manner that best suits your course. While it is important to be clear about policies and course expectations, you will want to consider the tone that you use to convey your expectations. If the syllabus reads like a list of what the students should *not* do and how they will be penalized, rather than encouraging them with positive examples of acceptable behavior, you may want to reconsider your wording choices. Syllabi should convey a student-centered focus to facilitate student learning and create a collaborative learning environment. Harnish et al. (2011) identified six characteristics of a "warm" syllabus: using positive or friendly language, providing rationale for assignments, providing positive self-disclosures, demonstrating enthusiasm, showing compassion, and using humor. Remember, the syllabus provides students with a first impression and insight into your teaching philosophy and interpersonal style. Give these characteristics some consideration as you prepare your syllabus and introduce the course to your students on the first day of class.

Chapter Summary

In this chapter readers were introduced to the key elements of curriculum development relevant to producing competent health professions graduates prepared to assume roles in the health care system. Here are some key points to consider as you participate in the curriculum development activities of your program:

- Faculty are responsible for developing, implementing, and evaluating the curriculum. It is a professional responsibility as an engaged member of the faculty to participate in curriculum development and identify essential concepts to integrate into the curriculum.

- The key elements of the curriculum include mission, philosophy, conceptual/organizing framework, end-of-program outcomes, competencies, course outcomes, learning experiences, and evaluation of student outcomes.
- The curriculum framework is a roadmap for the learner, leading to successful achievement of end-of-program outcomes and acquisition of the competencies necessary for safe practice as a health care professional.
- A well-designed curriculum framework logically organizes and sequences the requisite knowledge, skills, and attributes of a competent health care professional into a coherent, meaningful structure that leads to the achievement of program outcomes.
- Curriculum program outcomes (end-of-program outcomes) can be defined as statements that broadly represent what the graduates of the program have been prepared to do as they successfully complete the program's curriculum and assume their practice roles.
- When writing your course outcomes, it is important to remember that the level of verb chosen sets the expectation for the desired student learning outcomes and guides faculty in selecting appropriate learning experiences and evaluation strategies.
- Bloom's taxonomy (1956), revised by Anderson and Krathwohl in 2001, is used to frame the cognitive, psychomotor, and affective domains at the levels in which students need to demonstrate competency.
- The course syllabus is a contract with students, setting forth the course requirements that students must meet to successfully complete the course.

References

Anderson, L. W., & Krathwohl, D. R. (2001). *A taxonomy for learning, teaching, and assessing: A revision of Bloom's taxonomy of educational objectives.* Longman.

Bloom, B. S., Engelhart, M. D., Furst, E. J., Hill, W. H., & Krathwohl, D. R. (1956). *Taxonomy of educational objectives: The classification of educational goals. Handbook 1: Cognitive domain.* David McKay.

Dave, R. H. (1975). *Developing and writing behavioral objectives* (R. J. Armstrong, Ed.). Educational Innovators Press.

Harnish, R. J., McElwee, R. O., Slattery, J. M., Frantz, S., Haney, M. R., Shore, C. M., & Penley, J. (2011, Jan.). *Creating the foundation for a warm classroom climate. Observer.* https://www.psychologicalscience.org/observer/creating-the-foundation-for-a-warm-classroom-climate

Hoque, M. E. (2016). Three domains of learning: Cognitive, affective, and psychomotor. *The Journal of EFL Education and Research (JEFLER)*, 2(2). www.edrc-jefler.org

Indiana University School of Nursing. (2022). *BSN Program Outcomes.* https://nursing.iu.edu/academics/programs-degree/bsn/traditional-track/index.html. (Accessed 8 December 2022).

Institute of Medicine. (2001). *Committee on Quality of Health Care in America. Crossing the quality chasm: A new health system for the 21st century.* National Academies Press. https://doi.org/10.17226/10027

Institute of Medicine. (2003). *Health professions education: A bridge to quality.* National Academies Press. https://doi.org/10.17226/10681

Interprofessional Education Collaborative. (2016). *Core competencies for interprofessional collaborative practice: 2016 update.* Washington, DC: Interprofessional Education Collaborative.

Krathwohl, D. R., Bloom, B. S., & Masia, B. B. (1964). *Taxonomy of educational objectives: The classification of educational goals* (Vol. II). David McKay Co.

National Academies of Sciences, Engineering, and Medicine (NAM). (2021). *The Future of Nursing 2020-2030: Charting a Path to Achieve Health Equity*. Washington, DC: The National Academies Press, https://doi.org/10.17226/25982.

Sullivan, D. T. (2020). An introduction to curriculum development. In D. M. Billings & J. A. Halstead (Eds.), *Teaching in nursing: A guide for faculty* (6th ed., pp. 103–134). Elsevier.

Valiga, T. (2020). Philosophical foundations of the curriculum. In D. M. Billings & J. A. Halstead (Eds.), *Teaching in nursing: A guide for faculty* (6th ed., pp. 135–146). Elsevier.

CHAPTER 4

Common Issues Related to Curriculum Development

Developing and revising curriculum is an ongoing, ever-present responsibility of faculty; it is one that requires thoughtful and time-consuming consideration with input from multiple stakeholders. Faculty spend many hours addressing curriculum matters and participating in curriculum change. There is the old adage, "It is easier to move a cemetery than to change a curriculum." It is true that curriculum change can be a complex and somewhat lengthy, occasionally frustrating process. This chapter addresses some common issues about curriculum change that affect the faculty role, including faculty dynamics in response to curriculum change, navigating the curriculum approval process, and understanding the legal and ethical implications associated with curriculum implementation.

Curriculum Development and Faculty Dynamics

Faculty dynamics surrounding curriculum change can be intricate. According to Velthuis et al. (2018), curriculum change is more likely to be successful if curriculum change leaders understand complexity theory, organizational change, and change leadership. In their study addressing how to successfully navigate change in an undergraduate medical curriculum, Velthuis et al. (2018) identified three major themes related to leading curriculum change: (1) managing the multiple perspectives of many stakeholders, (2) dealing with faculty resistance to change in the curriculum, and (3) the act of leading the change process in curriculum. These identified themes illustrate the complexity of curriculum change and that undertaking curriculum development activities is not accomplished in isolation but requires the input and collaboration of key stakeholders. While it is unlikely that you will be leading curriculum change in your first year or two of teaching, you can anticipate participating in curriculum development activities. Understanding the curriculum change process will help you be a productive contributor.

MANAGING MULTIPLE PERSPECTIVES IN CURRICULUM CHANGE

In any given curriculum change there are many diverse stakeholders who are vested in the outcome of the process. Each bring their own perspectives to the discussions, informed by their unique beliefs, experiences, and specialty area expertise, and how they perceive the proposed curricular changes will affect them. Many will be personally and professionally vested in the curricular outcomes. Potential stakeholders include not only faculty but also students, clinical partners, administrators, and academic departments that provide science and general education courses for the curriculum, as well as regulatory and accreditation bodies. It will be important that the change process is designed to seek the input from these stakeholders early in the process and that their feedback is carefully considered in the discussions.

It is a positive situation to have multiple perspectives being shared during the curriculum change process. Genuinely encouraging divergent thinking can lead to a richer curriculum, one that respects the diversity of those who will be affected by the outcomes. Of course, seeking input from multiple parties does take time, which is one reason why curriculum revisions can take longer than you might expect. However, the revisions will be more readily accepted when individuals believe that the curriculum change process was a transparent one and their ideas and concerns were heard and received due consideration.

How does all this impact you as a participant in the process? First, anticipating the need to seek multiple perspectives and acknowledging the value that it brings to the discussions, even while knowing it may take time, can provide you with a realistic understanding of what to expect and lessen your frustration in the process. Box 4.1 provides some additional steps that you can take to become a valued and productive participant in the curriculum revision process.

COPING WITH RESISTANCE TO CURRICULUM CHANGE

Resistance to curriculum change is not uncommon. In practically any significant curriculum revision, some faculty become resistant to the proposed changes and may be even actively trying to negate the need for any change. They may even try to sway others to their way of thinking, waylaying others in the hallways or by the drinking fountain. New faculty members may become

---

BOX 4.1 ■ Getting Started: Being a Productive Participant in Curriculum Revision

- Read all the provided background literature; bring additional relevant literature to the attention of the curriculum leaders for possible dissemination to others.
- Remain knowledgeable about the forces affecting curriculum and the impetus for change.
- Commit to listening to multiple perspectives.
- Be open to and respectful of divergent opinions.
- Understand the timelines for completing curriculum revisions and meet any deadlines for requested input.
- Maintain an open-minded attitude and ground your responses in evidence-based curriculum practices whenever possible.
- Be an active participant in the discussions, bringing ideas and any potential concerns or questions to the table where they can be debated by all.

BOX 4.2 ■ Common Causes for Faculty Resistance to Curriculum Change

- Belief that it is an administratively driven process, rather than a faculty driven one
- Fear of becoming irrelevant in the new curriculum, with expertise no longer needed, resulting in loss of status/position
- Hold genuinely different philosophic beliefs about the direction/nature of change
- Concern about the effort it will take to make the required changes, considering other role commitments, feeling overwhelmed
- Fear of becoming outdated and viewed as incompetent, unable to acquire new teaching skills that the curriculum revisions may require
- Concern about resources needed to implement changes

---

uncomfortable and even feel threatened by these tactics, especially if the faculty who engage in these behaviors are more senior and have significant influence on the faculty. How should you respond if this happens to you?

First, it is important to understand that there are varied reasons that resistance to curriculum change can emerge, and any number of these reasons can be present simultaneously within the faculty. Box 4.2 identifies some common causes of resistance. These reasons can be significant and valid to those who hold them. It would be a mistake to discount the very real concerns that are associated with most episodes of resistance. Those who are leading the curriculum change should carefully consider the reasons for the resistance, as ignoring it rarely works. Those who are participants, such as yourself, should also carefully consider the concerns that are being raised. It is very possible that the naysayers have points that need to be addressed by the entire faculty.

You can respond to these concerns by respectfully listening to the thoughts that are voiced by others, allowing them an opportunity to share their views in appropriate venues. The hallway and drinking fountains are rarely considered to be appropriate venues, so when approached on the side, so to speak, it would be acceptable to listen but not engage in detail and encourage the individual to bring the concerns forward in meetings or other forums so that all can hear and respond to them. The curriculum change leaders are responsible for building consensus among the faculty and negotiating changes as determined by ongoing discussion. It is your responsibility as a participant in the process to respond in good faith, lending your input to the ongoing dialogue.

But what if *you* are the resister? If that becomes the case, you will want to do a careful self-assessment to uncover why you might be resisting the proposed changes. Are you uncertain about what it means for the courses you teach? Are you concerned that you lack the knowledge to implement the new curriculum? Or do you lack the skill to implement any new teaching strategies? Are you worried that you will not have access to needed resources to implement the change successfully? Or do you hold philosophically different beliefs about the changes needed? The underlying cause for resistance guides the steps that you need to take.

In many cases, respectfully giving voice to your concerns and asking for assistance in addressing them will be the best strategy to take. Talk to a trusted mentor. Share your concerns with the curriculum leaders in a positive manner, in which you are not blocking change but seeking opportunities to learn and engage in professional development so you can best implement the new changes. You will be most successful when you can identify the cause for your concerns and take steps to proactively address them.

LEADING AND PARTICIPATING IN THE CURRICULUM CHANGE PROCESS

Leading and participating in the curriculum change process requires a certain set of skills. As a new faculty member you likely will not anticipate leading curriculum change; however, it is possible that you will be asked to serve on curriculum committees or task forces that are charged with curriculum revision, and understanding the change process is important to the success of those initiatives. Even if you do not have a formal leadership role, you may well serve as an informal leader among your colleagues, so developing an understanding of the change process and being a productive contributor is an important skill to develop in your faculty role. Being comfortable with change is a skill that will serve you well in all aspects of your faculty role, not just with curriculum revision.

Curriculum change is complex and cannot be approached in a haphazard manner. As we have already discussed, many faculty are uncomfortable with change, especially curriculum change. To be successful in revising the curriculum, the process needs to be carefully considered and implemented by the leaders and participants. Walkington (2002) identified four stages of curriculum change (Box 4.3). These four stages clearly establish that curriculum change is not a quick process but one that typically takes several months to years to achieve, concluding with a systematic plan for ongoing evaluation of the new curriculum.

Preparing for curriculum revision is an important first step for faculty to take. From their perspective, Lachiver and Tardif (2002) addressed the conditions that need to be established for curriculum change to occur (Box 4.4). Strong leadership, clear and transparent communication, solicitation and consideration of feedback, and building consensus among the faculty for the need to change are all critical elements necessary to successfully implement

---

BOX 4.3 ■ Stages of Curriculum Change

- Stage 1: Establishing a need for curriculum change
- Stage 2: Defining the extent of needed change along with clarity of goals and desired outcomes
- Stage 3: Designing proposed curriculum revisions
- Stage 4: Implementing and evaluating outcome of curriculum revision

From Walkington, J. (2002). A process for curriculum change in engineering education. *European Journal of Engineering Education, 27*(2), 133–148.

BOX 4.4 ■ Setting the Stage for Curriculum Change

- Have a clear vision for change aligned with program/institution mission and guided by strong leadership
- Develop a general acceptance among faculty that change is needed
- Solicit input from program stakeholders
- Understand the interrelatedness of curriculum elements and how change in one element can affect others

Adapted from Lachiver, G., & Tardif, J. (2002, Nov. 6–9). Fostering and managing curriculum change and innovation. Proceedings of the ASEE/IEEE Frontiers in Education Conference, Boston, MA.

---

revisions. Opportunities for faculty to come together and brainstorm ideas for change and innovation should be integrated throughout all stages of the change process. Such brainstorming sessions can best be supported by conducting environmental scans of factors affecting the curriculum, reading seminal reports, examining evidence-based literature, reviewing professional standards, and disseminating information for faculty review and discussion prior to beginning revisions. Holding focus groups to gather input from the perspective of multiple stakeholders is another effective strategy to support change. Additionally, decisions should be made based on data that have been gathered about the effectiveness of the current curriculum. Using such data allows faculty to determine how extensive any changes need to be, as well as what aspects of the curriculum should be retained. Some faculty may find the nature of curriculum change to be frustrating, as curriculum development is rarely a linear process. It is decidedly nonlinear in nature (Walkington, 2002), requiring faculty to keep the program outcomes in mind, while drilling down into leveling competencies across the curriculum and developing course level outcomes. The curriculum development process is very much a reiterative one to ensure that the curriculum elements remain congruent and concepts are integrated throughout the curriculum. Faculty also need to keep in mind the resource implications of any proposed revisions as they make final implementation decisions in terms of clinical experiences, instructional resources, faculty numbers, among other things.

The obvious goal of any curriculum change is to positively impact and improve student learning outcomes. The development of a curriculum evaluation plan to measure the effectiveness of the new curriculum will be an important part of the change process and should be developed concurrently with the curriculum. As a participant in the curriculum development process you will also be engaged in developing a plan to evaluate the curriculum. Curriculum evaluation is discussed in Chapter 5.

As you can see, many aspects must be considered when faculty undertake curriculum revision. Understanding the change process associated with curriculum revision can help you gain confidence in your ability to contribute in a meaningful manner without being overwhelmed by the complexity of the process.

Navigating the Curriculum Approval Process

All institutions and programs have a curriculum approval process in place for new or revised curricula. You may be asked to develop a new course or to identify areas that require revision in courses that you are assigned to teach. In either case faculty must seek the approval needed to make the proposed curriculum changes. Understanding how to navigate the curriculum approval process will assist you in being successful in having your proposals approved for implementation.

The first step in any curriculum approval process is to understand the program and institutional review paths that your proposal will need to travel to be granted the necessary approval. The steps to the curriculum approval process are documented in your institution's policies and procedures. There are usually very specific timelines associated with each step of the approval process. If faculty do not meet the identified due dates for proposal submission, they may need to wait a considerable time before the next submission date.

The policy will also outline which aspects of the curriculum require the approval of others before faculty can make changes. For example, in most institutions changing the course title, course description, credit hours, and course objectives require approval not only within your program's academic unit but also at the university level. Changing lesson plans, course assignments, textbook selection, and teaching and evaluation strategies are frequently left to faculty discretion. However, in a team-teaching situation or in a program where faculty have identified essential/critical learning experiences or collectively established how certain student learning outcomes must be demonstrated and evaluated, those elements may require you to seek approval of program faculty to make changes at that level as well. Also, if you are proposing changes that require additional resources to implement, your request will require administrative approval.

The next step is to prepare the proposal, grounding your request for change upon supporting evidence that documents the need for the proposed revisions. Be clear about the proposed changes by explaining how these changes will improve student learning outcomes and how you will evaluate the outcomes related to the changes. Summarize the current literature, share data that you have collected that supports the changes, and cite stakeholder input in the proposal. Document any associated resource needs that will be required for successful implementation and describe how those resources will be obtained. Also, keep in mind that the curriculum revisions will likely be reviewed by curriculum committees composed of faculty who are not from your discipline. For this reason, you will want to avoid jargon that is discipline specific and provide background information to clarify your request for the reviewers. Most importantly, remember that seeking the input of stakeholders, especially administration and those faculty who will be impacted by any changes you may be proposing, is an essential step to ensure your success in gaining approval for request. Strive to be transparent in your request for change, understanding that the curriculum belongs to the collective faculty and that changes you are proposing may affect other courses as well. Begin these essential conversations before writing the proposal for change to avoid any element of surprise.

Legal and Ethical Implications Related to Curriculum Development

There are legal and ethical implications associated with curriculum development that faculty need to keep in mind as they engage in curriculum development activities at the program and individual course levels. While institutions and programs reserve the right to change the curriculum as needed, it is paramount that they do so in ways that do not inflict harm on students who are currently enrolled in the program. Faculty also reserve the right to make changes to their courses; however, be aware that putting a statement on your course syllabi that says you have the right to do so does not automatically protect you from student challenges that may result from changes that you make while they are enrolled in the course.

When the program publishes its program outcomes, number of credit hours required to graduate, grading scales, and required coursework to meet degree requirements, these publications are a form of contract with the admitted student. This does not mean that program outcomes, credit hours, and required courses cannot be changed; rather, it means that they cannot be changed without providing students with adequate notice and ensuring that students are not disadvantaged by the changes. The same is true of policies that govern student admission, progression, and dismissal from the program. Policies can be changed, but the program needs to provide adequate notice to the students prior to implementing the change.

For example, if a program moves to increase the number of credits or changes the required coursework that is required to receive an academic degree, then the implementation of such a change should be managed to take effect for all students newly admitted after a specific date. To change or increase requirements for students who are already admitted to the program that requires them to take additional coursework or extend their time within the program causing them to incur additional tuition costs and delay graduation may be legally challenged.

Health professions programs also have the responsibility to follow legal requirements that may be set by regulatory boards. To adopt a curriculum that does not conform to regulatory and licensure requirements could disadvantage students, potentially denying them the opportunity to obtain licensure to practice. Faculty must always stay cognizant of regulatory requirements that impact curriculum decisions.

At the course level, the syllabus is a contract with the student for the semester and should not be changed once the course starts unless necessary due to unexpected circumstances; the COVID-19 pandemic is a recent example of circumstances that dictated significant, unanticipated changes. However, typically course assignments, class and clinical hours, grading scales, evaluation strategies, and dates for examination should be set prior to the beginning of the semester so that students have a clear understanding of what they are agreeing to do when they enroll in the course. Even a seemingly minor change (e.g., pushing back a test date by 1 week) can create issues for students who have planned work and child care around the originally published schedule. If changes need to be made it is important to consider the implications for students and avoid disadvantaging them because of the changes.

Another potentially significant curricular area with legal and ethical implications is providing accommodation for students who have a documented disability. While students must demonstrate that they can meet the established learning outcomes, programs are legally required to provide reasonable accommodation for students who have a documented need. You will want to familiarize yourself with the institution's policies associated with following the Americans with Disabilities Act (ADA), which is legally mandated.

Legally and ethically, faculty are responsible for ensuring that the curriculum is inclusive and does not demonstrate bias toward students (e.g., based on racial, ethnic, gender, and LGBTQ identities). Bias can be insidious, and faculty must always be alert and sensitive to creating learning environments that are inclusive and respectful of the diverse nature of learners in their classrooms.

Chapter Summary

In this chapter readers were introduced to some common issues about curriculum change that affect the faculty role, including faculty dynamics in response to curriculum change, navigating the curriculum approval process, and understanding legal/ethical implications associated with curriculum implementation. Here are some key points to consider as you prepare yourself to be a participant in the curriculum development efforts taking place in your program:

- Faculty dynamics surrounding curriculum change can be intricate and are more likely to be successful if faculty understand change theory, complexity theory, and organizational change (Velthuis et al., 2018).
- Faculty may seek the input of multiple stakeholders when engaging in curriculum change to ensure the curriculum is relevant to contemporary health care and meets the needs of diverse learners.
- Curriculum revision decisions should be made based on data that have been gathered about the effectiveness of the current curriculum, to help faculty determine how extensive changes should be, as well as identify what aspects of the curriculum should be retained.
- Faculty resistance to curriculum change is common. Box 4.2 identifies some of the most common causes of resistance. If you are experiencing feelings of uncertainty and resistance, conduct a careful self-assessment to determine your underlying concerns and discuss your concerns with a trusted mentor.
- Before developing any proposals for curriculum revision, prepare yourself for the process by reviewing the curriculum approval policies that are in place in your program and institution.

- The implementation of the curriculum is subject to legal and ethical considerations that protect the rights of students. Regulatory agencies and the federal government also promulgate rules, regulations, and laws that impact curriculum implementation. It is your faculty responsibility to remain aware of such ethical and legal requirements.

References

Lachiver, G., & Tardif, J. (2002, Nov. 6–9). Fostering and managing curriculum change and innovation. Proceedings of the ASEE/IEEE Frontiers in Education Conference, Boston, MA.

Velthuis, F., Varpio, L., Helmich, E., Dekker, H., & Jaarsma, A. (2018). Navigating the complexities of undergraduate medical curriculum change leader's perspective. *Academic Medicine, 93*(10), 1503–1510. https://doi.org/10.1097/ACM.0000000000002165

Walkington, J. (2002). A process for curriculum change in engineering education. *European Journal of Engineering Education, 27*(2), 133–148.

CHAPTER 5

Curriculum Evaluation Strategies

Curriculum evaluation is an integral component of any curriculum develop-ment plan and should be addressed proactively as curriculum is designed and implemented. Evaluation strategies are used to determine if the curriculum is being implemented as planned and achieving the expected outcomes. Without regular, ongoing evaluation faculty are not able to document curriculum effec-tiveness to determine if the program is achieving the expected outcomes as envisioned by the faculty. For example, are students demonstrating expected program outcomes upon graduation? Are there curricular areas that could be improved upon to strengthen the achievement of outcomes? The purpose of this chapter is to introduce the curricular evaluation strategies that faculty may use to gather data about curriculum effectiveness. A complete discussion of program evaluation, including curriculum, can be found in Part 5.

Introduction to Curriculum Evaluation

Curriculum evaluation is one component of a program's systematic evaluation plan (SEP). A SEP provides faculty with a framework by which to assess all ele-ments of the program, by gathering data to analyze and determine program ef-fectiveness. A typical SEP identifies the elements that are to be evaluated, how often the evaluation will occur, what quantitative and qualitative data will be collected, what evaluation methods will be utilized, who will be responsible for conducting the evaluation, and how findings will be disseminated and used by faculty to support program decision making. The curriculum is one program element that is subjected to regular review by faculty, and you can anticipate assisting in data collection and participating in curriculum review activities.

The purpose of curriculum evaluation is to determine the extent to which the curriculum is being implemented as conceived by faculty and producing the outcomes that faculty have identified for the program. Even the best designed curriculum will have areas that need revision, and ongoing evaluation strate-gies will assist in identifying those areas. Of course, evaluation also helps fac-ulty identify the strengths of the curriculum. The first step toward being an effective participant in curriculum evaluation activities is to locate the pro-gram's SEP and review the part of the plan that is focused on the curriculum.

In addition to faculty input, there are other entities that will influence the curriculum evaluation plan and what elements of the curriculum are to be evaluated. Regulatory bodies such as state or national licensing and certifica-tion bodies may have regulations that indicate the elements of the curriculum

---

BOX 5.1 ■ Curriculum Evaluation Elements

- Mission and philosophy
- End-of-program curriculum outcomes
- Major concepts, professional standards
- Curriculum design and sequencing
- Level competencies
- Course outcomes
- Teaching and learning strategies
- Student learning outcomes

TABLE 5.1 ■ Evaluation Plan Template

Curriculum Element to Be Evaluated	Expected Outcome	Review Timeline	Data to Be Collected/ Method of Analysis	Responsibility for Data Collection and Analysis	Dissemination and Action Taken
List the curriculum elements to be evaluated. Each curriculum element should be addressed separately within the evaluation plan.	What is the desirable outcome for this element? How will you know when you have achieved this outcome?	How often is this element to be reviewed? Is there a particular time in the academic year in which the review will be most relevant?	What data collection strategies will be utilized? Which program stakeholders will be asked to provide data? How will the collected data be analyzed?	Who will be responsible for data collection and analysis? For example, is the responsibility assigned to a committee or a particular individual or position within the program?	How will results of data analysis be shared with stakeholders? How will decisions be made based on data analysis? Where will decisions be documented?

requiring evaluation. Program accrediting agencies also have criteria that address curriculum design, implementation, and evaluation. The institution may also have general education evaluation requirements that programs incorporate into their evaluation plans. Box 5.1 lists the curricular elements that are typically evaluated. Table 5.1 provides a template that can be used to create a curriculum evaluation plan. Faculty can use this template to guide evaluation activities at all levels of the curriculum, including your assigned courses.

Evaluating Curriculum: Program Mission and Philosophy

MISSION

The program's mission, philosophy, and outcomes are three curricular elements that are evaluated for continued congruency with the institution's mission and goals. It is expected by accrediting agencies that the program's mission remains aligned with the institution's mission. Typically, the institution's mission does not change very often, as an institution's mission is foundational to the institution's identity and reason for existence. For this reason, mission statements are not formally reviewed annually as other elements of the curriculum might be. Mission statements are usually reviewed about every 3 to 5 years to determine continued relevance to stakeholders and to capture evolving societal trends that affect mission implementation. Similarly, your program's mission statement should be evaluated within these timelines or whenever a change occurs at the institutional level to ensure continued alignment. Table 5.2 provides a sample evaluation plan for the program's mission.

PHILOSOPHY

The program's philosophy statement is a document that expresses the faculty beliefs and values related to human beings (persons), the health profession discipline, health and health care, teaching and learning, and any other concepts faculty deem relevant to how they enact their role (Valiga, 2020). It is not

TABLE 5.2 ■ Evaluating Mission and Philosophy

Curriculum Element to Be Evaluated	Expected Outcome	Review Timeline	Data to Be Collected/ Method of Analysis	Responsibility for Data Collection and Analysis	Dissemination and Action Taken
Mission	Program mission demonstrates congruency with institution mission.	Every 3 years, or when indicated by changes in institution mission.	Program mission will be compared to institution mission for examples of congruency. Comparison statements documented in table as evidence.	Faculty Dean/ director	Outcome of review shared with external and internal stakeholders. Any mission revisions approved by faculty and documented in faculty committee minutes. Necessary updates made to website and publications.
Philosophy	Philosophy statement reflects faculty beliefs and values. Philosophy is congruent with program mission.	Every 2 years	Faculty conduct review and confirm continued alignment with faculty beliefs and program's mission.	Faculty	Outcome of review documented in faculty meeting minutes. Revisions are disseminated to faculty.

likely that the faculty's philosophic belief system will shift radically in these areas, requiring major revision. However, a periodic review of the faculty's philosophic beliefs helps ensure that faculty maintain a consensus with how they conceptualize the curriculum, the teaching-learning process, and their interactions with students. Periodically reviewing the philosophy as a faculty and discussing how the stated beliefs affect the implementation of their role is a meaningful outcome from the evaluation process. Table 5.2 provides a sample evaluation plan for philosophy.

Evaluating Curriculum: Program Outcomes and Competencies

The program's end-of-program outcomes will not undergo frequent revision, as any substantive revisions to the program outcomes would require the curriculum competencies and the courses to undergo review and possible revision. The program outcomes should be reviewed for continued relevance every few years or so. However, reviewing the program outcomes for continued relevance is just one of the evaluation components related to program outcomes. Faculty not only want to know whether the program outcomes are relevant to practice but also ways to evaluate how successful students are at achieving the outcomes and demonstrating the associated competencies in practice upon graduation. Evaluating the achievement of program outcomes and competencies requires faculty to seek the perspective of multiple stakeholders, such as students, graduates (alumni), clinical practice partners, and employers.

Faculty also gather data to determine if the program outcomes and competencies remain relevant to health care practice or should be revised. Table 5.3 provides a sample evaluation plan for program outcomes and competencies. Faculty gather data from their students upon graduation as well as alumni who have been in practice and can provide retrospective feedback. Clinical practice partners provide rich data regarding what competencies are needed of health care professionals, and employers share feedback on graduate performance in the workplace. Graduate pass rates on professional licensing examinations and a careful analysis of graduates' performance that identifies strengths and areas for improvement also provide faculty with data when considering possible curriculum revisions.

However, the evaluation of program outcomes is more complex than just the measurement of student performance upon graduation. The curriculum program outcomes represent the program's end goal and culmination of the students' learning experiences. A comprehensive curriculum evaluation plan requires faculty to thoughtfully consider the leveling of competencies across the curriculum, as well as the curriculum design and course sequencing to achieve those competencies. Does the curriculum, as designed and sequenced, provide the students with the necessary competencies in the form of knowledge, skills, and attributes to achieve the program outcomes? Faculty also need to consider any revisions to program outcomes and competencies that might be necessitated in response to revisions in professional standards or

TABLE 5.3 ■ Evaluating Program Outcomes and Competencies

Curriculum Element to Be Evaluated	Expected Outcome	Review Timeline	Data to Be Collected/Method of Analysis	Responsibility for Data Collection and Analysis	Dissemination and Action Taken
Program outcomes Competencies	Program outcomes are reflective of contemporary health care practice and professional standards. Graduates possess requisite practice competencies. Graduates perform above national average on professional licensing examinations.	Annually	Comparison of expected program outcome relevance to professional standards and emerging health care trends. Qualitative feedback from focus group meetings with clinical partners. Survey graduates and alumni (1-year postgraduation) to determine student perceptions of preparation. Professional licensing examination pass rates. Employer satisfaction survey Employment rates	Faculty Dean/ director	Data shared with faculty, advisory committee, clinical partners, students Discussion and action taken documented in faculty meeting minutes.

accreditation standards and new reports from the discipline's professional organizations. Such evaluation requires an ongoing, systematic approach from faculty, one that touches on every course within the curriculum. Your role in curriculum evaluation as a new faculty will primarily be at this level, ensuring that the courses you teach remain aligned to the overall curriculum design and support student achievement of learning outcomes ultimately leading to achievement of program outcomes.

Evaluating Curriculum at the Course Level

One of your responsibilities as a teacher is to evaluate the effectiveness of the courses that you teach. This is an expectation of all faculty regardless of their teaching experience. Evaluating your courses will help you determine if they are facilitating the achievement of student learning outcomes at the appropriate level for where the course is situated within the program's curriculum. There are several ways to evaluate your course's effectiveness. Box 5.2 provides strategies on how to approach the evaluation process for your course.

Course evaluations completed by students are an essential aspect of measuring the quality of the educational experience—so much so that most

---

BOX 5.2 ■ Getting Started With Course Evaluations

- Consider course evaluations to be an opportunity to identify course strengths as well as areas of improvement.
- Design evaluation strategies that allow for formative evaluation of the course throughout the term as well as summative evaluation so that adjustments can be made as needed.
- Understand the rationale for each set of data you are collecting and how you intend to use it to improve your course.
- Discuss the value of course evaluations with your students emphasizing how you will use their feedback to improve the course.
- Approach evaluation proactively considering how you will evaluate the elements of your course *before* you begin teaching the course.
- Share your course evaluations with your mentor or other peer who can help you process and gain insight about the feedback received.

---

institutions and programs have policies in place that address the time in the term when evaluations should be conducted, how often courses should be evaluated, and often identify a core set of course evaluation criteria that all faculty are expected to use, in addition to faculty selected criteria. Course evaluations provide students with an opportunity to provide feedback about their experiences in the classroom or clinical setting.

It may also be an expectation that the outcomes of your course evaluations be shared with administration where they may be factored into your annual performance evaluation. It can also be the case that a summary of your course evaluations (excluding the evaluation of your personal teaching effectiveness) is to be shared with other faculty as part of the overall curriculum evaluation plan. So, the first step when getting started with course evaluation plans is to understand the course evaluation policies that are in place within your institution and program. Many new faculty (and even experienced ones!) are intimidated by the thought of having their course evaluated by others. However, a well-constructed evaluation plan for your courses yields valuable data that you can use as part of a continuous quality improvement plan to enhance the quality of your course.

What elements of your course should you include in your course evaluation plan? There are several different aspects of the course that you will want to evaluate. While student evaluation is one essential aspect of your evaluation plan, it should not be the sole evaluation strategy. Table 5.4 provides a comprehensive listing of the various aspects of course evaluation that you will want to consider, including strategies to measure their effectiveness. Faculty use multiple strategies to carry out the evaluation process, including survey tools, focused student inquiries, and student outcomes associated with various assignments. This is where proactive consideration of how to conduct evaluation of your courses will be beneficial, giving you time to prepare evaluation strategies.

You should consider when, how, and from whom you will you gather evaluation data. Faculty gather data from several sources. Your primary stakeholders

TABLE 5.4 ■ **Course Evaluation Elements and Associated Evaluation Strategies**

Course Elements	Evaluation Strategies	Frequency
Course design • Course outcomes • Course competencies • Course syllabi • Content/concept placement	• Review course outcomes for continued alignment with level outcomes and program outcomes. • Review course outcomes for relevance to contemporary practice (e.g., peer review, clinical practice partners' feedback). • Review course competencies with faculty peers to determine competencies reflect the requisite knowledge, skills, and attributes and the sequencing assigned to the course's placement in the curriculum. • Review course syllabi for all required elements, clarity, and "tone" of syllabi instructions. • Map content, inclusion of professional standards, and major course concepts through use of crosswalks, concept maps, etc. to demonstrate curriculum integration of course content.	• Annually
Teaching, learning, and evaluation strategies • Course assignments • Teaching strategies • Evaluation methods	• Review course assignments for alignment to course outcomes. • Seek student input on usefulness of assignments in achieving expected student learning outcomes through formative and summative feedback. • Review teaching strategies for effectiveness in facilitating achievement of student learning outcomes (e.g., formative and summative evaluation; peer review, student feedback). • Evaluate adequacy of instructional resources to achieve course outcomes (e.g., student feedback). • Review reliability and validity of course examinations. • Review end-of-course evaluations for course strengths and areas for improvement.	• Each course offering

are your students, so their input is important to consider when planning any revisions to your course. Additionally, you may find it beneficial to invite input from health care practice partners to assure the currency and relevance of the course to health care practice. Peer evaluation can provide faculty with feedback on course structure, teaching-learning strategies, and evaluation measures such as assignments and examinations.

It is equally important to conduct your own evaluation of your courses and examine evidence on how the course is achieving the intended learning outcomes. For example, have you reviewed the literature to identify evidence-based strategies to incorporate into your course? Staying current on the literature in your discipline, including how to effectively teach the discipline's knowledge base, is an expectation of all faculty. Are you able to trace all your course assignments back to the course outcomes (objectives) and competencies? Do the course outcomes and competencies remain aligned to the program's end-of-program course outcomes? If you cannot determine the relationship between your course's learning experiences, the course outcomes and competencies, and the end-of-program outcomes, you will want to reconsider the design of those experiences.

The timing of course evaluation strategies depend on what you hope to achieve with the evaluation data. For example, a formative evaluation plan, in which you carry out some evaluation strategies as student learning is unfolding within the course, can be a valuable source of just-in-time evaluation data. Formative evaluation strategies allow you to be proactive and responsive (Stufflebeam & Coryn, 2014), making adjustments in the course while you are still teaching it, thus possibly benefiting students who are currently enrolled. The use of a summative survey, administered at the end of the course, provides you with an opportunity to gather data that you can analyze and use to make revisions for any future offerings of the course, thus benefiting future students. You will find a combination of formative and summative evaluation to be most effective in providing you with useful data. Table 5.4 lists suggested evaluation strategies.

Student course evaluations can be accomplished through a variety of strategies. Quantitative and qualitative data are both useful in course evaluation. The typical end-of-course surveys that are required by institution and program policy are usually quantitative Likert scales that provide students with an opportunity to respond along a continuum of strongly agree to strongly disagree. There is also usually an open-ended section to the survey, allowing students to provide free-form responses as they desire. In addition to the standardized institutional course evaluation criteria, faculty have the freedom to develop their own evaluation surveys, allowing them to gather data that are specific and unique to their own courses.

It is important to remember that completing evaluation surveys can be intimidating to students if they believe their feedback is not anonymous and could in some manner impact their course grades. For this reason, the end-of-course surveys are usually administered at the end of the course, and the completed surveys are not directly submitted to the faculty but instead collected by a centralized institutional testing center, ratings compiled, and then returned to the faculty following grade submission. This method of administration separates the evaluation and grading processes, minimizing the potential for influence on the feedback received. Another common scenario is that students may experience evaluation fatigue at the end of the semester as they are asked to evaluate all their courses. For that reason, your evaluation tools should be concise and targeted to evaluate the most important components of your course. It is also important to always share with students how you use their feedback to improve your courses, so students understand that their feedback is thoughtfully considered.

Using Evaluation Data to Revise Your Course

Once you have gathered and analyzed your course evaluation data, the next step is to determine how to best use the data to make informed decisions about course revision. Using the data to assist in curricular decision making closes the evaluation feedback loop (Halstead, 2019). This final step of using data to support decision making in the revision of your course completes the evaluation process.

The data review process begins as faculty set aside time to carefully consider the data and identify trends or themes in the feedback. You will want to conduct this review in a timely manner that allows you to incorporate changes based on feedback received prior to the next time the course is taught. With student course evaluations, make note of what seems to have worked well in the course and areas that deserve further refinement. If comments seem to be outliers or unduly critical, then set them aside. Seek the objective advice of your mentor and colleagues for assistance on how best to interpret the comments, especially if they indicate a degree of dissatisfaction with the course. While this discussion has been focused on the evaluation of your course and not your own teaching performance, students do not always make that distinction, and it is inevitable that some comments will be directed toward your teaching abilities. Once again, look for themes in the feedback and seek assistance when developing any continuous quality improvement plans for your teaching skills.

When you make course revisions, remember to share this information with your students. By telling students what changes you have made based on their feedback, you are letting them know that you take their feedback seriously. This increases the likelihood that they will take their own evaluation responsibilities seriously.

Finally, remember that your role in course evaluation is part of the program's larger curriculum evaluation plan. For a curriculum to remain integrated in all its elements, faculty must accept the reality that their courses exist in an interdependent relationship with other courses in the curriculum. This means that faculty will likely be expected to share some of the course evaluation data you have collected with the rest of the faculty at large. In this manner the faculty collectively can make informed decisions about curriculum revision at the macro level of program outcomes and competencies.

Chapter Summary

In this chapter readers were introduced to curriculum evaluation strategies and how to prepare themselves to participate in the curriculum evaluation in their program and course. Here are some key points for you to consider as you prepare to be a participant in your program's curriculum evaluation efforts: Regular ongoing curriculum evaluation is used to determine if the curriculum is being implemented as planned and achieving expected program outcomes.

- Curriculum evaluation strategies should be addressed proactively as curriculum is designed and implemented.
- The curriculum elements that are regularly evaluated are mission and philosophy; end-of-program curriculum outcomes; major concepts, professional standards; curriculum design and sequencing; level competencies; course outcomes; teaching and learning strategies; and student learning outcomes.
- Curriculum evaluation requires the faculty to seek input from multiple stakeholders and consists of quantitative and qualitative data collection strategies.

- You will want to embrace course evaluation as an opportunity to identify areas for improvement and strength in your courses as part of your continuous quality improvement plan for your teaching role.
- When reviewing evaluation feedback, it can be helpful to seek the guidance of your mentor or other trusted colleagues to assist with interpretation of the feedback.
- When seeking evaluation feedback from students, share with them the importance of their feedback in making course improvements.

References

Halstead, J. A. (2019). Program evaluation: Common challenges to data collection. *Teaching and Learning in Nursing, 14*(3), A6–A7. https://doi.org/10.1016/j.teln.2019.04.001

Stufflebeam, D., & Coryn, C. (2014). Overview of the evaluation field. In *Evaluation theory, models, and applications* (pp. 3–43). Jossey-Bass.

Valiga, T. (2020). Philosophical foundations of the curriculum. In D. M. Billings & J. A. Halstead (Eds.), *Teaching in nursing: A guide for faculty* (6th ed., pp. 135–146). Elsevier.

PART 2

Teaching in the Classroom

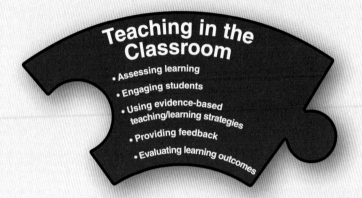

Teaching in the Classroom
- Assessing learning
- Engaging students
- Using evidence-based teaching/learning strategies
- Providing feedback
- Evaluating learning outcomes

For many new health professions faculty, teaching a course in the classroom is the first responsibility they are assigned in their new role as educators. Many experienced clinicians are accustomed to lecturing to groups about their area of expertise, so this aspect of teaching may seem familiar to you. However, developing and coordinating learning modules and activities for an entire course, as well as selecting the evaluation strategies to be used to measure student achievement of the course's learning outcomes, are likely to be new experiences for you. Part 2 is designed to prepare you to teach in the classroom environment. Chapter 6 introduces you to your role as faculty in the classroom. You will learn about the competencies necessary to function in this role, and you will have an opportunity to identify the competencies you already have acquired and those you will develop as you begin your teaching career. Chapter 7 provides the information you need to get started teaching in the classroom, including reviewing the curriculum and courses, meeting your colleagues, understanding the learning needs of students, being clear about the ethical and legal aspects of teaching, and knowing how to create a welcoming and inclusive classroom. Chapter 8 introduces you to a variety of teaching-learning strategies and activities that you might use in your course. Chapter 9 discusses assessment and evaluation strategies that are used to assess and evaluate students' attainment of course learning outcomes and your teaching effectiveness. Appendix B provides a list of the documents, policies, and procedures you should review as you are getting started teaching in the classroom.

CHAPTER 6

Introduction to Teaching in the Classroom

You may have decided to become a faculty member because you wanted to shape clinical practice for the next generation, or you may have had an inspiring (or not so inspiring) experience as a student and you have decided to be that person who inspires students, or you may have developed clinical expertise that you wish to share with students. You may have just completed an advanced degree and have accepted a faculty position as a researcher but also will have teaching responsibilities. You may also be entering the faculty role as a part-time faculty member while maintaining your clinical practice. Regardless of your reason for deciding to become a faculty, this handbook will serve as your guide to teaching in the classroom. In this chapter you will learn about the roles and responsibilities of being a faculty member who is teaching in the classroom. You will become acquainted with the requisite competencies for teaching and have an opportunity to assess what you already know about teaching and what skills you will continue to develop as you begin your journey teaching in the classroom.

Faculty Role and Responsibilities When Teaching in the Classroom

The faculty role is complex, and while the full role includes teaching, providing service to the school, campus, clinical agencies, and the profession, and conducting scholarly activities and research, this chapter focuses on the faculty role as a teacher in the classroom (Caputi & Frank, 2019; University of Michigan, n.d.). Our experience and the findings from a recent study about the transition from a role as a clinical expert to a beginning faculty member (Grassley et al., 2020) note that faculty in their first few years of teaching face many challenges. Grassley et al. (2020) found faculty new to the role felt unprepared because they did not have an educational background for teaching or had not been adequately oriented to the role. Also, there are differences between the cultures of academia and clinical practice. Because you have been a student and viewed a variety of faculty from that perspective, you may be surprised about what is involved in the faculty role. Faculty new to the world of academia have told us that they were amazed about the workload requirements and the behavior of the students, and overall they felt like a novice. Although you, too, may experience these situations, know that with preparation and a bit of experience you will become a competent faculty member!

Educator Competencies for Teaching in the Classroom

The competencies required to teach in the classroom are complex and may take several semesters of teaching experience to acquire. As you begin teaching in the classroom you should familiarize yourself with the mission and goals of the academic program, the overview of the curriculum, the specifics of the course(s) you will be teaching, and the administrative structure of the school. You should also develop an understanding of your students and how they learn. You will be responsible for establishing an inclusive and productive learning environment and must be familiar with policies related to student behavior and legal aspects pertaining to students' privacy and progress throughout the curriculum. Most of all, you will become competent in choosing and using strategies to facilitate student learning and then be able to assess and evaluate students' attainment of course learning outcomes. You will also learn how to use the technology such as a learning management system and digital learning resources used in your course (see Part 4). These faculty competencies described next are followed by a self-assessment guide to help you determine *your* competencies as you get started teaching in the classroom.

COMPETENCIES RELATED TO UNDERSTANDING THE ACADEMIC PROGRAM, CURRICULUM, COURSE, AND ADMINISTRATIVE STRUCTURE OF THE SCHOOL

A helpful starting point for preparing to teach for the first time, or to teach a new course, is to step back and review the purpose of the academic program and its relationship to the college or university. Next review the overall curriculum and determine how your course fits with the courses that precede and follow the one(s) you will be teaching (see Part 1). Also, you will find it helpful to understand the administrative structure of the school. Be sure that you know the person responsible for the course you are teaching. Part of your role will also include participating in the faculty governance activities of the school and broader campus. Box 6.1 provides specific competencies.

BOX 6.1 ■ Competencies Related to Understanding the Academic Program, Curriculum, Course, and Administrative Structure of the School

- Understand the relationship of the school to the governing body (college, university, health care agency), the mission of the school, the overall curriculum, and the administrative structure.
- Understand the course structure, syllabus, policies, teaching, assessment, and evaluation plans.
- Participate in governance activities of the school and campus such as committees that focus on student appeals, curriculum, faculty affairs, or appointment/promotion/tenure.
- Work within the curriculum framework, policies, and guidelines of the academic institution.

COMPETENCIES RELATED TO STUDENTS AND HOW THEY LEARN

The students in your classroom will likely be diverse in age, gender, racial and ethnic background, and preferred use of learning style; you will need to understand how this diversity influences learning and how to support students as they progress through your course. You may also have students with identified learning disabilities that require accommodation to support their learning. How students learn has been studied for many years, and you will benefit from understanding a variety of learning theories and frameworks that you can draw on as you use various teaching-leaning strategies. Box 6.2 provides specific competencies.

BOX 6.2 ■ Competencies Related to Students and How They Learn

- Understand how the diversity of your students—including their cultural, racial, ethnic background, learning style preference, previous learning experiences—influences their learning.
- Provide accommodations for students' special learning needs and health problems.
- Help students maximize their own learning styles.
- Understand the theoretical foundation of how students learn

---

COMPETENCIES RELATED TO MAINTAINING AN INCLUSIVE AND PRODUCTIVE LEARNING ENVIRONMENT

A significant aspect of your role as an educator is to establish a learning environment in which all students have access to learning and feel welcome in your classroom. You will do this by understanding and appreciating the diversity of your students and recognizing and managing disruptive behavior. Box 6.3 provides specific competencies.

BOX 6.3 ■ Competencies Related to Maintaining an Inclusive and Productive Learning Environment

- Create a positive learning environment that fosters a free exchange of ideas.
- Serve as a role model for legal, ethical, moral, and caring professional behavior.
- Socialize students to the discipline.
- Be accessible, enthusiastic, respectful, fair, and nonjudgmental.
- Demonstrate empathetic and civil interpersonal communication; communicate effectively verbally and in writing.
- Manage conflict and incivility in the classroom.
- Monitor classroom attendance according to course policies.
- Assess and respond to students' diverse needs and abilities.
- Establish relationships with students that foster productive learning.
- Prevent, intervene, and manage student academic and professional misconduct.
- Establish an inclusive classroom that promotes learning for all.

COMPETENCIES RELATED TO OBSERVING LEGAL AND ETHICAL PRACTICES WITH STUDENTS IN THE CLASSROOM

Teaching in the classroom is guided by a set of policies protecting the legal rights of students. Several of the policies are derived from federal laws designed to protect the privacy of the student and promote fair and equitable access to an education. These policies are observed by the college/university/ health care agency offering the program as well as at the school. The policies should be referenced in the course syllabus, and you will have the responsibility to inform/remind the students of these policies as you orient the student to the course. Box 6.4 provides specific competencies.

BOX 6.4 ■ Competencies Related to Observing Legal and Ethical Practices With Students in the Classroom

- Observe students' rights to due process.
- Observe the students' rights to privacy and confidentiality.
- Use the student appeal (grades, abuse of rights) process as needed.
- Support students who require accommodations for physical and mental disabilities according to the Americans with Disabilities Act (ADA) and campus and school policy.

COMPETENCIES RELATED TO CHOOSING AND USING TEACHING-LEARNING STRATEGIES

Likely, you are most interested in understanding how to implement the teaching-learning strategies described in the course syllabus. Typically, you will be teaching a course that is already developed, and the teaching-learning strategies may already be specified in the syllabus and imbedded in the course. In this situation you will need to become familiar with how you will use these strategies, and, as you become more experienced or are in a role of developing a course for the first time, you will understand the evidence that underlies the choice of the strategy, the attributes of each strategy, and how the strategy facilitates learning for the students in this course. Box 6.5 provides specific competencies.

BOX 6.5 ■ Competencies Related to Choosing and Using Teaching-Learning Strategies

- Facilitate learning based on educational theory and evidence-based practice.
- Develop a lesson plan.
- Use your clinical expertise to develop practice-based learning activities.
- Choose/use appropriate teaching strategies to facilitate students' attainment of course competencies.
- Choose/use appropriate classroom teaching/learning strategies to foster clinical reasoning/ judgment.
- Connect classroom learning with clinical practice by providing real-world learning experiences.
- Guide students to develop multiple thinking skills with an emphasis on making effective clinical judgments.
- Demonstrate and model inquiry and scholarship.
- Socialize students to the profession and value of lifelong learning; help students develop a professional identity.

COMPETENCIES RELATED TO CHOOSING AND USING TECHNOLOGY AND DIGITAL LEARNING RESOURCES

Educational technologies to structure and manage a course such as learning management systems make the course accessible to learners at a distance. Digital learning resources are now commonplace components of institutions of higher education and are used in the health professions as case studies, clinical excursions, and three-dimensional anatomic experiences. Although the competencies for using these technologies are universal, you will learn those used at your school and in your course. (For a complete discussion of teaching in an online classroom, using and choosing learning software, and choosing and assigning digital learning resources, see Part 4). Box 6.6 provides specific competencies.

BOX 6.6 ■ Competencies Related to Choosing and Using Learning Technology and Digital Learning Resources

- Use a learning management system (e.g., Blackboard, Desire to Learn, Canvass, Sakai).
- Use classroom technology, including computer projection systems.
- Develop or revise digital presentations (e.g., PowerPoint).
- Integrate multimedia and digital learning resources into learning experiences.

COMPETENCIES RELATED TO USING ASSESSMENT AND EVALUATION STRATEGIES

Throughout the course you will be assessing the extent to which students are attaining the course learning outcomes, helping students understand their progress, and ultimately evaluating student learning outcomes and assigning a grade. As you review the course syllabus you will note the evaluation/grading plan, and, because the syllabus is a contract with the student, you must use the assessment and evaluation strategies noted in the syllabus. Box 6.7 provides specific competencies.

BOX 6.7 ■ Competencies Related to Using Assessment and Evaluation Strategies

- Use assessment strategies to determine students' progress toward attaining course learning outcomes.
- Develop and/or use evaluation strategies (e.g., tests, written papers, presentations, digital video) to evaluate students' attainment of course learning outcomes.
- Conduct postexam review and item analysis with faculty and exam review with students.
- Assign grades.
- Use (if needed) the grade appeal process.

Self-Assessment of Competencies Related to Teaching in the Classroom

As you are getting started on your journey of becoming a faculty member, reflect on the knowledge, skills, and professional experience *you* bring to the role. Use the self-assessment guide (Table 6.1) to identify your competencies at this point and to identify where you will need to obtain information and experiences to build your teaching/evaluation expertise.

TABLE 6.1 ■ Self-Assessment

Consider to what extent you feel comfortable performing the following competencies, then check the appropriate box. After you complete the checklist, develop a plan to gain skill in the competencies in which you have less experience. Share your plan with your mentor for additional feedback.

Educator Competency	I Have No Experience	I Have Some Experience	I Have Much Experience
Know the purpose of the college/university/clinical agency and the school.			
Know the curriculum and the relationship of the course I am teaching.			
Understand the syllabus and course expectations.			
Understand campus, school, program, and course policies.			
Recognize diversity of students, age, gender, culture, race, learning styles.			
Understand the theoretical foundation of how students learn.			
Understand my own culture, learning style, racial/ethnic/gender biases.			
Create an inclusive learning environment in which all students feel welcome.			
Demonstrate empathetic and civil interpersonal communications with students and colleagues.			
Recognize and manage student academic and professional misconduct and implement appropriate policies as necessary.			
Promote civil communications inside and outside of the classroom.			
Follow the course syllabus as a contract with students.			
Develop/follow a lesson plan.			
Use lecture, discussion, reading assignments to facilitate student understanding of course content.			

TABLE 6.1 ■ **Self-Assessment** (Continued)

Educator Competency	I Have No Experience	I Have Some Experience	I Have Much Experience
Use case studies, reflection papers to facilitate student learning as they learn to apply course content to clinical practice and make safe clinical decisions/judgments.			
Use teamwork and collaboration activities to facilitate inter- and intrapersonal and interprofessional communication skills.			
Use assignments such as papers and presentations to help students learn written and verbal skills.			
Use strategies such as service learning, study abroad experiences, and participation in community events to guide the students' development of cultural humility, global appreciation, and their responsibility for civic engagement.			
Serve as a role model for academic and professional integrity.			
Observe policies related to student due process.			
Observe policies and practices related to maintaining student privacy and confidentiality.			
Implement students' requests for accommodations for learning and evaluation in the classroom.			
Use a learning management system.			
Use computer projection systems in the classroom.			
Develop and use PowerPoints.			
Review and assign digital media–related course learning outcomes.			
Use assessment strategies to monitor student learning progress (e.g., practice tests, 1-minute paper, teaching prompts/questions, case studies).			
Use exams to evaluate student learning outcomes (e.g., develop exam items, administer and proctor exams, provide exam security, grade tests, review item analysis reports, post results to gradebook, conduct postexam review with students).			
Develop/use/grade written assignments (develop/use rubrics to evaluate and grade).			
Develop/use/grade oral presentations (develop/use rubrics to evaluate and grade).			

Continued on following page

TABLE 6.1 ■ **Self-Assessment** (Continued)

Educator Competency	I Have No Experience	I Have Some Experience	I Have Much Experience
Assign final grades (follow student appeal process if needed).			
Conduct student evaluations of the course and teaching effectiveness (participate in self-reflection, administrative, peer review).			

Chapter Summary

In this chapter you have read about the competencies expected of a faculty member teaching in the classroom of a health professions school. You have assessed the skills you bring to the role of educator, and now you have an idea of what other competencies you will need as you begin teaching in your own classroom. Here are key points for you to consider as you begin your journey:

- Begin every course you teach by understanding the overall program mission and goals, the curriculum, and where the course you will be teaching fits within the structure of the program.
- Students are the focus of the course, and your role is to facilitate their learning. To be most helpful to students, understand who they are, their learning needs, their learning abilities, how they learn best, and what they most need from you as they progress through the course.
- Learning theories and frameworks describe the domains and dimensions of learning and provide a foundation for understanding how you can facilitate student learning for your students.
- Student learning is influenced by the learning environment. You have significant responsibilities to establish and maintain a productive and inclusive learning space for all students. Review campus and school policies that pertain to academic expectations of your students and the consequences you must invoke if necessary.
- There is a variety of teaching-learning strategies that you can use to facilitate student attainment of learning outcomes in your course(s). You will use strategies that help students learn the course content, but, equally important, you will use strategies that will require the students to be actively engaged in their learning and apply the course content to clinical practice.
- Students have legal rights to due process and privacy and for accommodations for diagnosed learning disabilities or health problems; familiarize yourself with the campus and school policies that ensure these rights and your responsibilities to protect them.
- Teaching in the classroom is supported by educational technologies and digital learning resources. As needed, become oriented to the learning management system used at your school, classroom projection systems,

and technology-supported teaching and learning activities such as Power-Point, digital polling systems, and digital case studies.

- The teaching-learning process includes a step for assessment that provides students an opportunity to assess their learning before they are evaluated and graded. The final step of the process is to evaluate students' attainment of course outcomes and assign grades. Be familiar with the variety of strategies used to assess and evaluate student learning and follow the evaluation plan in the syllabus, which is the learning contract with the students.

References

Caputi, L., & Frank, B. (2019). Competency I, facilitate learning. In: J. A. Halstead (Ed.), *NLN core competencies for nurse educators*. Wolters Kluwer.

Grassley, J., Strohfus, P., & Lambe, A. (2020). No longer expert: A meta-synthesis describing the transition from clinician to academic. *Journal of Nursing Education, 59*(7), 366–374.

University of Michigan Master of Health Professions Education. (n.d.). https://medicine.umich.edu/dept/lhs/education/degree-programs/master-health-professions-education-mhpe/curriculum

CHAPTER 7

Getting Started With Teaching in the Classroom

As you prepare to teach your course(s), you will find it helpful to spend time familiarizing yourself with the academic setting, the course, and your colleagues and students. This chapter provides you with background information to help you be successful! You will learn the importance of understanding the academic program, the courses in which you will be teaching, and the colleagues, staff, and student services that support you and your students. A successful classroom experience depends on understanding your students and knowing how to establish an inclusive and productive learning environment, and in this chapter you will learn how to facilitate student engagement in the classroom and academic environment. The chapter concludes with suggestions for meeting your students on that important first day of class.

Understanding the Academic Program, Curriculum, and Your Course

Before you begin to teach your course(s), start with the big-picture overview of the purpose of the academic program in which you are teaching, the curriculum in which your course is situated, and the course itself. Having this context will help you understand your contribution to the overall success of your students.

THE ACADEMIC PROGRAM

The program in which you are teaching is a part of the larger college, university, or health system. Familiarize yourself with the purpose, mission, and values of the organization. You can find information about the program on the program's website or in printed materials that may be included in a faculty orientation program.

THE CURRICULUM

The curriculum is the course of study your students will follow. Begin by looking at the overall curriculum. What competencies are the students to attain by the end of the program? How many semesters does it take the student to complete the degree? Where does the course(s) you will be teaching fit within the curriculum plan? What courses do the students take before they enroll in yours? Are these required prerequisite courses? Which courses follow the one(s) you teach? What courses do the students take at the same time they are enrolled in the course(s) that you are teaching? Do any of these courses link with your course (e.g., if you are teaching the didactic component of a clinical course)? Are the students enrolled in concurrent courses, and are you expected to integrate content from those courses into yours? Answering these questions will help you understand where your course fits in the overall curriculum plan and how you can prepare the students to attain overall curriculum goals.

THE COURSE

Start by reading the course syllabus and the student handbook. Be sure to follow up by asking your colleagues to provide additional information as needed. While faculty have their own ideas and preferences for teaching-learning and evaluation strategies, or how to implement course policies, the course you are about to teach has been designed within the broader framework of the program outcomes and curriculum, and you must follow what is included in the syllabus and shared with the students. If you are considering changing any aspect of the course, be sure to check with the course leader or administrator responsible for the course.

You may be one of several faculty who are teaching the same course. In this case, you are a part of a teaching team and must be consistent in how you implement the syllabus. Generally, when faculty are teaching as a team, there will be a course leader/coordinator who is responsible for ensuring that teaching and evaluation is equitable across the course. Be sure to contact this person if you have questions about your teaching practices.

It is also possible that the course you are teaching has a clinical component in which students are expected to connect the classroom (didactic) content to clinical practice. In this situation, you may be assigned to teach the clinical course, or if you are not also teaching the clinical component of the course you may need to coordinate with the faculty who is teaching that course. In some programs, the final grade requires the student to obtain a passing grade in *both* the classroom and clinical components of the course, and you will collaborate with the clinical faculty in assigning the final grade.

The Course Syllabus

The course syllabus is your contract with the student and once distributed to the student cannot be changed for the current semester. The syllabus is the guide to the course for both you and the student and sets expectations for learning, evaluation, and acceptable academic and professional behavior (see Part 1).

As you review the syllabus, note how many credits the student will receive and how many hours of class time and weeks in the semester are allocated to your course. Next, look at the course learning outcomes and associated course competencies. These are the knowledge, skills, and abilities/values the students should attain at the end of the course. The learning outcomes are the roadmap to the course, and all course activities are designed with these in mind.

The syllabus also specifies course assignments and learning resources. These may be included in a course schedule that includes a week-by-week or lesson-by-lesson list of assignments such as readings in the textbook, readings from professional journals, workbook pages to complete, PowerPoints to review, quizzes/pretests to complete, or digital media case studies to view. The most important thing you can do to be prepared for teaching the course is to familiarize yourself with the assigned material to understand the background students should have prior to coming to class and how you will integrate this preparatory information into the lesson plan for each class. Read the assigned material through the eyes of the student. Where will students need help understanding the content? What is the most important information they should learn? How will the students use the content during the class session and in clinical practice? How long does it take students to complete the assignments? Is this a realistic and beneficial use of their time?

The syllabus also describes the course evaluation plan, including evaluation strategies and the grading scale that will used to assign the final grade. This is a significant part of the syllabus, and you may need to refer to it if the student is not clear about course requirements for the grade or disputes the grade you assign. It is helpful to see examples of previous students' work that is used in the evaluation plan such as papers, case studies, presentations, or exams and to note how the previous faculty graded the assignment. This will help you address the information as you are teaching the course. Learn where and when you should post grades from exams, papers, or other graded assignments.

Student Handbook

This handbook describes student expectations for behavior in the classroom and the consequences that will be applied if expectations are not being met. The handbook may apply to all students on the campus or be specific to your school. Parts of the handbook may also be included with the course syllabus and listed as "policies" or may include a link to the school or campus website. Be sure to locate the handbook used by your students, and, as you review the policies, note those that pertain to the management of your course(s) such as class attendance, expectations for civil and professional behavior, and grading policies. Also review policies related to academic behavior, sexual harassment, bullying, accommodations for disabilities, and the student appeal processes. At the first meeting with students, it is your responsibility to ensure that the students understand the policies and consequences of not following them.

FACULTY ORIENTATION PROGRAM

Some schools conduct a faculty orientation program that may be held several days before classes begin and/or throughout the semester. Orientation programs may include information about (1) the school and its organizational structure, (2) the school culture and differences from the culture in a clinical service setting, (3) teaching and evaluation methods, (4) the faculty role, (5) faculty policies including academic conduct, and (6) academic policies that pertain to the student. If your school does not have a structured orientation program, it is appropriate to ask the course leader or department chair for information about these topics.

During the orientation you may be assigned a mentor or a faculty guide. Newly appointed faculty who participate in an orientation program and have a mentor are likely to continue in the faculty role, be better teachers, and report being satisfied with the role of being a faculty member. Faculty new to teaching tell us that it is also helpful to observe someone teaching your course or a course with similar students and teaching activities or meet the person who has taught the class previously to obtain a practical understanding of how to approach the course. If there is not a structured orientation program, request that a faculty member be available to give you information about the course.

Meeting Your Colleagues, Staff, and Student Support Services Personnel

Teaching, although a solo event when you are in the classroom with the students, is supported by a team of teaching colleagues, course and department coordinators/leaders/administrators, administrative support staff, technical support staff, and student support services. You should meet the members of this team and understand their roles as you are getting started teaching your course.

COORDINATORS, ADMINISTRATORS, AND MENTORS

Most schools are organized with a hierarchic structure depending on the size of the faculty and student body. There may be a course coordinator (course leader) who is responsible for coordinating sections of a course or several courses within the semester. This is the person you should approach first with questions about the course, suggestions for handling an issue with a student, or reporting student misconduct. Be sure you have contact information for this person!

In large schools there may be an administrator, usually a department chair who is responsible for courses and faculty in that area. The dean or program director is the person who has ultimate responsibility for the welfare of the students and faculty and provides leadership and direction for the school. Be mindful of following the chain of command as you manage issues of concern.

Mentors are faculty colleagues who volunteer or are assigned to assist newly employed faculty. They help new faculty become familiar with the program, course, and students. If your program does not provide someone to serve in this role, you can request that someone be available to you, or seek out a faculty colleague who seems willing to answer your questions. Newly appointed faculty find that having a mentor eases the transition to the faculty role, is available to answer questions about the course and your teaching responsibilities, and provides guidance about the informal culture of the school (Ephraim, 2021).

TECHNOLOGY SUPPORT STAFF

Technical staff manage the technology in the classrooms, offices, student lounges, and elsewhere on campus. This staff also will establish an email account for you and other accounts you will need to access to teach your course. If the campus or school uses a learning management system (LMS) or videoconferencing system and if you will be using learning technology, there will also be staff at the school or campus to assist with course design. Your classroom should be equipped with an internet connection, a projection system, and access to media that you may wish to use in your course. Know how to contact technical support services for assistance or to plan for technology support for you and your students.

STUDENT SUPPORT SERVICES

Depending on the size of the school, these services may be housed at the school or on the campus and organized in various ways. In larger programs, the school will have an office of student services dedicated to the needs of students. This office facilitates student recruitment, registration, recording grades (registrar), counseling, and academic advisement. This office may also organize peer tutoring and other learning support services such as a writing center of assistance for students for whom English is an additional language. Large schools may have their own offices of diversity, equity, and inclusion and an office of global affairs to support faculty and student recruitment, retention, and study-abroad programs. Be familiar with the resources these offices offer and consult with them or refer students to their services as needed.

Services that may be offered at the campus include a writing center, which assists students with technical aspects of writing a paper, and an office for students with disabilities (students with diagnosed disabilities must register at this office before they can request accommodations for taking tests or adapting learning activities for their needs). Many campuses also have a center for teaching and learning that provides support and workshops for faculty about designing courses, teaching online, developing assessments and tests, and using innovative teaching strategies.

Understanding Your Students

The students are the reason you have decided to be a teacher! Try to learn as much about them as you can before you meet them in the classroom. Begin by understanding where they are in the academic program. For example, students for whom this is the first course in the professional program may still not know how to read the syllabus, how to find or use resources required in the program such as library, use the LMS, or use required software such as accessing the textbook or related resources online and will need extra orientation to be successful in the course. On the other hand, your students may be in the last semester of the program and are more knowledgeable about using student resources.

Although you may not have detailed information about the students who will be in your course, you can find out about the student body at the school in a general way. The college or your school may have a general profile of the students that indicates the percentage of students who attend classes full or part time; the racial, gender, and age composition of the student body; the percentage of students who are employed; the percentage of students for whom English is not their first or only language; and the percentage of students who are the first person from their family to attend college. This information may help you anticipate how to structure class activities, identify students who may need learning support services, and how you will develop and implement course norms and policies.

Understanding Legal Implications of Teaching in the Classroom

Before you begin teaching in the classroom (and in the clinical or online setting!) you should be aware of several federal laws and policies that protect students, and the process students can use to appeal grades or file grievances. Students have the right to due process, fair treatment, and privacy/confidentiality. These policies are available at the university and the school, and if they are not discussed in an orientation program, then locate them and familiarize yourself with the implications for your role as teacher.

DUE PROCESS

Students have the right to fair treatment. This right includes fairness when faculty apply penalties for infractions as defined in the academic standards and the Student Code of Conduct policy of the university. These academic standards are specified in the course syllabus. Students have the right to procedural fair treatment and the right to present their side of the story as noted in a student appeals policy. Students also have constitutional rights to privacy and due process. Your role is to make sure students understand course and behavior expectations and the consequences that will be applied, and to advise students about the university/school student appeals process when students dispute grades or your observations of their behavior. If you are in a situation with a student where due process is an issue, first remove the student from the setting and then discuss the situation with the student in private. If necessary, discuss with the course leader or first line administrator while respecting the student's privacy (Box 7.1).

STUDENT APPEAL AND GRIEVANCE PROCESS

Even though you may have followed due process guidelines, it is possible that the student views the situation differently and will appeal your actions. Each college/university and school have a written appeal and grievance process that students must follow. The process begins with you and the student discussing the situation to see if it can be resolved. If the situation is not resolved, the student can file a written appeal, which is directed to the administrator or chair of the appeals committee according to the policy, and is then heard by the appeals committee who decides the case. If the issue is not resolved with the school, the appeal can continue through university

---

BOX 7.1 ■ General Guidelines for Managing Inappropriate Student Behavior While Observing Due Process and Student Privacy Guidelines

- Remove student from situation.
- Identify the unacceptable behavior or academic misconduct.
- Discuss situation with student while observing privacy and confidentiality laws and policies.
- Verify that what has occurred is unacceptable behavior or academic dishonesty.
- Review expectation (per course, school, and or university policy).
- Link student behavior to expectation.
- Plan with the student to remediate the behavior or invoke consequences per policy guidelines.
- Record the situation in anecdotal notes without using identifying information; save all tests, written work, clinical performance evaluations.
- Report the situation to the appropriate administrator without identifying the student if the student has not waived their right to privacy.
- Follow student due process and appeal guidelines.
- Document all interactions and actions.

---

channels and to court action. Locate the student appeal policy at your school and familiarize yourself with the process and your responsibilities.

CONFIDENTIALITY AND PRIVACY

The Federal Educational Rights and Privacy Act of 1974 (FERPA) directs that students can have access to their records and give consent to who else can view their records. This law also indicates that students can contest information that is in their academic record. Students have the right to have interactions with faculty and information about class attendance, course behavior and progress, and records and grades held in confidence and discussed with the student in private. *Unless the student waives the rights to confidentiality and privacy* (gives permission to discuss information with others), you cannot (1) post grades in public places; (2) share lists of students in the class; or (3) discuss course attendance, behavior, or grades with others, including other faculty or administrators, students' parents, spouses or partners, or attorneys. There may be situations in which you need to discuss a student situation with a colleague or administrator, and you can do so by describing the general situation and withholding the student's name or other information that would link the student to the discussion. You may discover that faculty at your school share information about specific students and the students' experiences in previous courses, keep a database of student behavior that all faculty can access, have informal conversations naming students, or ask another faculty to observe a student's clinical performance or review written work and indicate what grade they would give. These are violations of FERPA, and you should avoid engaging in these situations.

AMERICANS WITH DISABILITY ACT (ADA)

The ADA provides opportunities for students to receive reasonable accommodations for physical impairment (e.g., vision or hearing impairment), mental impairment (e.g., bipolar disorder, posttraumatic stress disorder), or learning disability (e.g., attention-deficit disorder, anxiety disorder) that limits life activities; in the context of higher education, it limits the ability to participate in learning and evaluation/testing activities (ADA Testing Accommodations, 2014). Learning disabilities are the most common types and may require accommodations (such as extra time, quiet space). To be eligible for an accommodation, the student must provide a record of the impairment, usually diagnosed by a health care provider or submitted as a record of previous accommodation.

This law also directs universities/colleges/schools to provide reasonable accommodations for students with disabilities. Your university has an office of student services or student disability services that works with students and faculty to arrange these reasonable accommodations. In general, students must first inform the university that they have a condition requiring accommodation and provide proof that the diagnosis has been made by a qualified health care provider. It is then each student's responsibility to notify the faculty and the university student services office about the need for accommodation. The student disability services office then confirms to the faculty that the student is eligible for accommodation. It is then the responsibility of the student disability service to arrange the reasonable accommodations. The process of assisting students with disabilities varies for each school, and you should identify what process is in place at your school and university and be familiar with the types of resources provided (Yarbrough & Welch, 2021).

When teaching in the classroom, you may be involved in assisting students to make accommodations for participating in your course (Box 7.2). For example, to facilitate learning in the classroom, students can request a note taker. Students with hearing impairment can request the use of assistive technology such as having the faculty use a microphone that amplifies sound to a student's device or uses a voice captionist to display the spoken word to the student's computer. Students with low vision may need enlarged print examinations and handouts. In online courses there are ADA standards for using appropriate font size and style.

Students can also request accommodations when taking a test. The most common accommodation is to increase the time to take the test. When students

---

BOX 7.2 ■ Faculty Responsibilities for Assisting Students Requesting Accommodations

- Place information about procedures for requesting and implementing accommodations in the syllabus and review with students during the orientation to the course.
- Review letter from student disability services explaining the request for accommodations and make plans with the student before the need for accommodation arises (e.g., before the test).
- Honor reasonable accommodations.
- Verify who is responsible for implementing the accommodations (i.e., you or the office of student disability services).
- Implement accommodations fairly and consistently.
- Avoid inquiring about the nature of the disability.
- Respect the student's privacy by not discussing the situation with others.
- Refer the student to other support services (such as counseling, tutoring) as needed.
- Focus on the student's strengths.
- Document your interactions with the student and further actions.

request this accommodation, determine in advance if you will be the one to supervise this student or if that is a service of the office of disability services. Other requests for accommodations may involve making changes to the testing environment such as allocating a quiet and separate space to take the test, providing devices such as screen reading technology, having a person read the test item to the test taker or serve as a scribe, taking the test in a distraction-free room, or providing wheelchair-accessible testing stations. If you have questions or concerns, check with your course leader and the office at the school or campus that provides support to students with disabilities who need accommodations.

Establishing an Inclusive and Productive Classroom

One of the biggest challenges faculty new to teaching face is understanding what to expect from the students both inside and outside the classroom. As you prepare to teach, it is helpful to consider what you can do to establish an inclusive, welcoming, caring, and safe learning environment, as well as being able to recognize, prevent, and manage student misconduct and academic dishonesty so that all students are treated fairly and have an equal opportunity to be successful in your course.

ESTABLISHING AN INCLUSIVE CLASSROOM

The students in your classroom will likely be of all genders, ages, and generations; represent varied racial and ethnic groups; use varying learning styles and approaches to learning; and may be learning English as a second language. Your role is to ensure that *all* students in your classroom have access to and support for maximizing their potential as learners (Box 7.3).

BOX 7.3 ■ How to Establish an Inclusive Classroom

- Use universal design for learning (UDL) principles in the curriculum, course, and lesson plans. UDL involves creating an environment in which the needs of all learners are supported by presenting information in a variety of ways; using a variety of teaching, learning, and evaluation strategies; and giving students options for learning and evaluation. Ensure images reflect the diversity of your classroom and assignments encourage diversity of opinions and viewpoints. Create assignments that provide options for learning, assessment, and evaluation.
- Recognize your own culture and how it contributes to your understanding of other cultures and perspectives. Recognize your biases. Develop empathy and cultural humility.
- Be aware of words you use that may be interpreted as offensive by others.
- Encourage students to share their perspectives in a nonjudgmental environment. Narratives and storytelling are useful strategies to elicit and illuminate varying perspectives.
- Build community at the onset of the course. Provide an opportunity for you and the students to know each other's names and a few sharable and relatable details that open discussion. Use the course LMS to create options where students can post names, photos, gender pronouns, or other personal information they wish to share in a protected space in the LMS.
- Plan to arrive early and stay after each class to have informal conversations with students. Establish office hours for personal interaction with groups or individual students.
- Use inclusive pedagogy. Embrace diversity, be flexible, encourage collaboration, and use agreed upon classroom norms and policies and apply consequences fairly.

MAINTAINING A PRODUCTIVE CLASSROOM

You can establish a productive classroom by demonstrating respect for all students, recognizing your own culture and beliefs while appreciating the values and beliefs of all students in the classroom. Your role is to facilitate learning by creating opportunities that encourage participation in the way each student feels comfortable, giving voice to all students and recognizing and managing the inevitable situations with students that can disturb the learning environment.

Students can disrupt the classroom learning environment for their classmates by coming to class late, submitting assignments past the deadline, or making requests to take a test or submit a paper later. Students can offer a variety of excuses for these situations, and it may be difficult to determine the validity of the excuse and decide how to handle the request. You have a responsibility for holding all students to the agreed upon polices as noted in the student handbook and in the course syllabus. If you make exceptions for one student, you must make them for everyone. Before you meet your students, be sure you understand the policies that contribute to classroom management and how the faculty at your school interpret them across all courses. At the same time, policies may need to be designed for flexibility and offer options for common issues such as making up class work during an absence or taking a test at another time. Your course may offer these options, or if you plan to offer some flexibility, discuss your plans with the course leader before you make any changes.

Students lead busy lives, many have families, and most of your students will have jobs, either part or full time, and many other responsibilities besides being a student. Students may not have access to the technology needed to participate in class or broadband or Wi-Fi access to complete assignments or take tests remotely. With all these pressures, students are stressed and may not be able to comply with course expectations. Students are also under pressure to succeed. They may have a scholarship that requires obtaining and maintaining a certain grade point average or passing the course to be able to continue in the program. Parents and partners may also have expectations for the student to succeed. This pressure often manifests itself in frustration, anger, and aggression and is particularly evident when students do not receive the grade they believe they should.

You should anticipate how you will handle these situations before they occur and be familiar with course norms and policies that communicate appropriate behavior to the student. At the same time, you will need to balance the time required to invoke consequences against the time spent in facilitating student learning. If possible, discuss possible classroom management issues with the course leader or your mentor, and understand how you will manage them if they occur. Table 7.1 provides potential class management issues that can occur and suggestions for how to handle them.

TABLE 7.1 ■ Maintaining a Productive Learning Environment: Potential Issues and How to Manage Them

Classroom Management Issues	How to Manage
Students are late to class.	Follow policies and consequences for arriving late. There are many legitimate reasons for being late, and you will need to weigh how to implement consequences. Classroom norms for late arrivals often indicate that the student should avoid disrupting others and sit in the back of the room. You must be fair and consistent in applying any consequences for behavior related to tardiness.
Students are not prepared for class.	Explain your expectations that students prepare for class and link the preparation to what they need to know to participate in class. Guide the preclass preparation by highlighting what to learn. Have students submit worksheets at the beginning of the class. Divide students into teams, and have each team be responsible for preparing and presenting key information; all students will hear and learn during class; use the LMS for students to submit a short assignment or complete a mastery, ungraded pretest. Allow brief in-class time for students to read or locate key information needed to participate in class activities.
Students talk out of turn.	Remind students that it easier to hear when just one person talks; establish and refer norms for how students should indicate they wish to speak such as raise their hand; when several students raise their hand, tell students you will call on each of them, and then proceed to call on each student one at a time.
Student challenges you or asks a question for which you do not have an answer.	Acknowledge the question and admit you do not have an answer. Ask the class how they would find the answer. If students have access to computer, ask someone to volunteer to look up the answer. Serve as a role model for seeking information.
Student leaves and returns to the classroom frequently.	Establish norms and post in syllabus about leaving class; indicate students who need to leave should sit near exit on aisle to minimize disruption. If occurs frequently, consider if this is a problem and discuss with student.
Students do not participate in class discussion.	Some students learn best by listening, others may fear being criticized or bullied (during and after class); fear giving an incorrect answer; require additional time to formulate a response; or cultural norms are to listen to and respect the teacher. You can accept these possibilities, and not call on students directly. You can also make eye contact with students who may be about to participate and get a sense if they are ready to be called on. Some students may feel more comfortable participating in a small-group activity such as think-pair-share or by submitting their thoughts in a written activity such as a 1-minute paper. To encourage all voices, you can incorporate these strategies in your lesson plan.
Students are aggrieved, believe they have been treated unfairly.	This behavior typically occurs following receiving a grade on a test or paper. The student may have excuses, ask for sympathy. You can listen, understand, assist the student reflect on the behavior and the fairness of the situation. Help the student focus on problem solving and understanding how to study and achieve desired grades. Unless there is an error, do not change the grade; any changes made for one student must be made for all students.
Students monopolize discussion.	Ask the class if others have a comment; engage others by asking a follow-up question.

Continued on following page

TABLE 7.1 ■ Maintaining a Productive Learning Environment: Potential Issues and How to Manage Them (Continued)

Classroom Management Issues	How to Manage
Students are angry, aggressive.	Use deescalation techniques: Remain calm; speak slowly and softly; remain respectful; listen actively, indicate you are available to help; indicate you have heard the student's frustration; ask for clarification; use empathetic statements; be respectful; set limits and tell student you will continue to discuss the issue when the student is calm. Tell the student you need to check with the appropriate administrator. Work to resolve the issue; refer as necessary to professional resources; document and report to administrators.
Students do not participate in group/teamwork, change groups to be with friends, or prefer to work alone. During group/team assignments one or two students do most of the work.	At the beginning of the course, establish norms for group/teamwork, including expectations for participation; if results of group work will be graded, consider giving points or asking students to sign a form indicating their contribution; use a variety of strategies for forming groups such as asking students to form own group, numbering off for the size of the group; making random assignments; making assignments that ensure diversity of the group.
Students have emotional reactions to class discussion.	A variety of topics such as social injustice, death, or health problems can trigger a student's emotional response to class discussion or assignments. During class, students may become angry, frustrated, or sad. Assess the situation and determine if it is best to handle during the class or privately after class. If the student expresses the response to the entire class, you should acknowledge the student's feelings, and, if appropriate, pause the class and use the moment to engage the class in further discussion.
Students make derogatory or uncivil remarks.	Be familiar with school and campus polices about incivility. If appropriate, pause the class and intervene. Refer to class norms for appropriate behavior during class discussion. As appropriate, use the moment to help all students learn appropriate communication skills.
Two or more students chat during class.	The noise of chatting disrupts students nearby. State the problem, explain how the chatting is bothering others, and ask that everyone listen. If there are established norms, follow the agreed upon norms. Ask if there are questions that all need to hear so all can have the answer. It is usually not necessary to call attention to the students involved by asking them to be quiet or calling on them. If the behavior persists, discuss with students privately. Consider revising norms.
Students ask to submit work or take a test on another day than the due date.	Responding to students' request to change due dates is difficult balance between being accommodating and holding students responsible. Refer the student to course policies (or establish them at the outset of the course) about late papers and allowable circumstances for postponing a test. Exceptions made for one student must be made for all students.
Students want to be your friend; asking for health care or other advice; asking for exceptions.	Know that your role is that of the student's faculty member. Be friendly, but not a friend; offer support, but not advice; clarify norms and rules for behavior, but be consistent, fair, and equitable when making exceptions for one student and not all students.

Recognizing, Preventing, and Managing Student Misconduct and Academic Dishonesty

The classroom learning environment can be disrupted by students who do not observe guidelines for appropriate conduct and ethical behavior. Maintaining a culture of integrity (Moore & Gaviola, 2018) requires you to recognize, prevent, and manage student's behavior that violates the school and university codes for academic conduct. These expectations are defined in student handbooks developed by students, faculty, and administrators at any school and university.

Student misconduct is defined as behavior that disrupts the teaching, learning, and research environment. The student handbook at the campus or school defines appropriate conduct and misconduct as well as the student responsibilities to the academic community. Student misconduct can escalate in a continuum from annoying to criminal. Your responsibility as a teacher is to recognize the behavior and discuss it with the student to prevent escalation, and then, as necessary taking steps to manage the behavior as indicated in the relevant policy.

Academic dishonesty refers to dishonest acts related to teaching, learning, and research such as cheating, plagiarism, fabrication or falsification, and sabotage. Academic dishonesty can include lying, perjury, stealing, cheating, texting answers to test questions, charting information not obtained or observed, copying or not citing published works, assisting classmates or other students with their work, copying a test or using a copied test, and submitting other students' papers that were obtained/purchased online (McClung & Schneider, 2018). Studies of college students at varied types of institutions indicate that as much as 90% of students cheat and that most students report having witnessed academic dishonesty (McClung & Gaberson, 2020; McClung & Schneider, 2018).

Students do not always understand what constitutes academic dishonesty or what behaviors are, in fact, dishonest. You can socialize students to their responsibilities for demonstrating professional and ethical behavior by defining dishonesty and related behaviors and reviewing academic policies, expectations, and consequences at the beginning of each course. Some colleges and schools have orientation programs or online modules to ensure students understand the expected behaviors and consequences. While these behaviors typically do not occur during the first few weeks of the course, they are often precipitated by a confluence of events and student stress that increases over time. It is your responsibility to recognize the behavior before it escalates (Table 7.2) and take the steps to manage the behavior while respecting students' privacy and due process (see Box 7.1).

The First Day of the Course

Anticipating the first day of class is both exciting and anxiety provoking. Careful planning for this moment will go a long way to starting your course on

TABLE 7.2 ■ Recognition, Prevention, and Management of Student Misconduct in the Classroom

Behavior	Definition	Recognition	Prevention	Management
Cheating	Unauthorized use of information such as stealing an exam or copying test answers or submitting papers written by another student.	During exams: Student looks at another students' paper; passes notes; eyes wander; looks at phone, paper, hands. Before exams: Student is found copying tests; accessing hard drive where tests are stored. After exams: Student is sharing answers, selling tests, etc.	Establish a culture of integrity; orient students to definition of cheating and associated behaviors; use a written honor code and have students sign; offer a short online module about what constitutes cheating and the consequences that will be applied. In the classroom, use proctors; in an online environment use cameras, software, and other monitoring devices. Collect all exam papers and, if returned to student, monitor use; protect access to computers where exam questions are stored. Update test after each administration.	Verify cheating with student; follow school/university procedure; report to administrators; follow student handbook policy.
Plagiarism	Taking someone else's work and claiming as own; using someone else's work without acknowledgment or citation	Written work appears not to give credit for work or ideas that are not the student's. Use digital plagiarism checking programs such as Turnitin.	Include a definition of plagiarism and examples in the syllabus; make expectations clear and specific such as what percentage of the paper that that has been plagiarized constitutes plagiarism; explain consequences for plagiarism as noted in the school and/or campus policies; teach students how to cite other people's ideas and work. Make assignments that emphasize original work; read preliminary drafts of written work and give feedback before grading. Change assignments each semester to minimize cheating or plagiarism from easy access to previous semester's assignments.	Once discovered and confirmed, discuss with student, report to administrators, and follow course, school, and campus policies.

Incivility	Making rude, annoying, unprofessional, impolite, disrespectful comments. Behavior can range from disruptive to violence. Lateral incivility: student-student; faculty-faculty; nurse-nurse. Hierarchic incivility: administrator-faculty; faculty-student; nurse-student	Minor: Eye rolling, sarcasm; racial/ethnic slurs; microaggression. Students can send uncivil comments through email rather than in person. Major: Intimidation, threatening; physical violence to faculty, classmates	Include code of behavior in course syllabus; conduct information sessions on recognizing and managing incivility.	Do not engage or escalate in dialogue with student. Calmly discuss with student and follow course, school, campus, agency policies. Discuss email incivility in person or telephone. Frame responses in terms of program goals for professionalism.
Bullying	Five types: physical, verbal, social, cyber, sexual School/campus: Verbal, social, psychologic, or physical confrontations, intended to dominate or humiliate. Online: Cyberbullying occurs in online courses and social media: texts, emails to taunt or give false information; sexting.	Intimidating remarks, threats, physically threatening or assaulting; excluding student from peer or group work.	Establish norms and policies; refer to state and federal legislation. Zero tolerance.	If you witness bullying: speak up and call out the behavior; if safe, calmly confront the bully; support the victim; write anecdotal note or make video; report to administrators.
Impaired behavior	Behavior not typical for student or appropriate for being in the classroom	Student is dizzy and stumbling; slurring words; may be aggressive or volatile, irritable or agitated, flying into a rage. May be caused by substance abuse, student anxiety, medications, health problems.	State policy in syllabus and student handbook.	Remove student immediately from the situation. Discuss with student; refer as needed to health services; follow up with report to course leader/administrator.

a positive note. Your planning for this first day began when you reviewed the curriculum and course syllabus; learned about the mission, program outcomes, and structure of the school; met your administrators and colleagues; gained an understanding of your students; and learned how to establish and maintain an inclusive and productive classroom.

Before class starts, it is helpful to visit the classroom. Stand in various parts of the room to get a feel for how the students view the room and will be able to participate in planned learning activities. Will the classroom accommodate the size of your class? Is the classroom a theater-style lecture hall with a lectern at the pit and facing the students? Can the chairs be rearranged? How will you conduct small-group work? What technology skills do you need to use the computer and projection screen? How do you call for technology or other assistance?

Now, as the class is about to begin, you are ready to meet your students! Keep in mind that you should (1) introduce yourself to the students and the students to their classmates, (2) establish a welcoming and inclusive classroom, (3) collaborate with students to determine what will make a productive learning environment for all and confirm norms for behavior, (4) explain the course and review the syllabus, (5) suggest strategies to be an effective learner in the course, and (6) end on a positive note!

Both students and faculty enter the course on the first day wondering about each other, and beginning the class with introductions is a great way to start the class. If students have access to the course before it starts through a LMS or other mechanism for communicating with each other, you can post a short introduction and ask the students to do the same. You can also conduct an anonymous survey within the LMS to find out about students' interest in the course, what they expect to learn, their experience with technology, their clinical experience, what you can do to facilitate learning, and other information that would be helpful to know about your students. Then, when you meet the students in the classroom, consider greeting students as they enter the room and introduce yourself and chat as time allows. Having students wear name tags and/or using a name placard on their desk will help you and the students learn each other's names.

As the class begins, you will introduce yourself. What will you say? Students like to know a bit about how you wish to be addressed (Dr., Professor, Ms./Mr., or by first name), your educational background, your interests, experiences, and expertise with the subject matter. Students enjoy knowing your passion for the course topic, and they can benefit from your expertise. Basically, students value a faculty who is enthusiastic, fair, caring, patient, flexible, collegial, and knowledgeable about clinical practice. Be authentic and let your personality shine.

After you have introduced yourself, encourage students to introduce themselves to you and their classmates. In a small class you can ask students to introduce themselves individually and tell the group something that will help others know a bit about them, such as why they are taking the class or what they most hope to learn in this course. In large classes you can have students form a small group (standing in a circle, or by moving desks into a circle) and meet each other.

Students will also be curious about course expectations. You will need to ensure that all students are familiar with the syllabus, course learning outcomes, course assignments, grading criteria and grading scale, and use of technology (e.g., can students bring computers to class or is class information posted in a LMS?). Where should students go to seek learning support? What are the class norms and where can students find the student handbook? While you must be sure students have reviewed all these documents, it does not need to be a boring event! You can create a questionnaire, or a treasure hunt, or break the class into small groups and ask them to highlight significant information and what it will mean to them and their classmates. Where possible, ask the students if they have suggestions for norms that will make the class productive for their learning. Use your creativity, engage the students, and keep it fun. Allow sufficient time for these activities, as this class session sets the tone for the rest of the course.

Most students like to meet with their faculty outside of classroom time to ask questions or to have a further dialogue. Holding office hours may be a requirement of all faculty and can be held in person on campus or using meeting technology for students at a distance. Be sure you build in time before and after class as well as office hours. Tell the students how you wish to interact with them and when. Tell students how and when you will return assignments and test grades (using the LMS? in class? from your office?). Inform students about how you can be contacted for course-related issues. It is appropriate to set limits so students do not expect you to be available 24 hours a day! Be sure students know how to contact you in an emergency (by phone, text, email).

Chapter Summary

This chapter has presented a preview of the role of a faculty member to prepare you for what you should do before you enter the classroom and what you can expect once you begin teaching. You are now ready to get started teaching in *your* classroom with *your* students! Here are key points to remember as you begin teaching your course:

- Understand your course in the context of the campus, academic program, and curriculum.
- Meet your colleagues before the course begins. Know who you can contact for questions, and find a mentor if one is not assigned to you. Meet and obtain contact information for the course leader and/or department chair. Meet your support staff, the people in the student services office, and the technology support team.
- Knowing your students will help you facilitate their learning. Take time to learn their names and their expectations for the course.
- Be prepared to establish a productive learning environment that welcomes all students. Students appreciate faculty who are fair, friendly, and equitable; follow established policies and procedures as described in

the syllabus. Be able to identify and manage disruptive behavior and ask for assistance from the course leader/department chair as needed.
- Above all, get ready to enjoy your role as a faculty member. Your greatest satisfaction will be knowing that you are preparing the next generation who will continue to advance the profession.

References

ADA Testing Accommodations. (2014). https://www.ada.gov/regs2014/testing_accommodations.html

Ephraim, N. (2021). Mentoring in nursing education: An essential element in the retention of new nurse faculty. *Journal of Professional Nursing, 37*(2), 306–319.

McClung, E., & Gaberson, K. (2020). Academic dishonesty among nursing students. *Nurse Educator, 46*(2), 111–115.

McClung, E., & Schneider, J. (2018). Dishonest behavior in the classroom and clinical setting: Perceptions and engagement. *Journal of Nursing Education, 57*(2), 79–87.

Moore, H., & Gaviola, M. (2018). Engaging students in a culture of integrity. *Journal of Nursing Education, 57*(4), 237–239.

Yarbrough, A., & Welch, S. (2021). Uncovering the process of reasonable academic accommodations for prelicensure nursing students with learning disabilities. *Nursing Education Perspectives, 2*(1), 5–10.

CHAPTER 8

Using Teaching and Learning Strategies in the Classroom

Before you begin using specific teaching and learning strategies, it will be helpful to understand the theoretical underpinnings of how students learn. This chapter introduces you to the dimensions and domains of learning, offers general principles for facilitating learning, and explains common theories that provide the evidence for choosing teaching-learning strategies. This chapter also provides an overview of a teaching-learning process and how to develop and use a lesson plan.

Knowledge Dimensions and Domains of Learning

The body of knowledge that you will be helping your students learn can be described in terms of the dimensions and domains of learning. Understanding the dimensions of knowledge and the domains of learning will help you choose and organize appropriate learning (and assessment and evaluation) strategies.

KNOWLEDGE DIMENSIONS

The knowledge dimension of learning refers to the type of knowledge to be learned and applied. One framework (Anderson & Krathwohl, 2016) differentiates four different types of learning: (1) factual—basic information needed to solve problems; (2) conceptual—relationships between the facts and the larger application of the facts; (3) procedural—skills and techniques; and (4) metacognitive—students' awareness of their own thinking processes. Teaching involves integrating these four dimensions of learning into learning activities as appropriate.

DOMAINS OF LEARNING

Bloom et al. (1956) classified learning into three domains of learning with levels of varying complexity (Fig. 8.1). The cognitive domain refers to knowledge, the psychomotor domain pertains to attaining skill competency, and the affective domain explains how students develop attitudes and values. Each domain is further described by sequential levels. This taxonomy is used extensively in health professions education to guide writing learning outcomes, choosing teaching-learning strategies, and aligning these with evaluation strategies, particularly exam items.

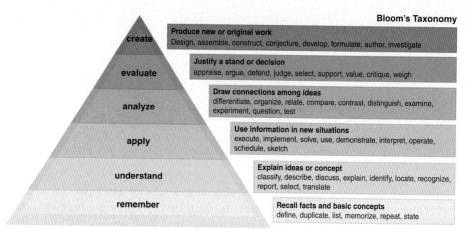

Fig. 8.1 Bloom's taxonomy. (Modified from Armstrong, P. [2010]. *Bloom's taxonomy*. University Center for Teaching. https://cft.vanderbilt.edu/guides-sub-pages/blooms-taxonomy/)

How Students Learn

Understanding how students learn is the foundation for successful teaching and learning. While your role is to identify what students should learn (learning outcomes/competencies) and to collaborate with students to determine how they can best attain the learning outcomes (learning activities), it is the students' responsibility to take an active part in their learning. In the health professions, faculty draw on theories of how students learn and use evidence-based practices for guiding students' learning. The following principles about how students learn, drawn from relevant learning theories from higher education (Ambrose et al., 2010; Chickering & Gamson, 1987) and health sciences literature, will provide a starting point as you begin your teaching journey. General principles about how students learn are summarized in the next paragraphs.

Learning occurs in both lower and higher levels of the learning domains. As noted in Fig. 8.1, students must first understand and remember the content they need to provide safe patient care; teaching-learning strategies such as reading assignments, study guides, and lecture help the student form a foundation of the knowledge base of the profession. At the same time, students must be able to apply, analyze, and evaluate the content to provide safe patient care. You can help students develop these higher-level cognitive skills by using teaching strategies that require the student to analyze data from a variety of sources such as the patient's health record, laboratory reports, or medication logs; use clinical information to draw conclusions about the patient; evaluate care outcomes; or create a plan of care.

Students' culture and previous life experiences affect how they learn. Students come to your classroom (online or on campus) and clinical experiences with beliefs, attitudes, and knowledge that may facilitate or hinder learning. Students must reconcile their own culture and life experiences with those experienced in the curriculum, courses, and with their patients. Faculty help students build these bridges by acknowledging and respecting what students bring to the learning experience and guiding students to reflect on how their beliefs and experiences intersect with those of their faculty, classmates, and patients.

Previous experience with learning guides current learning. By the time students enter professional programs they have had experience with how they learn. Students vary in their preferences for how to learn; for example, they may approach learning from a concrete or abstract perspective, or prefer to learn in a group or alone, or find it more effective to receive information in a visual, kinesthetic, or auditory format. While you can offer options that appeal to a variety of learning styles, students are also able to adapt their learning style to the nature of learning in your course.

Students' motivation determines how they approach learning. Motivation can be intrinsic (the desire to become a health professional) or extrinsic (the desire to pass the course). When students see value in the course content, understand how learning activities contribute toward their goals, and perceive support from faculty and peers, they are motivated to learn.

Adults learn differently than children; young adults learn differently from older adults. Recent research provides evidence that the age of the student has an impact on how they approach learning and how the faculty can use that information to facilitate learning. Malcom Knowles (1980) is known for his work in explaining the ways that adult learning (andragogy) differs from that of children (pedagogy). Adults are generally self-motivated and have life experiences to use as a basis for learning. Faculty draw on these characteristics when respecting what experience the adult student brings to the classroom and empower students to determine their own path to learning. Studies from neuroscience indicate that young adults take a multidimensional approach to learning as opposed to linear learning and focus on information that is relevant in the moment, as opposed to older adults who process information more sequentially. While both approaches to learning lead to similar outcomes, faculty can design learning activities that can be accomplished in a variety of ways.

Repetition and feedback reinforce learning. Skinner (1953) and other behaviorists believed that learning is observed through behavior, and behavior can be shaped by feedback. Feedback can be given by the faculty, by classmates, and by the students themselves. This theory is particularly useful when teaching skills where students are developing proficiency and in the classroom by giving student an opportunity for deliberate practice with an assignment in which they can receive feedback.

Learning occurs in an environment with others. Sociocultural theorists such as Vygotsky (1962), Piaget (1973), and Bandura (1977) believe that learning is an interactive process that occurs when students are interacting with their classmates, their faculty, and their patients. Your role is to structure learning activities in which students are working with each other and then to follow up with an activity in which the student can reflect and solidify the learning.

Developing professional expertise occurs in stages. Benner (1982) proposed that developing expertise involves passing through five stages from novice, advanced beginner, competent, proficient, to being an expert. As you work with your students it is helpful to be aware that students likely are at the novice stage of developing clinical knowledge and expertise and will require several years in clinical practice to become proficient or reach the expert stage. Knowing this can help you manage your expectations of how long it takes for students to become proficient or expert and the need to provide as many opportunities as possible for students to practice and use their knowledge and skills.

Thinking, reasoning, and judgment skills are essential to providing safe patient care. Developing judgment and reasoning skills requires students to use a consistent framework that is integrated into every patient encounter to develop a level of competency and mastery that ensures patient safety. Each discipline has a preferred iterative process, which in general guides students to gather patient information, analyze that information, make plans for patient care based on information, implement plans of care, and evaluate care outcomes.

What is learned can be stored in short- or long-term memory. Often described as surface versus deep learning, surface learning occurs when students memorize facts and content (short-term memory); deep learning, however, involves relating the facts to how they will be applied (long-term memory). Students who learn information just for the exam (surface learning) may not be able to retrieve the needed information in clinical practice (deep learning). You will be involved in helping students develop deep learning by providing opportunities for application in a real-world context with sufficient and deliberate practice.

Learning must be meaningful and have a context. Students will be more interested in learning when they understand why what they are learning will be essential to providing safe patient care. Teaching strategies in the classroom such as solving case studies or unfolding case studies, and using clinical scenarios that provide the context for learning and link the learning to clinical practice provide meaning to learning the facts.

Students learn most when they understand how they learn and can monitor and adapt their approach to learning (metacognition). Metacognition occurs when students are aware of how they think and evaluate the processes they are using to learn material. When students understand how they are learning, they can identify their own learning style preferences, modify how they are learning if needed, and tailor learning approaches to the task at hand. You can help students develop metacognitive skills by using teaching questions/ prompts to ask students how they came to certain conclusions or made specific clinical judgments and then follow up by drawing the student's attention to their development of metacognitive skills and increasing their awareness on how to use these skills.

Learning increases when faculty incorporate several ways students learn into each lesson plan. Chickering and Gamson (1987) reviewed literature about student learning in higher education and synthesized the findings into a practical framework called "Seven Principles of Good Education." These include (1) high expectations, which are communicated by establishing high-level learning outcomes and expecting success; (2) time on task, which is necessary for students to learn and apply course materials; (3) active learning, which occurs when students engage with the course content; (4) rich and prompt feedback, provided by faculty, peers, and students' own reflections on their learning; (5) interaction with classmates through class discussion and group projects; (6) interaction with faculty (role models) during office hours and school-related social events; and (7) faculty respect for student diversity, which is exhibited through a welcoming and inclusive learning environment. These seven principles can be integrated into each lesson plan.

The Teaching-Learning Process

Teaching in a classroom setting (as well as online and in clinical settings) is a process or a series of steps that are iterative. The process begins with establishing program, course, and lesson learning outcomes, which are then activated when you select evidence-based teaching strategies that align with these learning outcomes. Teaching strategies are the techniques faculty choose to guide learning, while learning activities are student centered and designed to promote student engagement in learning. After participating in learning activities, students must then have an opportunity to practice and apply what they are learning to patient care and receive feedback from you, their classmates, or from themselves as reflective learners. Next, you and the students must ensure that learning has occurred by using assessment strategies that provide sufficient feedback to master the learning outcome. The last step is evaluation, which results in measuring the students' learning and assigning a grade. You will use this process intentionally and intuitively each time you develop a lesson plan and teach your course.

The Lesson Plan

Faculty develop a lesson plan for each teaching session. A lesson plan communicates in writing learning outcomes, preclass assignments, teaching-learning activities, and assessment techniques that will take place during the class session (Box 8.1). The lesson plan serves as a guide for both you and the student about the expectations for what will be accomplished during the class session. Lesson plans can be included in the course syllabus or distributed to the

---

BOX 8.1 ■ Elements of a Lesson Plan

1. Introduction. Provide an overview of the session. Indicate the time frame for each activity. Gain students' attention. Use short videos, images, stories to provide context for what students will learn.
2. Learning outcomes. Review the outcomes with students by highlighting knowledge, skills, and attitudes/abilities they will attain at the end of the class session; communicate your high expectations for their learning!
3. Teaching-learning strategies and learning activities. A lesson plan includes preclass, in-class, and postclass learning activities. Preclass activities give students information they will need to understand and remember when they participate in the class session (see strategies to help students understand and remember). In class, choose teaching-learning strategies that

Continued on following page

BOX 8.1 ■ Elements of a Lesson Plan (Continued)

integrate preclass assignments and previous learning to help students apply what they have
learned in a clinical context (see strategies to help students apply, analyze, create content
and think critically, collaborate or work in teams, use verbal or written presentation skills,
or develop a professional identity). Assign postclass activities that give students opportunities to practice and apply course content and receive feedback before they are evaluated.

4. Practice and assessment. Give students time in class or after class to apply concepts in
   real-world situations, practice, and receive feedback. Specify how learning will be assessed
   (e.g., practice test questions or a short paper).
5. Summary. Conclude the lesson by reviewing key points related to lesson outcomes.
6. Evaluation. Evaluation and grading of student learning usually occurs after the student
   completes the lesson (see Chapter 13). Indicate what aspects of the lesson will be included
   in the evaluation plan.
7. Preview the next lesson; clarify assignments.

---

students before the class begins. Review the lesson plans for your course or
develop your own.

Teaching-Learning Strategies

Teaching-learning strategies are used to promote student engagement and
active learning. Choose strategies to help students achieve course outcomes
to help students (1) learn and remember course content, (2) apply the content to clinical practice, (3) collaborate and work in teams, (4) develop verbal and written presentation skills, and (5) acquire a professional identity.
Teaching-learning strategies can be used across all settings, including the
classroom, clinical practicum, learning resources/simulation centers, and in
online courses. This chapter discusses the teaching-learning strategies used
the classroom. For more information about their use in the clinical setting or
in online courses, see Parts 3 and 4. Most teaching-learning strategies can
also be used as evaluation strategies and graded; see Chapter 13 for how to
use these strategies to evaluate students' attainment of course outcomes.

Teaching-learning strategies are used not only to help students learn the
content (understanding and remembering) but also to ensure that students can
apply what they have learned to giving safe patient care (applying, analyzing,
evaluating, and creating). It may be helpful to think of using a variety of
teaching-learning activities at three distinct time periods: before the class,
during the class, and after the class. Preclass assignments prepare students to
participate in active learning during class. Here, you can use strategies such
as reading assignments, worksheets, pretests, or a digital lecture to highlight
important concepts. During class, students will apply the information using
strategies such as case studies, role play, or small-group work. Other strategies
can be used as postclass follow-up such as reflections, written papers, or
completed worksheets that may or may not be graded.

It is likely that the first time you teach in the classroom you are using an
already developed syllabus, and the teaching-learning strategies will have been

selected and assigned to the students. As you gain more experience, however, you can adapt the strategies to your own emerging teaching style. Teaching in the classroom should be creative and fun for both you and the students!

STRATEGIES TO HELP STUDENTS UNDERSTAND AND REMEMBER COURSE CONTENT

The following strategies are typically used *before* the class so students have a basic understanding of terminology and foundational material that they will then use *during* class. Students may come to class expecting to hear a lecture and receive the content and thus do not prepare by reading the textbook or completing assignments. To ensure that students are prepared to participate in class, you may require students to pass a pretest or submit an assignment before they come to class.

Reading Assignments

Most courses use a textbook to provide foundational information related to course content. The assigned readings are noted in the syllabus, and you should read the assigned readings so to know (1) what knowledge to expect from the student, (2) how much time it will take the student to complete the assignment, (3) what important content the student should obtain from the assignment, (4) how you will integrate the readings into your lesson plan, and (5) what additional information you will need to provide to ensure students' success. Students in the beginning courses in the curriculum may have difficulty identifying essential information and determining how to apply it in a clinical context. When developing your lesson plan, consider what other teaching strategies you can use to help the students learn how to obtain information and then apply it to patient care.

Lecture

A lecture is an organized presentation about a specific topic and is often accompanied by visual enhancements such as PowerPoints. Lecture allows faculty to present a large amount of foundational information in a short time but has the disadvantage of being a passive learning activity. Some students rely on faculty to provide this baseline information, and students for whom English is not their first language find it helpful to review important information when it is available in an outline or visual format such as from a recorded or narrated presentation such as PowerPoint (see Part 4).

Previous course faculty may have lecture material you can adapt for your use. Textbook publishers often provide lecture outlines, learning activities, and PowerPoints. If you are using lecture notes or other teaching materials developed by another faculty or provided by the publisher, you first must evaluate these for accuracy, completeness, fit with the course, and the amount of time allocated to the topic. Also, you must evaluate all materials that you are using in the course to ensure that the information aligns with course learning outcomes/competencies and the exam.

You can enhance the use of the lecture to engage students by giving a micro lecture (a short burst of content) and then asking the students to apply the content to solve a case study or intersperse practice test questions or polling questions so students can assess their understanding of the content. Another way to use the lecture strategy is to create a narrated PowerPoint lecture and place it in the course learning management system (see Part 4). You can use this prerecorded lecture as a preclass assignment.

STRATEGIES TO HELP STUDENTS APPLY, ANALYZE, EVALUATE COURSE CONTENT AND TO THINK CRITICALLY AND MAKE EFFECTIVE CLINICAL JUDGMENTS

Students will ultimately use course content in a clinical context that requires them to think critically and make effective clinical judgments. You can use the following strategies to meet this teaching goal.

Class Discussion

Discussion, when guided by high-level questions that go beyond factual knowledge, helps students think, articulate their knowledge or views, broaden their views by listening to other viewpoints, make judgments, evaluate ideas, and apply class content. Discussion gives you an opportunity to correct misunderstandings and provide feedback. You can conduct a discussion in a large class, but breaking the class into small groups gives students more opportunities to participate. Discussion can be combined with other strategies such as lecture or case study.

Case Study/Clinical Scenario

Case studies are representations of clinical situations. The cases integrate class content such as health history, lab values, health care provider's orders, or clinical notes, but they also require students to use thinking and judgment processes to determine appropriate actions for patient care.

While you or your students can design a clinical case, you may also find already developed cases to use or adapt from the textbook resources or online faculty teaching websites. Before you use the case study with the students, review the key teaching points that you will highlight. You can use the case with individuals, small groups, or the entire class working to solve the case. Your role is to use teaching prompts to elicit student's thinking and ability to draw on the course content, to enrich the discussion with additional information, and give feedback.

Reflection Papers

Reflection papers, journals, and blogs are written or electronic comments about the students' experience that relates to the content of the lesson or course. Structure these papers so the student applies course material and reflects, analyzes, or critiques their participation in the experience. You can have students share their reflections with their classmates and receive feedback. You can also grade these papers.

Role Play

Role play is a short, acted out scenario or situation in which students assume various roles (patient, health care provider, manager, family member) in a variety of situations such as giving a shift report, confronting incivility, teaching a patient, or interacting with a disturbed, confused, anxious, or psychotic patient. Role playing gives students an opportunity to assess and respond to the situation. The role play promotes empathetic communication, clinical judgment, and application of knowledge. Learning from a role play takes place during a guided debriefing in which students reflect on what occurred during the role play, what went well, and what can be improved.

Your responsibility is to design or use an existing role play. Be sure you have clear learning outcomes and have identified the key points you want students to learn from the experience. You can have several students enact the scenario while the other students observe and participate in debriefing. You can also have students form groups with each student participating in a role, and one student serving as the facilitator to guide the debriefing. This strategy uses your creativity and is a quick and fun way to engage students.

STRATEGIES TO HELP STUDENTS LEARN TO COLLABORATE AND WORK IN TEAMS

An essential skill for all health care professionals is to be able to work in teams. The following strategies can be used to set the stage for students to work with each other in a classroom setting, and if you have students from a variety of disciplines in the class, these strategies help students develop intra- and interprofessional teamwork.

Think-Pair-Share

This simple strategy pairs two or three students, who first think (i.e., develop their own answer to the task at hand), then pair (come together) to exchange their response with their classmates to form a more complete answer or solution, and finally share (present) their refined answer to the larger class. This strategy can be accomplished in 5 minutes for thinking and pairing, and, depending on the size of the class, 10 to 15 minutes for sharing. The ultimate learning outcome is for students to learn the skills and appreciate the benefits of collaboration.

Collaborative Learning

Collaborative learning involves students working together to solve a clinical situation, write a paper, develop a poster or presentation, or make a video. Each student must contribute to the effort of the group and at the completion of the learning activity reflect on the group process. Some students prefer to work alone, and some students may contribute little effort to the learning activity. As needed, you may decide to require students to submit a group reflection on the collaboration process or ask students to identify what they contributed individually to the group effort. You can also assign roles and/or points for participation.

Games

Games promote cognitive and affective learning in a competitive environment usually with two or more students, although students individually can compete within the game to improve their own score or time to solve a task. Games can also be used to simulate a clinical scenario. You may develop your own game or locate online games, such as Jeopardy-style or scenario-style games. You can help students solidify learning with a short debriefing session that focuses on the process of collaboration and teamwork.

STRATEGIES TO HELP STUDENTS DEVELOP VERBAL AND WRITTEN PRESENTATION SKILLS

Health care professionals must be able to communicate effectively in both verbal and written formats. You can integrate the following strategies into class activities that develop these skills.

Student Presentations

Presentations help students develop skills of organizing and presenting content professionally. In the classroom you can assign a group of students (or students can form their own groups) to develop a presentation or a poster related to the content and concepts of the lesson. Your role is to define the elements that should be included in the presentation, establish time limits for the presentation, prompt presenters to amplify or clarify their presentation, and reflect on the contribution this strategy made to the lesson and course learning outcomes.

Debate

A debate involves an argument and defense of a position. This strategy helps students develop critical thinking and logical reasoning skills as well as verbal skills for stating their position. You can organize the debate to be completed by two people with the class observing and serving as judges or by having all students in the class pair up and conduct the debate. You can also assign teams of students to develop the argument and defense and present the various positions to the class. The topic for debate should align with a learning outcome and have enough different viewpoints to encourage a discussion.

Written Papers

Students must be able to communicate effectively in writing. You can provide opportunities for students to write short papers that, for example, connect concepts, present a teaching plan, or persuade public officials to take action about a health care concern. Longer papers can be used to develop a care plan, present a community assessment, or analyze a health care system. When assigning written papers, particularly if they are lengthy, it is helpful to establish a time frame that gives you an opportunity to review an outline, parts of the paper as they are completed, or a full draft so that you can give feedback prior to grading the paper.

STRATEGIES TO HELP STUDENTS DEVELOP A PROFESSIONAL IDENTITY

The curriculum in which you are teaching likely has end-of-program and end-of-course learning outcomes/competencies for students to become socialized to the profession and develop a professional identity. These competencies may be more relevant in some courses than others, and at various levels of the curriculum, but as appropriate, the following strategies can be designed to help students attain these competencies. These classroom activities facilitate application to clinical practice when the student is enrolled in the clinical course that may be aligned with this course.

Role Play

You can use role play (see earlier) to help students develop ethical and professional behavior. For example, the students can enact situations that involve difficult conversations, such as a scenario that involves a medication error or a conversation with a family considering end-of-life issues. When using this strategy be sure the learning outcomes are clear to the student and use the debriefing session to elicit a range of issues related to the topic.

Case Studies

You can also design or locate relevant case studies (see earlier) that can be used to engage students in attaining program outcomes that relate to professionalism and professional identity.

STRATEGIES TO DEVELOP CULTURAL HUMILITY, GLOBAL APPRECIATION, AND CIVIC RESPONSIBILITY

While a large part of the curriculum is devoted to developing the students' ability to provide safe patient care and perform specific clinical skills, many health sciences programs have program outcomes/competencies to develop students' cultural humility, global appreciation, and civic responsibility. Cultural humility is the process of understanding one's own culture to understand another's culture. Acquiring a global appreciation involves understanding the need for improving health and ensuring health equity worldwide. Civic responsibility refers to engaging in activities that improve the community through volunteer efforts. The program in which you are teaching may have specific teaching-learning activities to help students develop the values of service, global awareness, and civic responsibilities. Three common learning activities that contribute to the formation of these values are described next.

Service Learning

Service learning is a structured learning activity designed to facilitate students' learning about cultural and social values of communities and populations through establishing a partnership that benefits the community or population requesting the service while providing students an opportunity to develop cultural humility, continue to develop a personal and professional identity, and appreciate the value of service (Dombrowsky et al., 2019). Service learning experiences take place in the community and involve collaboration with the community but are connected to program and course learning outcomes. Service experiences are distinct from clinical experiences that are designed for students to apply knowledge and skills, in that the service experience focuses on developing students' affective skills. The service experiences may be either integrated into courses across the curriculum or linked but distinct from a specific course. A service learning experience may be included in the course you are teaching. Teaching a service learning course requires specific orientation and training, and if you are asked to teach a service learning course be sure you understand the intended learning outcomes and how to facilitate the students' experience.

Internationalizing the Curriculum and Study-Abroad Programs

Global health focuses on improving the health status of all people worldwide. Several organizations and higher education associations have developed competencies and goals for global learning that can be used to guide experiences for health professions to use in local and global populations. Global health experiences can be integrated throughout the curriculum, known as internationalizing the curriculum (Indiana University–Purdue University at Indianapolis, 2022), to prepare students to live and work in local and global communities and enhance multicultural understanding and communication skills. In other models, colleges/universities/schools offer students an opportunity to meet goals of global understanding through a credit-bearing experience in another community or country. Teaching in these programs requires a specific set of skills, a complete orientation, and support from the campus such as legal and travel support and guidelines for expectations of students' behavior while traveling abroad. If you are interested in participating in these programs discuss your interest with the people involved in offering them.

Civic and Community Engagement

Many health care agencies, colleges, and universities have a mission for engaging with the community and providing service in areas such as food insecurity, homelessness, health teaching programs, or environmental action. Participating in these programs may be a course requirement for your students to attain campus and school learning outcomes that are designed to help students develop values for community engagement. More likely students will volunteer in programs in areas of their interest.

Chapter Summary

Teaching in the classroom is the most significant role of the faculty. While it will take several semesters before you have mastered the competencies necessary to be an effective classroom teacher, each class you teach will be different, and you will learn as much from your students as they will learn from you. This chapter has provided an overview of learning, the teaching-learning process, and teaching-learning strategies. Here are key points:

- Learning is described in dimensions and domains. Bloom's taxonomy of learning domains (cognitive, psychomotor, and affective) can be used to align assignments, teaching/learning, and evaluation strategies.
- Students learn in different ways. There are a variety of theories/frameworks that explain how students may approach learning in your course. Use these theories to choose/use appropriate teaching-learning strategies.
- Teaching and learning include establishing program and course outcomes, using evidence-based teaching-learning strategies, structuring time for deliberate practice and assessment with feedback to the students, and evaluating students' attainment of the learning outcomes and assigning a grade. Using an iterative teaching-learning process model describes the elements and sequence of effective teaching.
- Lesson plans describe what is to be accomplished during a defined time frame. Learning improves when students know exactly what they are to accomplish and if they have done so.
- Teaching-learning strategies are selected to help students attain the desired course learning outcomes/competencies.

References

Ambrose, S., Bridges, M., DiPietro, M., Lovett, M., & Norman, M. (2010). *How learning works*. Jossey-Bass.

American Association of Colleges & Universities. (n.d.). *Global learning VALUE rubric*. https://www.aacu.org/value/rubrics/global-learning

Anderson, L. W., & Krathwohl, D. R. (Eds.). (2016). *A taxonomy for learning, teaching and assessing: A revision of Bloom's taxonomy of educational objectives*. Longman.

Bandura, A. (1977). *Social learning theory*. Prentice Hall.

Benner, P. (1982). *From novice to expert*. Addison Wesley.

Bloom, B., Englehart, M., Furst, E., Hill, W., & Krathwohl, D. (Eds.). (1956). *Taxonomy of educational objectives*. Longmans, Green.

Chickering, A., & Gamson, Z. (1987). Seven principles for good practice in undergraduate education. *Wingspread Journal, 9*(2), 1–7.

Dombrowsky, T., Gustafson, K., & Cauble, D. (2019). Service-learning and clinical nursing education: A Delphi inquiry. *Journal of Nursing Education, 58*(7), 381–391.

Indiana University–Purdue University at Indianapolis. (2022). *Curriculum internationalization*. https://international.iupui.edu/global-learning/curriculum-internationalization/index. html#:~:text=Benefits%20of%20Curriculum%20Internationalization%201%20Provides% 20exposure%20to,students%20in%20internationally%20informed%20research%20More% 20items...%20

Knowles, M. (1980). *The modern practice of adult education*. Follet.

Piaget, J. (1973). *To understand is to invent: The future of education*. Grossman.

Skinner, B. F. (1953). *Science and human behavior*. Macmillan.

Vygotsky, L. (1962). *Thought and language*. MIT Press.

CHAPTER 9

Evaluating Teaching and Learning in the Classroom

The fourth and fifth steps of the teaching-learning process are to assess and evaluate the students' attainment of course learning outcomes and assign grades. This chapter explains these steps and describes related strategies. The chapter concludes with a discussion of evaluating course and teaching effectiveness and provides examples of how you, your students, administrators, and peers can provide feedback for teaching improvement.

Assessment, Evaluation, and Grading

As noted in previous chapters, assessment is formative in nature and uses techniques to give students an opportunity to practice what they are learning while receiving feedback. Evaluation, on the other hand, is a summative activity in which judgment is made about students' attainment of course competencies. Evaluation ends in a grade. Two grading philosophies guide the assignment of grades: criterion referenced and norm referenced. Criterion-referenced grading is based on the premise that all students can meet the criterion (learning outcome). With criterion-referenced grading all students can potentially master the content and achieve 100% of the points used to determine a grade. When using norm-referenced grading, the students' scores are placed on a curve and a certain percentage (usually 10%) of students will attain the top grades and also the lowest grades, and the remaining scores will be equally distributed on the curve. Criterion- referenced grading is typically used in the health professions because it is important that all students who pass the course have attained the course outcomes. When you are assigning grades, you will follow the evaluation plan, which includes the evaluation strategies and the grading scale, which links the cumulative score to a course grade (Fig. 9.1). The evaluation plan and grading scale are posted in the syllabus; you must use this plan and the grading scale to assign grades fairly and equitably.

Strategies to Assess Student Learning

Assessment strategies are learner-centered, teacher-directed activities that give both you and the student information about how well the student understands course concepts (Angelo & Cross, 1993). The activities are used to improve both the students' learning and your teaching. Assessment strategies are short and

Example of an evaluation plan and grading scale

Evaluation Plan

The student's performance in the course will be measured as follows:

- Exam #1 (25 Points)
- Exam #2 (25 Points)
- Exam #3 (25 Points)
- Assignments (concept paper, 10 Points; 3 case studies, 5 Points each (25 Points Possible)

Evaluation consists of three (3) in-class multiple choice examinations (see test blueprint) 1 concept paper (see grading rubric) and 3 case studies (see grading rubric). Students must achieve a minimum final course grade of 75% for successful completion of the course. Exam scores are not rounded up. There is no extra credit offered.

Grading Scale

Grade	Percentage
A+	96% to 100%
A	93% to 95.99%
A minus	90% to 92.99%
B+	87% to 89.99%
B	84% to 86.99%
B minus	81% to 83.99%
C+	78% to 80.99%
C	75% to 77.99%
C minus	72% to 74.99%
D+	69% to 71.99%
D	66% to 68.99%
D minus	63% to 65.99%
F	62.99% and below

A grade of "C" is the cut-off for a passing grade in this didactic course.

Fig. 9.1 Example of an evaluation plan and grading scale.

easy to administer. They are not graded, but faculty, students, and student peers give feedback to improve learning. Two easy-to-use classroom assessment techniques are practice test questions and 1-minute papers. Both can be used in on-campus and online courses.

PRACTICE TEST QUESTIONS

Practice test questions are similar in style and level of the domain to those that might appear on an exam but are used for learning, not grading. These questions can be embedded in a PowerPoint, administered using the testing software of a learning management system as a nongraded quiz (see Part 4), used as polling questions in the classroom, or generated by students for practice in small groups. Faculty provide feedback to the students' answers by discussing the rationale for the correct and incorrect answers.

1-MINUTE PAPERS

These papers prompt students to apply course content in a short (1 minute!) paper. Faculty pose a question that requires the student to use higher-order thinking skills such as apply, analyze, or make a clinical judgment using the information that has just been discussed in class. Students then write a quick response. Students can share their answers and receive feedback from faculty and classmates. You can also collect the papers, usually without student identification, and review them to identify common misconceptions that you can use to determine if additional teaching/learning is necessary.

Strategies to Evaluate Student Learning

Evaluation strategies measure the extent to which the student has attained course learning outcomes/competencies. They must align with the learning outcomes/competencies of the course. The strategy should also align with the teaching strategy (see Chapter 8) so students can learn in the way they will be evaluated. Using a variety of evaluation strategies addresses the variation in domains of learning as well as students' preferred learning style.

Evaluation strategies must also be valid, reliable, and easy to use. Above all, faculty must use the strategy and grade all students equitably and fairly. The results of the evaluation strategy are used in assigning a grade to each student as specified in the evaluation plan and grading scale.

In courses with large enrollments, there may be several sections of the course. If the same syllabus is designed to be used in each section taught by different faculty, it will be important to ensure that all faculty use the same teaching and evaluation strategies and grading scale. Having frequent course meetings to discuss student progress it is imperative to ensure fairness and equity in assigning course grades across all sections of the course; if needed, it may be helpful to have a meeting to establish interrater reliability (see Part 3) by having a faculty teaching in the course grade all assignments, discuss the results, and consider how to harmonize the grading so the grade is comparable across each section.

STRATEGIES TO EVALUATE STUDENTS' UNDERSTANDING OF COURSE CONCEPTS

Exams

An exam is a common way to evaluate student learning outcomes. While exam items are time consuming to write, once well developed, exams can be used to sample a large amount of learning in a short amount of time. A benefit of using exams with prelicensure students is that this testing format may be like the exam that students may experience when they take a licensing exam.

You may be asked to develop exam items, but more likely you will be responsible for administering and proctoring the exam as well as participating in exam review sessions or meeting with the students to discuss the exam results. Before participating in any aspect of using exams as an evaluation strategy, you should understand the key elements of exam development, administration, and scoring.

Types of Exam Questions. There are a variety of types of exams such as essay, matching, or fill in the blank, but the most common exams are multiple choice and structured option, in which the answers are provided for the student and the student must choose the correct answer.

Exam Blueprint. Designing an exam begins with making an exam plan or blueprint. The blueprint ensures that all learning outcomes that will be evaluated on the test are included, and that the relative importance of the content is ensured (Fig. 9.2). A simple blueprint includes a two-way grid with learning outcomes on one axis and content to be tested on the other. The number of items per learning outcome is presented in the appropriate cell. Blueprints can also be three or four dimensional to include other components of learning that faculty wish to emphasize such as the steps of a clinical judgment model, level of the domain of learning, or components of a framework for a licensing or certification exam.

Exam blueprint for a 10-item test

Learning outcome	Content area A heart failure	Content area B arrhythmias	Content area C blood disorders	Content area D coronary artery disease
1. Know use and side effects of drugs used to treat patients with cardiovascular disorders	3 items	1 item		1 item
2. Perform a physical assessment for a patient with a cardiovascular disorder	1 item	1 item		1 item
3. Using data from patient's health history and physical assessment, identify patients priority health problem			1 item	1 item

Fig. 9.2 Exam blueprint for a 10-item test.

Developing a blueprint prior to developing test items ensures that the test is valid by representing relevant content. The blueprint also is used to guide student learning and preparation for the test. Faculty should share the blueprint with the students at the beginning of the course or prior to the administration of the exam.

Exam Items. Exam items are developed to determine students' attainment of the learning outcomes/competencies. Items include a scenario (clinical situation) that provides the context of the question and includes data the student must use to answer the question; a stem (question), which indicates what the student is being asked to do; and four or more options (answers) (Fig. 9.3, Box 9.1). One or more answers is clearly correct, and the others are plausible but clearly wrong.

In addition to items that are developed by course faculty, you should know that exam items are available online and in test banks from textbook publishers. It may be tempting to use these questions on your test, but before you do be sure each question does the following: (1) aligns with the course/lesson learning outcomes/competencies for your course, (2) is at the intended level of the domain, (3) is represented in the test blueprint, (4) tests information students have learned, and (5) requires the students to apply the information to patient care. Also know that students have access to exam items that are published in ancillary materials in a textbook and others that are posted online and shared widely.

Time Allocation for Administering an Exam. The amount of time allocated to administering a test has been traditionally determined by a rule of giving students 1 minute to answer each test item, but recent evidence indicates that students may need more time because exam items have become more complex, and more students have disabilities that require accommodation or for whom

---

Example of a multiple-choice exam item

Scenario: A client is receiving 1,000 mL normal saline with 40mEq KCL which is infusing at 125 mL/h. The client tells the nurse "My IV hurts".

Stem: What should the nurse do **first**?

Options:
1. Notify the health care provider.
2. Slow the infusion to a keep-open rate of 20-50 mL/h.
3. **Assess the IV insertion site for signs of extravasation.**
4. Check the solution and administration set for date when mixed.

Fig. 9.3 Example of a multiple-choice exam item.

BOX 9.1 ■ Guidelines for Developing Exam Items

Scenario

- Set the context by describing the patient (e.g., age, gender, race, ethnicity if pertinent); the clinical setting (e.g., home, clinic, intensive care unit, rehabilitation center); current contact with health professional/agency (e.g., on admission, postoperative; being intubated); health history; health assessment data; laboratory tests, medications, health care provider orders/prescriptions, radiographic tests as pertinent.
- Describe the problem the student is to solve (e.g., what to do first; what information to obtain; which health care professional to report information to; calculate a drug dose).
- Include relevant and irrelevant data to require students to determine what is most important and needs to be included in making a clinical judgment about care.
- Include information from the chart such as an admissions note, laboratory report, medication record that requires student to interpret the information to answer the question.

Stem/Question

- Ask one question per item.
- Ask questions that require application, analysis, evaluation, creation.
- Use action verbs at higher levels of the cognitive domain.
- Ask questions that require the student to consider various steps of a clinical judgment model such as gather information, determine the patient's problem, determine priorities, take action/implement a plan, evaluate outcomes.
- Write clear, direct questions. Students should not need to guess what the question is asking them to do.

Answers/Options

- Write the correct answer(s) first.
- Identify the source for the correct answer (textbook, reading assignments, discussion in class) for the correct answer. Students may challenge the answer and you must be able to refer them to the source.
- Write the incorrect answers next. Consider points where students may be confused or could make an error. All incorrect answers must be plausible. The incorrect answer should be clearly distinct from the correct answer.
- All answers should be similar in style and length.

Style, Peer Review, and Proofreading

- Use simple, clear language. Avoid slang, jargon, cultural references unless that is the focus of the item.
- Have one or more colleagues review the exam items for style and accuracy.
- Proofread, proofread! Check spelling and punctuation.

English is not their primary language. A preferred testing practice is to consider the student and test complexity, obtain data about the number of students who finish the test in the time allotted, and then add half as much additional time for students who need it. Birkhead (2018) found that giving students the option of extended time reduced their stress and did not impact exam grades or program outcomes.

Administering and Proctoring an Exam. One of your responsibilities may be to administer and/or proctor the test. The test can be administered in a format using a hard copy of the test and a Scantron answer sheet or can be administered

---

BOX 9.2 ■ Guidelines for Proctoring an Exam in a Classroom or Computer Center

1. Review college and school policies regarding academic honesty with particular attention to procedures for (a) identifying the students who are to be taking the exam, (b) identifying signs of cheating, and (c) knowing what to do when cheating is suspected.
2. Ensure that bookbags, phones, notes, hats, and other items are placed at the front or outside of the room.
3. Ensure that seats are spaced at a distance, and that each student has a comfortable seat for taking the exam. Some courses may require assigned seating.
4. Distribute the tests and answer sheets to each individual student; use alternative forms of the test as per course practices.
5. Ask students to sign academic honesty pledges if required.
6. Remind students of procedures that will occur if cheating is observed.
7. When you suspect a student is cheating (eyes on classmate's test; referring to notes), move the student to another part of the room. After the student has submitted the exam, discuss the incident with the student and follow up as needed with the course leader or other administrator.
8. Two faculty always should be in the classroom to ensure exam security. Move around the room and observe that students are focusing on the test in front of them.

---

online. Faculty administer the hard copy test in a classroom and administer computer-generated tests either in an onsite computer center or a remote testing center. In some situations, students may take the exam on their own computer or mobile device at their home or remote location, often using remote proctoring systems to ensure academic honesty.

Regardless of how the test is administered, you are responsible for maintaining exam security and an environment of academic honesty. Using proctors is the most effective way to ensure exam security and academic honesty when the exam is given in the classroom or computer center (Box 9.2). When exams are deployed to the students' personal computer, faculty may use test protection software and/or cameras (see Part 4). If you have access to the test file or a test bank, you must protect the security of the exam when it is maintained on a computer or removable hard drive.

Postexam Review, Item Analysis, and Item Revision With Faculty. Following the exam, course faculty meet to review the exam results and assign grades. Most schools use a test scoring service that provides an analysis for each question and overall data about the test such as mean, standard deviation, effectiveness of test options, measure of reliability, item difficulty, and item discrimination (McDonald, 2018) (Box 9.3). For additional information about these statistics talk to the consultants at the test scoring service used at your school.

After conducting the item analysis, faculty may note errors in the test such as items in which an error was made when entering the correct answer on the answer key or significant typographic errors that confused students. Faculty may decide to eliminate questions in which there was teacher error and rescore the test before giving students their scores. Item analysis will also reveal which questions most students did not answer correctly (note by

BOX 9.3 ■ Exam Item Analysis

Validity. An exam is valid when it samples students' knowledge of *relevant content* in the discipline. This means the test questions related to content students learned and expected to be on the test. Valid exams test students' attainment of course learning outcomes/competencies and standards of best practice. Using an exam blueprint will ensure that the exam items are linked to course or lesson learning outcomes/competencies and the number of questions on the exam correlate with the amount of teaching and learning time in the course.

   Reliability. A reliable test measures student knowledge consistently. The Kuder-Richardson (K-R) coefficient assesses exam interitem consistency and is calculated and reported by the exam scoring service. This data point is used with others (see later) to understand the reliability of the overall test. Reliability is affected by the number of items on the exam and the number of students taking the test. Large numbers of test items and students improve the reliability of an exam, and this may not be practical for classroom tests in the health professions. Thus there is a wide range of what is considered an acceptable measure of exam reliability using the Kuder-Richardson coefficient or other similar measures.

   Range = 0–1
      Coefficient of .50 is acceptable.
      Coefficient of .60 is adequate.
      Coefficient of .75 is ideal.

   Mean. Average of scores. Compare this statistic to your grading scale to obtain an *estimate* of the grade most students attained on this exam.

   Standard deviation. Range of scores around the mean. A smaller standard deviation indicates most scores are close to the mean.

   Effectiveness of exam options (answers). The scoring service will provide a report of the percentage of students choosing *each* answer. This information is helpful in understanding which information students did not learn well (if most students choose the same incorrect answer) and in determining which options to revise. You can also use this profile of each item to determine if any option needs to be revised.

   Item difficulty. Percentage of students choosing the correct answer.

   Range = 0.1–1.0; ideal is .70 to .80

   Item discrimination. Indicates the extent to which students who scored well on the test differed from those who did not score well. The discrimination index is calculated as a point biserial correlation using the top 10% (or 15%, depending on the test scoring service) of the scores compared to the bottom 10% (15%) of the scores. The correlation can be positive or negative. A positive correlation indicates that students who scored well on the test answered the question correctly and students who did not score well on the test did not answer the question correctly. Conversely, a negative correlation will result when students who typically scored well in the exam did not score well on the question or students who did not score well on the exam answered the question correctly.

   While item difficulty indicates the percentage of students who answered the question correctly, it does not indicate how individual students scored. Item discrimination provides information about which students answered the question correctly. The item discrimination index can range from 0 (no correlation) to 1 (perfect correlation). The closer the index approaches 1, the stronger the item is in differentiating students who understood or did not understand the content on the exam. The following scale shows an estimate of a way to interpret the strength of the discrimination index.

   Range = 0–1
      ≥.30 is excellent.
      .20–.29 is good.
      .10–.19 is fair.
      ≤.09 is poor.

reviewing the item difficulty and the effectiveness of the options) or questions that may have confused students who typically knew the content on the exam (note by reviewing the item for a negative discrimination). Faculty may consider removing these items and rescoring the exam before returning results to the students.

At the end of the exam review, and before administering the same test items again, faculty should revise ineffective questions. Questions that should be revised include those that were too difficult or too easy, that did not have a strong discrimination index, were not written clearly, or in which there was a negative item discrimination indicating students who scored well on the other test questions were the students who scored low on this test question.

Postexam Review With Students. Students should have an opportunity to review their test to (1) determine why they missed a particular test item, (2) how to improve their test-taking skills, and (3) learn the correct answer. Box 9.4 provides guidelines for conducting a postexam review with students. Students may ask you to award points that will improve their score, and you must be fair and apply all course policies in a consistent way for each student.

BOX 9.4 ■ Conducting a Postexam Review With Students

1. Review the exam with students after the test by having students make an appointment with you or review the exam with the entire class as a group. If you conduct the review with a group of students, establish ground rules such as (1) grades will not be changed, (2) all exams must be returned, and (3) no notes or photocopying of the exam questions.
2. Before you conduct the postexam review, review the test and know the correct answer and rationale. Review the incorrect answers to be able to explain to the students why the answer was incorrect.
3. Ensure security of the exam. If exams are returned to students in a group, count the exams before and after the exam review. Observe students to ensure they are not photocopying the questions or making notes.
4. Keep the focus on learning the content and the process of answering test questions correctly. Students should leave the test review knowing (1) the correct answer, (2) the relationship of the amount of their exam preparation to the exam grade, and (3) why they missed the test question (such as not knowing the content, not reading the question carefully, guessing, not being prepared, or not understanding terminology).

Collaborative Testing

Collaborative testing is an assessment or evaluation strategy in which students work in teams to take an exam that may be used for students to assess their own learning, to review for a test, as a posttest review, or to take a test that will be graded to evaluate learning outcomes. There are several ways to organize the logistics of collaborative testing. One approach is to randomly assign students in groups of two to five. First, students take the test individually, then meet as a group to take the test again discussing the test item and agreeing on the correct answer and marking it on the one test, which is also scored. You will score both tests and award additional points to the individual test if the group test grade is higher than students' individual test grades. A simple approach to adjusting grades is to add 3 points to the individual test if the group test is graded as an A, 2 points if the group test is a B, and 1 point if the group test is a C. Typically, students improve their grade when scores from both tests are used.

Collaborative testing promotes teamwork and ultimately the ability to collaborate in clinical situations. Other benefits of collaborative testing include developing students' skills for giving peer feedback, being able to articulate a position, and developing critical thinking and clinical judgment skills. Collaborative testing can also decrease test anxiety in some students. One disadvantage from the faculty perspective is the time required to organize, administer, and grade the test.

STRATEGIES TO EVALUATE COMMUNICATION SKILLS

Written Work

Written work such as reflection papers, reports of projects, summaries of patient experiences, an analysis of a problem, a review of a clinical agency organization, or scholarly work can be evaluated and graded. Written work is graded using preestablished guidelines, or rubrics, which specify the number of points awarded for addressing each element of the paper (Box 9.5). Using rubrics will help you quickly evaluate the quality of the paper, identify the inclusion of the required elements in the paper, provide consistency as you grade all the papers for a group of students, and simplify the grading process.

BOX 9.5 ■ How to Develop a Grading Rubric for a Written Assignment

1. Identify the purpose and goal of the assignment.
2. Identify the key criteria/components to be included in the assignment.
3. Describe the performance for each level of the criteria using descriptions (excellent–poor), percentages (100%–0%), or letter grades (A–F).

Presentations

When evaluating student presentations, the focus is on the content as well as the ability of students to present their work to a group. The presentations may involve one student or a group of students who present information to their classmates, faculty, patients, or clinical staff. Presentations are easily graded using a rubric that specifies the criteria by which the presentation is judged.

Case studies/clinical scenarios/care plans

Case studies/clinical scenarios are used to evaluate students' ability to apply, evaluate, and create plans of care for patients and communicate the plan effectively. When used as an evaluation strategy, case studies/clinical scenarios are useful to determine that students can make safe clinical judgments. These are easily evaluated using a rubric.

Monitoring Student Progress

Both you and the student have responsibility for monitoring academic progress throughout the course. After each evaluation event that produces a course grade, you should note which students are not attaining satisfactory grades. These students can quickly become at risk for not passing the course. You should meet with each student who does not obtain a passing score on the first work submitted for evaluation. During the meeting, help identify why the student did not obtain a passing score. Possible reasons for the failing grade could include the student did not understand the content, did not understand the assignment, or underestimated the requirements. Some students have difficulty organizing their materials to study or may experience anxiety that blocks their effective thinking during an exam or when completing a writing assignment. Once both you and the student are clear about the cause of the lack of satisfactory progress, you and the student can develop a written progress plan or learning contract with action steps for improvement (see Part 3). Students should sign the learning contract and review progress on a regular basis. When necessary, you can refer the student to school or campus resources such as a writing center, study groups, or counseling.

Evaluation of the Course and Faculty Teaching Effectiveness

Course structure and faculty teaching effectiveness influence student learning and are improved by feedback from students, administrators, and the faculty. Most schools require faculty to obtain information from students about their perspective on the course and faculty teaching effectiveness. Results of these evaluations may be used to make decisions about course changes, renewing a faculty contract, or making decisions about faculty promotion, tenure, and teaching awards. You should retain all evaluation data in a teaching portfolio to use to document your teaching effectiveness and improvement over time.

STUDENT EVALUATION OF THE COURSE

Course evaluation by students can provide information for course improvements. Data about the course are gathered from anonymous surveys that ask specific questions about the course structure, the usefulness of assignments, use of learning resources such as multimedia and models, value of the textbooks, and time allotted for learning and evaluation (see, e.g., University of Wisconsin–Madison, n.d.). Data collected at midsemester can be used to make changes that will affect the students who are currently enrolled in the course, while substantive changes can be made from end-of-course data. Student evaluations are typically collected using a computer-administered evaluation instrument, are anonymous, and are reported as grouped data so that no student can be identified.

The results of student evaluations of your course will be returned for your review. You will find that students who were very happy with the course and those who have suggestions for improvement will provide the most comments, and thus many of the students may not respond to the survey. When you receive the feedback, reflect on the students' comments and your own perception of the course. Make notes about changes in course organization, assignments, or resources for the next time you teach the course.

The school (and campus) may require that the results of student course evaluations be shared with your course/leader or department chair or the curriculum committee who will help you interpret and respond to students' comments. Findings from course evaluations for all faculty may be reported at the campus level to determine student satisfaction with courses and instruction across all departments. Save each course evaluation report to use for administrative reviews, as evidence for contract renewal or promotion and tenure decisions.

STUDENT EVALUATION OF TEACHING EFFECTIVENESS

At the end of each course, students have an opportunity to evaluate the faculty's teaching effectiveness. The evaluation instrument may be developed by the school or can be one that is developed to be used by all students at the university to evaluate teaching effectiveness across all schools or departments. Typically, the instrument gathers information about faculty's use of teaching and evaluation strategies, number and usefulness of assignments, attainment of learning outcomes, knowledge and skill in helping students learn complex concepts fairness, and modeling of professional behavior. The instrument is administered by a neutral party such as a campus teaching center. Data collected from students are anonymous and returned to faculty aggregated. Review the evaluation instrument used at your school and the process by which you will receive the results.

Review findings from the student evaluations of your teaching when they are returned. The Vanderbilt Center for Teaching (n.d.) recommends that when you review the results of student evaluations of your teaching find a time and a private place to consider the results. As you read the comments, focus on both positive and negative ones—what went well and what needs improvement. Keep in mind that you may be new at teaching and still developing your teaching skills. Generally, student evaluations of teaching are more positive in classes with fewer students, electives, and when students do well; consider these findings in the context of the course you teach. Also know that all faculty receive negative and even rude comments from students; you are not alone! The purpose of student evaluations of teaching is improvement. Consider what you can do differently the next time you teach the course. Discuss the student evaluation with your course leader or department chair. If needed, most colleges have a center for teaching and learning and can provide suggestions for teaching improvement.

SELF, PEER, AND ADMINISTRATOR EVALUATION OF THE COURSE AND TEACHING EFFECTIVENESS

In addition to student evaluations of the course and instruction, you will have an opportunity to conduct your own self-evaluation. Here you can reflect on what went well and what needs to be improved and respond to students' suggestions for improvement. Write your self-evaluation and retain it for use during an annual review and to demonstrate improvement over several semesters of teaching. Peer review of teaching is a specific process and involves having a peer review the course syllabus, lesson, and evaluation plans and observing an actual class session (Danielson, 2012). If you choose (or are requested) to participate in a peer review, locate the policies and practices that describe how peer review of teaching is conducted at your school.

Chapter Summary

In this chapter you have learned how to evaluate student learning outcomes/competencies and how to receive feedback to improve your course and teaching effectiveness. Here are key points:

- Assessment of student learning provides information for monitoring student progress toward attaining course learning outcomes; evaluation strategies are used to determine students' attainment of learning outcomes and results in assigning a final course grade.
- Evaluation plans are published in the course syllabus and are a contract with the student. Evaluation plans include information about evaluation strategies used in the course, the grading scale, school and campus policies pertaining to academic honesty, procedures for appealing a grade, and curriculum policies related to course failure and continued progression in the program.
- There are a variety of strategies that can be used to evaluate student learning outcomes. These include, among others, exams, papers, and presentations.
- Exams are a common strategy for evaluating student learning. Exams sample a large amount of content, are easy to administer, but they are time consuming to develop. Exams are based on an exam blueprint and include test items (questions) that are aligned with the domain and level of the learning outcome.
- Faculty have responsibility for ensuring academic honesty when students take exams by following school and campus academic policies, using proctors, and protecting the exam when viewed by students and on the digital storage device.
- Faculty review exam results and conduct an item analysis (mean and standard deviation, validity, reliability, effectiveness of item options, item difficulty, and item discrimination) before sharing exam results with students.

- Postexam review with students helps students learn how to improve their test-taking skills and clarify their understanding of course content.
- Evaluation strategies must be valid and reliable. Valid strategies reflect common practice in the discipline; reliable strategies achieve consistent results when used over time.
- Grading must be fair and equitable. When evaluation strategies are used by multiple faculty teaching the same course, course faculty must ensure interrater reliability in use of all evaluation strategies.
- Course design and faculty teaching effectiveness influence student success in the course. Student evaluations, self-evaluations, administrative evaluations, and peer evaluations provide feedback for improving both the course and the teaching.

References

Angelo, T., & Cross, P. K. (Eds.). (1993). *Classroom assessment techniques: A handbook for college teachers*. Jossey-Bass.

Birkhead, S. (2018). Testing off the clock: Allowing extended time for all students. *Journal of Nursing Education, 57*(3), 166–168.

Danielson, C. (2012). Observing classroom practice. *Educational Leadership, 70*(3), 32–37.

McDonald, M. (2018). *The nurse educators' guide to assessing learning outcomes*. Jones and Bartlett.

University of Wisconsin–Madison. (n.d.). *Student learning assessment: Best practices and sample questions for course evaluation surveys*. https://assessment.provost.wisc.edu/best-practices-and-sample-questions-for-course-evaluation-surveys/#:~:text=Meaningful%20input%20from%20students%20is%20essential%20for%20improving,reflect%20and%20provide%20feedback%20on%20their%20own%20learning

Vanderbilt Center for Teaching. (n.d.). *Student evaluation of teaching*. https://cft.vanderbilt.edu/guides-sub-pages/student-evaluations/

PART 3

Teaching in the Clinical Setting

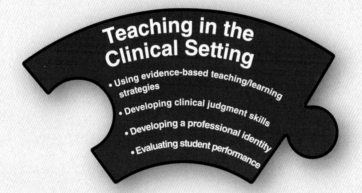

Teaching in the Clinical Setting

- Using evidence-based teaching/learning strategies
- Developing clinical judgment skills
- Developing a professional identity
- Evaluating student performance

One of the most rewarding aspects of being an educator in the health professions is helping students apply their newly acquired knowledge to the care of patients in the clinical setting. Through your clinical teaching you will have the opportunity to influence the practice of countless students during one of the most formative times of their career as they develop the knowledge, skills, and abilities of their profession. Part 3 is designed to prepare you to teach in the clinical setting. Chapter 10 introduces you to the role and responsibilities associated with clinical instruction. You will learn about the competencies necessary to function in this role and have an opportunity to identify the competencies you already have and those you will develop as you learn to share your clinical expertise with students. Chapter 11 provides information you need to get started teaching a clinical course, including reviewing the curriculum and expected course outcomes, meeting your colleagues, and understanding how to create an inclusive learning environment that meets the students' learning needs. Chapter 12 introduces you to a variety of teaching-learning strategies and activities you can use in your clinical teaching. Chapter 13 discusses assessment and evaluation strategies that are appropriate for evaluating students in the clinical setting. Appendix C lists the documents, policies, and procedures you should review as you are getting started teaching in the clinical setting.

CHAPTER 10

Introduction to Teaching in the Clinical Setting

Teaching in the clinical setting may be one of the most important aspects of your faculty role. You will be responsible for shaping the next generation of health care providers by helping students connect what they are learning in the classroom to caring for patients in the clinical setting. You may be employed to teach full time in clinical settings such as in acute care hospitals, outpatient facilities, clinics, community health agencies, and in patients' homes, or have an assignment that includes teaching in both the clinical setting and classroom. As a clinical instructor, you could also have a part-time faculty appointment with the focus on teaching in the clinical setting, or a joint appointment between a clinical agency and the college or university. Regardless of your appointment, you will be focusing on developing students for clinical practice. The purpose of this chapter is to provide you with the practical information you will need to begin your journey teaching in the clinical setting. In this chapter, you will learn about your role and responsibilities for teaching in the clinical setting and the competencies you will need in this role. At the end of this chapter, you can complete a self-assessment to identify the competencies you already have and those that you will need to acquire.

Faculty Role and Responsibilities in Teaching in the Clinical Setting

You likely have had experience working in a clinical setting and have developed the expertise to deliver safe and high-quality care. You are now embarking on your career as a faculty member and will build on your experience and expertise as you get started preparing the next generation of students for clinical practice. You will be making the transition from being an expert clinician to becoming a novice faculty as you shift your role from provider of care to facilitator of learning (Fisher, 2020; Halstead, 2019; Shellenbarger, 2019). Many expert clinicians are surprised at the complexities of the faculty role, and you may initially feel unprepared. You can anticipate that there will be differences in the culture between the clinical service environment and the academic environment; you will also find that your role as an expert clinician will change to being a novice faculty where you are once again in a learning mode. Initially you may feel overwhelmed and unprepared. If you have worked with students in your capacity as a clinician you may find that students have different levels of preparation for taking care of patients, need guidance, and may be dealing with a variety of academic and personal issues. You may find that you need a different skill set to facilitate their learning, and, because the student needs to be the primary caregiver, you will need to be able to step back. To anticipate and then manage this transition, Grassley et al. (2020) suggest you start by becoming oriented to the curriculum, teaching, and evaluation strategies. The authors also note that you will need to understand student behaviors and their role as learners. As you begin your journey you will find it helpful to find supportive faculty or even consider identifying a mentor. Do not hesitate to request assistance and advice from your course leader and other faculty. Do know that over time your confidence will increase, and you will find satisfaction in preparing the next generation of health care professionals.

Educator Competencies Related to Teaching in the Clinical Setting

Teaching in the clinical setting requires not only clinical expertise but also an understanding of how students learn, how to select and use teaching strategies that are appropriate for the students' experience and learning needs, and the ability to evaluate students' attainment of the course learning outcomes. In your role as an educator in a clinical setting, you will also draw on your knowledge of clinical practice there and collaborate with the staff to ensure a successful learning experience for your students. Your role will also require you to model the behaviors of professional, ethical, and legal behavior and to facilitate students as they develop their own professional identity. These attributes are referred to as competencies, or expected knowledge, skills, and abilities that are the foundation of a clinical educator's repertoire. Highlights of these competencies are described next and are followed by a self-assessment guide to help you determine your competencies and those you will need to acquire as you get started teaching in the clinical setting.

COMPETENCIES RELATED TO FACILITATING STUDENT LEARNING IN THE CLINICAL SETTING

Your most important role as an educator working with students is to help them acquire the knowledge, skills, values, and professional behavior of the profession. If your previous experience has been working in the clinical setting as a health care provider, you will find that your role will shift from providing care to helping others learn how to be the care provider. Box 10.1 lists skills you will develop as you focus on helping students learn.

> **BOX 10.1 ■ Competencies Related to Facilitating Student Learning in the Clinical Setting**
>
> - Work within the curriculum framework, policies, and guidelines of the academic institution.
> - Use your clinical expertise to guide students' learning.
> - Bridge the classroom content with clinical practice; integrate student learning into clinical practice.
> - Plan learning activities and clinical conferences that provide students opportunities to apply knowledge, skills, and values related to clinical practice.
> - Use appropriate teaching strategies to facilitate students' attainment of course competencies.
> - Use high-fidelity and digital simulations and standardized patients (volunteers, paid actors).
> - Facilitate student development of ethical, safe, and caring practice.
> - Use educational technologies and learning management systems to support course activities.
> - Recognize and manage student misconduct.
> - Establish an inclusive culture of learning with the school, students, faculty, and staff in the clinical agency.

COMPETENCIES RELATED TO ASSESSING AND EVALUATING STUDENT LEARNING IN THE CLINICAL SETTING

Part of your role as educator in the clinical setting is to assess (give feedback and coach) the progress of students as they are learning, then ultimately to evaluate how well they have attained the course competencies and assign a grade. As you implement this aspect of your role, you will need clear expectations of your students' performance at their appropriate level in the curriculum and the ability to make judgments about students' performance as novices in the profession, not at the level you would expect from staff. Box 10.2 lists competencies that *you* will need to assess and evaluate your students' clinical performance.

> **BOX 10.2 ■ Competencies Related to Assessing and Evaluating Student Learning in the Clinical Setting**
>
> - Understand evaluation and grading policies.
> - Use evaluation strategies to evaluate students' attainment of clinical course competencies.
> - Be respectful and fair; implement evaluation and grading guidelines consistently for all students.

COMPETENCIES RELATED TO BEING A ROLE MODEL

One of the most important ways that you help students learn is to serve as an example of what is expected of a licensed professional working in the practice setting (Box 10.3). You will be amazed by how much students are learning by observing your approach to patients and to team members in the clinical setting. Students observe your interactions, how you dress, and your patient care skills.

> **BOX 10.3 ■ Competencies Related to Being a Role Model**
>
> - Serve as a role model for legal, ethical, moral, and caring professional behavior.
> - Socialize students to the discipline and profession.
> - Socialize students to the value of lifelong learning.
> - Help students develop a professional identity.

COMPETENCIES RELATED TO ESTABLISHING RELATIONSHIPS WITH THE CLINICAL AGENCY AND STAFF WHEN TEACHING STUDENTS

When teaching in a clinical course, your classroom as such will be in a clinical setting, and you will be responsible for establishing effective relationships with the staff in the clinical agency. The success of the students' learning experience depends on your ability to communicate information about the students' learning needs to the agency staff and collaborate with the staff to ensure both patient safety and students' learning. Box 10.4 lists competencies you will use when working with staff and students in the clinical agency.

BOX 10.4 ■ **Competencies Related to Establishing Relationships With the Clinical Agency and Staff When Teaching Students**

- Collaborate with clinical staff and interprofessional teams to support student learning.
- Choose appropriate clinical sites, settings, and patient assignments; follow agency practice guidelines.
- Establish working relationships with personnel in the clinical setting.
- Use evidence-based practices for yourself, your students, and staff in the clinical setting.
- Use health care record/chart, communicate, retrieve, and use data to ensure safe and high-quality patient outcomes; use telehealth applications.
- Demonstrate empathetic and civil interpersonal communication; communicate effectively verbally and in writing.
- Prevent and manage conflict between and among patient, students, and staff.

Self-Assessment of Competencies Related to Teaching in the Clinical Setting

As you begin to think about your role as an educator in a clinical setting, now is a good time to reflect on the knowledge, skills, and professional experience you bring to the role. Use the self-assessment guide (Table 10.1) to identify your competencies at this point and to identify where you will need to obtain information and experiences to build your teaching/evaluation expertise.

TABLE 10.1 ■ Self-Assessment of Competencies Related to Teaching in the Clinical Setting

Consider to what extent you feel comfortable performing the following competencies, then check the appropriate box. After you complete the checklist, develop a plan to gain skill in the competencies in which you have less experience. Share your plan with your mentor for additional feedback.

Educator Competency	I Have No Experience	I Have Some Experience	I Have Much Experience
Demonstrate skills			
Use a simulation (setting up, observing, debriefing)			
Use standardized patients			
Use teaching questions, teaching prompts			

TABLE 10.1 ■ Self-Assessment of Competencies Related to Teaching in the Clinical Setting (Continued)

Educator Competency	I Have No Experience	I Have Some Experience	I Have Much Experience
Use case studies/scenarios/concept maps			
Assign written work such as reflection papers, care plans			
Coach; give feedback			
Conduct pre/post conference			
Use a course grading scale			
Use a checklist, rating scale, or rubric to evaluate clinical performance			
Grade a care plan, concept map, written paper			
Evaluate students' communication skills (interpersonal with patients, staff, classmates)			
Evaluate students' team and interprofessional practice skills			
Use Objective Structured Clinical Exams (OSCE)			
Make patient assignments			
Ensure students act professionally, observe policies related to appropriate academic and clinical behavior; follow guidelines for legal and ethical behavior			
Serve as role model			
Obtain and observe agency polices			
Establish productive relationships with agency staff			
Collaborate with staff at clinical setting to ensure student has a learning experience related to course learning outcomes			
Implement a preceptor model			
Collaborate with agency staff to select patients appropriate for student learning outcomes			

Chapter Summary

In this chapter you have read about the competencies you will need as you are getting started teaching in a clinical setting. You will draw on your experience as a health professional, and add to your clinical expertise the knowledge, skills, and values that you will use as you work with students in a clinical setting. Here are key points for you to consider as you begin your journey:

■ Build on your skills and experiences as a health care professional as you serve as a role model for your students.

- A variety of teaching-learning strategies are used when teaching in the clinical setting. Depending on the course and your students, be prepared to teach using simulated clinical experiences with high-fidelity manikins, standardized patients, or digital learning resources to prepare students for giving actual patient care, and to help your students learn when caring for actual patients.
- Establishing collaborative relationships with staff is the foundation of a successful clinical experience for your students. Become familiar with the clinical agency and their expectations for working with your students.
- Learn to use assessment strategies such as coaching and giving feedback to help students attain course learning outcomes.
- Learn to use evaluation strategies and the course grading scale. Evaluate students fairly as novices, not from expectations of expert practitioners.

References

Fisher, M. (2020). Teaching in nursing: The faculty role. In D. Billings & J. Halstead (Eds.), Teaching in nursing (6th ed.). Elsevier.

Grassley, J. S., Strohfus, P. K., & Lambe, A. D. (2020). No longer expert: A meta-synthesis describing the transition from clinician to academic. *Journal of Nursing Education, 59*(7), 366–367.

Halstead, J. A. (Ed.). (2019). *NLN core competencies for nurse educators: A decade of influence.* Washington, DC: National League for Nursing.

Shellenbarger, T. (2019). *Clinical nurse educator competencies.* Wolters Kluwer.

CHAPTER 11

Getting Started With Teaching in the Clinical Setting

Although you may be familiar with the clinical setting as a health care provider, you will also need to become familiar with your role as a faculty member who is teaching in the clinical setting. To help you make the role transition, this chapter offers information about understanding the academic program, the curriculum, and the course in which you will be teaching, as well as knowing about the colleagues, clinical staff, and students with whom you will be working. In your role as a clinical faculty you will also need to become familiar with the clinical setting in which your students will have their experience, including understanding the organizational structure of the clinical site and their policies and procedures, the types of patients your students are permitted to care for, and knowing which spaces are available for students to use such as lockers, conference rooms, and classrooms. The chapter concludes with suggestions for planning your first day as a clinical educator.

Understanding the Academic Program, Curriculum, and Your Course

THE ACADEMIC PROGRAM

As you assume your role as educator in a clinical setting, you should familiarize yourself with the overall scope of practice specific to your profession and the specific outcomes of the academic program (see Part 1 for further discussion of program outcomes). You should also become familiar with the professional practice standards that students will be expected to follow in clinical practice courses.

THE CURRICULUM

As you are getting started teaching in the clinical setting, one of the first things you should do is to obtain a copy of the overall curriculum plan (see Part 1). Review the program outcomes and competencies to understand how your course contributes to the expectations for knowledge, skills, and abilities at the end of the program. Find out what prerequisite courses students have had and what knowledge and skills you can expect students to bring to your course. Understand the curriculum competencies that students will develop during their clinical experience, such as using a clinical judgment model, developing a professional identity, and demonstrating the values of the program.

THE COURSE

Obtain a copy of the syllabus for the clinical course and, as needed, the syllabi for the prerequisite and corequisite courses, which provide the foundation for the knowledge, skills, and abilities the students will be expected to bring to your course. It may also be helpful to review courses that follow the one(s) you are teaching to be sure the students in your course are ready to progress. Review the course learning outcomes and competencies for your clinical course and the teaching strategies used to guide student attainment of the course outcomes. Familiarize yourself with evaluation strategies, evaluation tools, rubrics, and the grading scale for your course. Also know where to post grades (often in the learning management system [LMS]) and review the student appeal process. As you review the syllabus, understand the course credit allocation, which identifies the number of clinical hours, and, if appropriate, the balance of actual patient contact hours with the use of simulation and observational experiences. If there are assigned readings for your course, read these and be prepared to help students integrate the information into their clinical practice.

The syllabus will also include information about course polices for attendance and professional behavior such as being late or absent, appropriate dress code, requirements for immunizations, and background checks. The syllabus should also include information about how students will be notified when the clinical experience is cancelled or changed for situations such as inclement weather, civil emergencies, or agency closures.

The syllabus will refer students to the student handbook, which explains expectations for academic honesty and appropriate student conduct. The student handbook is usually found online, and you should review this document and bookmark the site. As is true in the classroom (see Part 2), students are held to standards of academic and professional behavior and must observe college, program, and course norms and policies as well as those of the clinical agency. You have a responsibility to recognize signs of unacceptable academic and professional behavior such as being late to clinical experiences, being unprepared to give safe patient care, demonstrating unprofessional behavior (with patients, staff, faculty, and classmates), or demonstrating signs of physical or mental impairment. Students must avoid behaviors related to academic dishonesty such as lying, making false reports, or charting information they did not obtain; disrespecting patient privacy by taking photo images of clinical records or divulging patient information (Health Insurance Portability and Accountability Act [HIPAA] violations); not reporting medication or patient care; and engaging in uncivil or racist behavior. Table 11.1 provides information about recognizing, preventing, and managing unacceptable student behavior in the clinical setting. Box 11.1 offers guidelines for managing the situation.

While you are preparing to teach a clinical course, you should learn about the faculty-student ratio for your course. The faculty-student ratio is

TABLE 11.1 ■ Recognition, Prevention, and Management of Student Academic Dishonesty and Professional Misconduct in the Clinical Setting

Behavior	Definition	Recognition	Prevention	Management
Student-faculty, student-student, and student-clinical staff relationships	While in role of student faculty you are the students' teacher; you are not friend, mentor, colleague, health care provider; students are in the clinical agency to learn, and should not form personal relationships with you, other students, or agency staff.	Student asks for favors, discusses personal issues, makes sexual advances; students may attempt to establish personal relationships with staff and staff with the students, or students with each other.	Clarify roles of student and faculty and staff; avoid interactions that are beyond your role or beyond the role of the student as learner in a clinical environment.	Maintain boundaries of student-faculty relationships. Discuss with student that while in clinical setting to maintain professional vs. personal relationships with faculty, staff, and classmates. Discuss with course leader/department chair as needed.
Misconduct	Behavior that interferes with the process of teaching and learning	*Minor disruptions:* Arriving late to clinical assignments, disrupting work of clinical agency staff, annoying classmates in the area, using electronic devices when not related to course activities *Serious disruptions:* Arguing with patients, staff, faculty, classmates; threatening verbally or physically; stalking; damaging property; carrying a weapon; sexual harassment	*Minor disruptions:* Provide written norms and behavioral expectations during clinical experiences in the student handbook and course syllabus; remind student of the norms if they are not being followed; discuss the behavior privately with the student (with a colleague or administrator as needed).	*Minor disruptions:* Discuss behavior with student privately (with colleague or administrator if needed); refer student to appropriate resources (behavioral management; counseling, health care provider) *Serious disruptions:* If occurs during clinical experience call security as needed; follow up with school and campus administrators.
Incivility	Making rude, annoying, unprofessional, impolite, disrespectful comments; behavior can range from disruptive to violence. *Lateral incivility:* Student-student, faculty-faculty, nurse-nurse *Hierarchic incivility:* Administrator-faculty, faculty-student, clinical staff-student	*Minor:* Eye rolling, sarcasm; racial/ethnic slurs *Major:* Intimidation, threatening; physical violence to faculty, classmates, clinical staff, or patient/family/visitors	Include code of behavior in course syllabus; conduct information sessions on recognizing and managing incivility.	Do not engage or escalate in dialogue with student; calmly discuss with student and follow course, school, campus, agency policies.

Continued on following page

TABLE 11.1 ■ Recognition, Prevention, and Management of Student Academic Dishonesty and Professional Misconduct in the Clinical Setting (Continued)

Behavior	Definition	Recognition	Prevention	Management
Anger, aggression	Typically precipitated by stress; student may respond to feedback or clinical grades with anger.	Is agitated, hostile; swears, threatens	Teach students stress reduction and anger management strategies as needed.	*Use deescalation techniques:* Remain calm; speak slowly and softly; remain respectful; listen actively, indicate you are available to help; indicate you have heard the student's frustration; ask for clarification; use empathetic statements; be respectful; set limits, such as you will continue to discuss the issue if the student manages the current behavior. Work to resolve the issue; refer as necessary to professional resources; document and report to administrators.
Unprofessional behavior	Student does not observe dress code; uses inappropriate communication with patients/families, staff, team.	Behavior is observed.	Review dress code with each group of students at the beginning of clinical; give examples of inappropriate attire; review professional communication strategies	Discuss with student and follow up.
Impaired behavior	Behavior not typical for student or appropriate for giving patient care (e.g., concentration abilities)	Student is dizzy and stumbling; smells of alcohol; slurring words; may be aggressive or volatile, irritable, or agitated, becoming enraged; may be caused by substance abuse, student anxiety, medications, health problems.	State policy in syllabus and student handbook.	Remove student immediately from patient care and clinical responsibilities. Discuss with student; refer as needed to health services; follow up with report to course leader/administrator.
Fabrication and falsification	Reporting, documenting information that is not true or was not obtained from the source (such as patient, staff).	Student reports or charts inaccurate information (e.g., recording vital signs that were not obtained; reports/charts medication or treatment as given that was not administered)	Observe student's work; validate reports and documentation.	Once discovered, confirm with student; report to administrators and follow school and campus policies.

BOX 11.1 ■ Managing Unacceptable Student Behavior in the Clinical Setting

- Remove student from situation
- Identify unacceptable behavior
- Discuss situation with student
- Verify behavior with student (avoid discussing with staff, preceptors, patient)
- Review expectations (per course, school, and/or university policy)
- Link student behavior to expectation and policy
- Plan with student to remediate the behavior or invoke policy guidelines (aka disciplinary)
- Refer to health services or community resources as needed
- Record situation in anecdotal notes
- Report situation to the appropriate administrator
- Follow student due process guidelines

---

established by the state regulatory agency and professional accreditation standards and may be determined by the clinical agency that specifies how many students they can accommodate and their expectation for the presence of a faculty member. The number of students with each faculty may also depend on the experience of the student, the nature of the learning experience, and the learning outcomes to be attained.

Information technologies are used to support patient care and student learning. Before you embark on your role as clinical faculty, you should become familiar with the technology used at the clinical site and in the course (see Part 4). Although you may not have responsibilities for using any technologies in your course, your students may have used them to prepare for the clinical experience. For example, there is software to teach students how to chart using simulated electronic health records, make care plans, or review procedures. Course information may be embedded in a LMS in which the syllabus, course materials, and gradebook are housed. Clinical courses may be linked with didactic courses or learning experiences that involve the use of skills practice laboratories or simulation centers. As you are oriented to the course, clarify your role with using these technologies with the students or expectations for students to use them in your course.

Meeting Your Colleagues, Staff, and Student Support Personnel

When teaching in the clinical setting you will interface with faculty colleagues, course leaders/coordinators, mentors, administrators, and support personnel from the academic setting as well as those from the clinical site. Ideally, you will have an opportunity to participate in a structured orientation program in which someone will introduce you to key people in both settings, but it is also appropriate for you to ask to meet them or introduce yourself to them. The people you should know from both the school/university and the clinical site are discussed next.

COURSE LEADERS/COORDINATORS, ADMINISTRATORS, AND MENTORS IN THE ACADEMIC SETTING

Most schools are organized with a hierarchic structure depending on the size of the faculty and student body; if possible, obtain a copy of the organization chart. There will be a course leader/ coordinator who is responsible for coordinating sections of a course, or several courses within the semester. This is the person you should approach first with questions about the course, to seek suggestions for handling an issue with a student, or to report student misconduct. Be sure you have contact information for this person.

In large schools there may be an administrator, usually a department chair who is responsible for courses and faculty in that area. The dean or program director is the person who has ultimate responsibility for the welfare of the students and faculty and provides leadership and direction for the school. You should know who these administrators are, and that student and faculty issues will ultimately be managed at these administrative levels as needed.

Mentors are faculty colleagues who volunteer or are assigned to assist newly employed faculty become familiar with the program, the course, and the students. If your program does not offer someone to serve in this role, you can request that someone be available to you, or seek out a faculty colleague who seems willing to answer your questions. Newly appointed faculty find that having a mentor eases the transition to the faculty role.

TECHNICAL SUPPORT STAFF IN THE ACADEMIC SETTING

Although your appointment as a clinical educator may involve teaching primarily in the clinical setting, you may also be teaching the didactic component of the clinical course either on campus or online. In either case, you should understand what technology you and the students will use and the technical staff who will be available to manage the technology in the classrooms, offices, student lounges, and elsewhere on campus (see Part 4). This staff also will establish an email account for you and other accounts you will need access to teach your course. If the campus or school uses a LMS or videoconferencing system, there may be staff to assist with course design. If you will be teaching in a classroom in addition to teaching your clinical course, you should learn how to use the technology such as an internet connection, a projection system, and access to media that you may wish to use in your course. Know how to contact technical support services for assistance or to plan for technology support for you and your students.

STUDENT SUPPORT SERVICES

These services may be housed at the school or on campus. Generally, the school will have an office of student services dedicated to the needs of the students at your school. This office facilitates student recruitment, registration, recording grades, counseling, and academic advisement. This office may also organize peer tutoring and other learning support services. Many schools now have their own offices of diversity, equity, and inclusion and international affairs to support faculty and student recruitment, retention, and study-abroad programs. Be familiar with the resources these offices offer and consult with them or refer students to their services as needed.

There are a variety of student support services at the campus that may be helpful to your students. Most campuses have a writing center, which offers students assistance with technical aspects of writing a paper. You may also have a student with a disability in your course and will be in contact with the office for students with disabilities, which handles students with diagnosed disabilities who must register at this office before they can request accommodations for participating in clinical assignments such as taking tests, managing anxiety, or managing a physical disability requiring specialized equipment or modifications of procedures (Levey, 2021) (see Part 2 for further discussion of teaching students with disabilities). Many campuses also have a center for teaching and learning that provides support and workshops for faculty about designing courses, teaching online, developing assessments and tests, and using innovative teaching strategies.

Understanding Your Students

Before you begin teaching in the clinical setting, you should learn about the students' academic background as well as their previous clinical experiences. Begin by understanding what courses the students have completed and are enrolled in concurrently. For example, students for whom this is their first course in the professionals program may still not know how to read the syllabus, how to find or use resources required in the program such as the library, the LMS, or required software such as accessing the textbook or related resources online and may not have had any or very little experience in a clinical setting. If possible, obtain information about what knowledge and skills the students who are in your clinical course bring to the course and what types of patient care assignments will be appropriate. Some faculty ask their students to complete a checklist to indicate what knowledge and skills they already have and what additional experiences they need.

You may also find it helpful to know general information about the students before your first meeting with them. For example, the school may have information such as the percentage of students who attend classes full or part time; the racial/ethnic, gender, and age composition of the student body; the percentage of students who are employed; the percentage of students for whom English is not their first or only language; and the percentage of students who are the first person in their family to attend college. This information is helpful in anticipating how to make clinical assignments or identifying students who may need learning support services. Although having background information about the students is helpful, the most useful information is knowing the clinical capabilities of each student in your course. This information is best obtained by carefully observing students during their first few patient care assignments.

Prior to participating in a clinical experience, students must meet several requirements of the school and the clinical site. These may include having approved background checks, being certified in basic cardiopulmonary resuscitation (CPR), having liability insurance, purchasing specified uniforms and equipment (e.g., stethoscope, scissors), having received required vaccinations/immunizations, signing a needlestick policy, and passing a drug test. If your school does not have a clinical placement coordinator, it may be your responsibility to verify that each student has completed these requirements.

When teaching in the clinical setting, it is also important to understand that learning to take care of patients is an anxiety-provoking situation for many students. This anxiety often is compounded by other stressors in their life and can lead to poor clinical performance and jeopardize patient safety. Cornine (2020) suggests that faculty can help students manage their anxiety by (1) conducting a thorough orientation to the course and the clinical agency, (2) making clinical assignments that allow students time to prepare for giving care to a specific patient, (3) making assignments where two or three students are working together, (4) using virtual and actual simulations as preparation for the clinical experience, (5) encouraging students to use mobile devices to access resources, (6) being aware of how faculty teaching styles can contribute to student anxiety, and (7) ensuring a productive learning environment by conveying respect, patience, and support. In addition, you can empower students to manage their own anxiety by teaching them stress and anxiety management techniques such as guided imagery, mindfulness meditation, and relaxation exercises.

Establishing an Inclusive and Productive Learning Environment

To establish a safe and productive learning environment when you are teaching in the clinical setting requires balancing the demands of both the academic and clinical settings. Your priority is to the students and ensuring they have an equal opportunity to develop clinical skills while observing the expected academic behaviors of both the campus and the clinical agency. While students and faculty are expected to follow agency policies while in the clinical setting, you are the person who is responsible for also ensuring that the students are following the policies prescribed in the student handbook. (See Table 11.1 for behaviors that are potentially disruptive to a productive learning environment and guidance about how to recognize, prevent, and manage these behaviors should they occur; see Box 11.1 for the steps to take when you manage the unacceptable behavior.)

Becoming Familiar With the Clinical Setting

The learning experiences in clinical courses take place in a variety of settings, including acute care hospitals, outpatient clinics, community-based settings (schools, worship centers, community centers, prisons, long-term care facilities), or patients' homes, and it will be important for you to establish positive relationships with the administrators and staff at the site where your students will have their learning experiences. You already may be familiar with the clinical facility and the unit where students will have experiences, or you may not know the facility, but the unit has been used previously and the staff are familiar with having students or, in other instances, you may be the one that needs to find appropriate settings in which the students can participate in learning activities that will help them attain course competencies. Hopefully the contract with the clinical facility is signed, but you may be employed at the facility and be expected to have access for your students. Regardless of the situation, you will need to (1) learn about the setting/clinical unit where students can have access to patients; (2) identify areas you and students can use for conferences and to store personal items; (3) review the policies and procedures of the agency; (4) orient the staff to course requirements, students' abilities, and your role; and (5) discuss how the clinical unit prefers that you or the student choose the patient and post the assignment. At this time, it may also be helpful to review the contract the school has with the clinical agency about the availability of space and access to patients.

SETTING

Prior to taking students to the clinical site, you should visit the site and meet the administrators and staff. It may also be helpful to view a copy of the organizational chart. The clinical setting may also involve a high-fidelity simulator or digital clinical simulations. The clinical setting may also be accessed by telehealth or digital devices.

LEARNING SPACES AND INTERNET ACCESS

Inquire about where you can meet with students. Many clinical sites have a classroom for use with students, which may be on the clinical unit or located elsewhere at the site. This classroom is where you can hold pre- and postconferences and have private meetings with students. Plan to visit the classroom and determine if there is internet access, cell phone service, and access to any other audiovisual resources or library resources you or the students may need. Clinical sites also have guidelines about accessing the internet. Will students be able to access the internet to look up information about medications or procedures, or use websites for patient teaching? There may be other spaces available to students such as lockers or changing rooms; however, students should be advised to not bring personal items or money to the clinical class. If the clinical site does not have facilities where you can meet with students, you may need to plan to meet at the school or in an online meeting room following the experience.

UNDERSTANDING POLICIES AND PROCEDURES

Before you begin teaching in the clinical setting, ensure that your students have met all requirements to be a student at the site. This information can be found in the contract the school has with the clinical site, which the dean of the school or clinical site coordinator has signed. This contract includes student requirements such as background checks, immunizations, dress codes, access to electronic health records, ability to administer medications and perform certain procedures, and the student-faculty ratio.

MODELS OF CLINICAL TEACHING

There are various models for teaching in a clinical setting and you should understand the ones used in your course and academic program. Although the traditional approach to teaching is to have one faculty member be responsible for the teaching and supervision of each student, in other situations faculty may use a paired model in which the student works primarily with the staff. It is also possible to use a dyad/triad model in which two or three students plan care for one patient, and the faculty member is responsible for students' care of the client. In other situations, the student may be assigned to work with a preceptor (see later). In the preceptor model, the student is assigned to work with a staff member during the times that the staff member is working. This model of clinical teaching is typically used as the students are nearing the end of the curriculum and preparing to transition to practice.

ORIENTING CLINICAL STAFF TO YOUR COURSE

Before you bring your students to the clinical site, take time to orient the staff who will be working with the students to the course. It is appropriate to share the syllabus and any other course documents with the staff who will be working with the students. Be sure to point out the focus of the learning outcomes and course competencies, the level and previous clinical experience of the students, and your expectations for the students' learning. Discuss how the staff should work with the students. Are they to work with the student, or should they direct the student to work only with you? Will the clinical site be providing a preceptor? If so, meet the preceptors and orient them to their role. Will the staff assigned to the patient be available to assist the student? To whom should the student report information about the patient and conduct handoff of care when the student leaves? Clarify that while the staff can report information about students to you, you will be the one evaluating the students' attainment of the course outcomes and assigning the grade. Box 11.2 offers suggestions for working with clinical staff.

BOX 11.2 ■ Suggestions for Working With Clinical Staff

- Explain the course expectations to all staff who will be working with students.
- Invite the leader/administrator of the agency/clinical unit to conduct an orientation to the clinical unit(s) where students will be having learning experiences.
- Clarify that the role of the student is to learn, not to serve as extra staff.
- Understand the roles of ancillary staff and explain the role of the student and what the staff should continue to do for the patient and what the student will do.
- Identify sentinel or adverse events (those situations that require immediate response involving patient safety or error in which the student is involved). Staff should be empowered to intervene when patient, staff, or student safety is at risk, and then immediately report the event to you. You are the one responsible for the student and will take appropriate action as described in Box 11.1.
- Clarify responsibilities for students' documentation, charting, handoff of care, and other responsibilities that interface with staff.
- Before leaving the clinical unit, report to the person in charge and summarize what the students did during their experience and highlight any care that needs to be completed or issues with patients.
- Thank the staff for their assistance; consider hosting a celebration with students and staff.

WORKING WITH PRECEPTORS

Preceptors are experienced staff members who are willing to teach students and who serve as role models, mentors, and facilitators of student learning as they connect theory to practice. Being a preceptor is usually a voluntary, unpaid role, but the school may compensate the preceptor with a title or tuition rebate or other ways of recognizing the value of the role. The preceptor model typically is formed as a triad, with the preceptor, student, and faculty having equal roles in teaching and assessing student learning, but you will have the final responsibility for evaluating the student and assigning the grade (DeMeester et al., 2017). Preceptor models are particularly effective in courses in which students are at the end of their academic program and preparing to transition to employment.

Before working with faculty and students, preceptors should participate in an orientation program that provides information about the role expectations of working with the student, information about strategies to help the student learn and how to give feedback, and the course materials. The preceptor orientation may be offered by the school, as a generic course, usually offered online, that may be offered for a fee, or a course offered by the professional organization such as the preceptor training course for respiratory therapy faculty offered by the American Association for Respiratory Care (AARC Preceptor Training Course).

Faculty have a significant role in developing and/or using a preceptor orientation course. For example, faculty are involved in identifying and approving preceptors (the state board of health professions may have specified the level of educational preparation of preceptors, usually one degree beyond the degree the student will receive or experience), orienting the preceptor to the course; clarifying roles of faculty, student, and preceptor; introducing preceptor/student; explaining to the student and preceptor their roles in assessment and evaluation; giving course materials (some schools give preceptors access to the course as a benefit of being a preceptor); and scheduling site visits (Chicca & Shellenbarger, 2021). At the conclusion of the course you, the preceptor, and the student will evaluate the experience (see Chapter 9). Help the student end the relationship on a positive note and thank the preceptor for contributing to the student's education. You and/or the school should acknowledge the preceptor's role in facilitating learning; some schools host a celebration and/or offer tuition reimbursement to enroll in courses.

The use of preceptors requires planning and follow-up. If you will be using a preceptor in your course, review the role description and contract. Although the student and preceptor will form a close relationship, you will meet with them often and assess both the student learning and the progress of the relationship.

MAKING PATIENT CARE ASSIGNMENTS

One of the most important activities you will do when teaching in a clinical course is to ensure each student can attain the clinical course competencies. The number of students for whom you will provide assignments and supervise is determined by the state board of health professions, the capacity of the clinical site, and the focus of the clinical experience.

Depending on the experience of the student, the nature of the course, and the availability and acuity of patients at the clinical site, either you, a staff member/preceptor, or the student can make the patient care assignment. The advantages of having the preceptor or staff make the assignment or suggest appropriate patients to you is that they are familiar with the patients, their care needs, and the willingness of the patient to have a student provide care. In other situations, it may be more appropriate for you to make the assignments because you will be familiar with the students' learning needs and capabilities and your ability to manage your time to provide adequate supervision of the student. Another approach is for you to choose the patients and inform the students of the assignment via secure email or within the LMS. In other instances, it may be valuable for the student to make the assignment. The major advantage of having students make their own assignments is that they can know ahead of time their patient assignment and will be better prepared for the experience. At the same time, some students may select a patient assignment that does not present an appropriate challenge. Regardless of who makes the assignment, ideally each student or dyad should have a patient assignment (which can include a team of patients; or an observational experience with a particular focus) prior to coming to the clinical experience, and you and the staff should be clear about which patients have students taking care of them and what their responsibilities are to you and the students.

You should plan to arrive on the unit 30 to 60 minutes before the students to finalize any last-minute plans or changes in patient conditions. You can also discuss alternative plans with the staff in case a patient will be having a test or surgery. If the clinical unit conducts a shift report, rounds, or handoff of care, it is helpful to listen to these reports so you can communicate any updates to the student.

Many faculty find it helpful to use a paper or electronic form to organize key information about the student and patient to set priorities for supervision and instruction and to make ongoing notes about the students' performance (Fig. 11.1). Keep note of the patient's initials, room number, status, and any procedures the student will perform that you will need to assist or supervise; also include the students' initials. This form can also be used to record quick notes, which you can use after the clinical experience as the basis for writing any anecdotal notes or a summary of the students' clinical performance.

Student name/initials				
Patient initials	Room number	Diagnosis	Meds (time) Procedures/treatment (time) Alerts/allergies/other	Notes

Student name/initials				
Patient initials	Room number	Diagnosis	Meds (time) Procedures/treatment (time) Alerts/allergies/other	Notes

Student name/initials				
Patient initials	Room number	Diagnosis	Meds (time) Procedures/treatment (time) Alerts/allergies/other	Notes

Fig. 11.1 Clinical experience worksheet.

Understanding Legal Implications of Teaching in the Clinical Setting

When teaching in the clinical setting you will follow the legislative and procedural guidance of both the school and the clinical site. Your role in supervising students is primarily guided by individual state practice acts, but in general (1) students are held to the same legal standards as registered practitioners, (2) the staff who is assigned to care for the patient is ultimately responsible for the care of that patient, (3) federal laws that protect patient safety and privacy such as the Health Information Privacy and Protection Act (HIPPA) prevail, and (4) you are responsible for observing and evaluating the students. The clinical agency may also have guidelines and standards regarding patient safety and standards of care that you and students should observe. Other information may be specified in the contract the school has with the clinical agency that you and the students should follow.

As noted in Part 2, issues of due process, appeal and grievance, confidentiality and privacy, and accommodations for disabilities (including learning disabilities, physical impairment, and issues with mental health) also pertain to teaching in the clinical setting. Of particular importance is protecting confidentiality and privacy regarding student performance; faculty may be tempted to pass on information about a student's clinical abilities or request information about a student from a previous faculty member. Unless permitted by the student, sharing this information is a violation of the student's privacy, and faculty can only use information that pertains to the student's abilities in the class that the faculty is teaching. You may also have students who need special accommodations for taking care of their patients such as ability to lift patients, hearing impairment, or visual impairment. Students and the office of student disability services at the campus should inform you about how to accommodate the student.

The First Day of Your Clinical Course

Now that you are prepared with some background about working with students in a clinical setting, the day has come when you will meet your students! In some situations, the first meeting may occur at the school, but usually the first day of the clinical experience occurs at the clinical setting; be sure, however, the students know where to meet you regardless. At this time you will meet the students, orient them to the course and the clinical setting, and tell them how they will be assigned to and plan care for their patients. Typically, the first meeting with the students is short and does not involve patient care. The first day for the students (and you!) is both exciting and anxiety producing, so your goal will be to help students maintain their enthusiasm while giving information to answer questions and ease concerns.

You will begin this first day by meeting your students. As per school and/or agency policy the students will have a name tag, which will help you match names and faces. At this time you can do a quick assessment of the students' previous experience, their expectations for the experience, and any concerns/questions they have. Some faculty ask students to complete a checklist indicating the skills and experiences they have had and their need for more practice and/or supervision. This information will help you know how to assign patients and how to prioritize your supervision of the students.

If you have not done so prior to meeting the students at the clinical agency, review the course syllabus with the students. Explain the learning outcomes, what experiences they will have to attain them, and how they will be evaluated. Review all course policies with attention to consequences for being late or absent, how to notify you if students will not be able to attend clinical, and how you will notify students if the clinical experience has changed or been cancelled.

On this first day you will also orient the students to the clinical agency and the area(s) in which the they will be taking care of their patients. Some faculty ask the unit manager or a staff member to welcome the students and explain the organizational structure of the agency and the staff expectations for the students. Students will also need an orientation to the physical aspect of the agency and the clinical unit where they will be located. While you can lead the students on a tour, some faculty use ice-breaker activities such as a scavenger hunt, during which students can locate key areas and equipment. If the students will be working with a preceptor, this is an ideal time to plan a meeting between these two.

Chapter Summary

In this chapter you have been oriented to the general information you will need as you get started teaching in the clinical setting. You will also meet with the course administrator and colleagues to obtain specific information about your course and the clinical site where your students will have clinical experiences. Here are key points for you to consider as you begin your journey:

- Review the program and course learning outcomes, and the syllabus to ground your understanding of expectations for your role teaching in a clinical course.
- Establish a caring, supportive, fair, and inclusive clinical learning environment. Understand the learning needs of your students. Obtain information about what you can expect students to know and do on the first day of their clinical experience. As soon as possible, identify students who need accommodations for health or learning disabilities or need extra support or supervision when providing patient care.
- Be familiar with expectations for students' academic and professional behavior. Review course policies and be able to recognize behavior that is unacceptable and know how to intervene. Follow legal and ethical guidelines of both the academic program and the clinical agency.

- Your "classroom" is in a clinical site. Understand the policies and establish effective relationships with staff. If your course uses a preceptor model, be sure to meet and orient preceptors to the course. Collaborate with clinical staff but know that you are the one who is responsible for student behavior and assigning grades.

References

American Association of Respiratory Care. (n.d.). *Preceptor training course.* https://www.aarc.org/education/educator-resources/preceptor-training-course

Chicca, J., & Shellenbarger, T. (2021). Nursing faculty roles in prelicensure baccalaureate clinical preceptorships. *Nursing Education Perspectives, 42*(2), 98–100.

Cornine, A. (2020). Reducing student anxiety in the clinical setting: an integrative review. *Nursing Education Perspectives, 41*(4), 229–234.

DeMeester, D., Hendricks, S., Stephenson, E., & Welch, J. (2017). Student, preceptor and faculty perceptions of three clinical learning models. *Journal of Nursing Education, 56*(5), 281–286.

Levey, P. (2021). *From classroom to clinic: Negotiating reasonable accommodations in clinical settings.* https://www.queensu.ca/rarc/sites/webpublish.queensu.ca.rarcwww/files/files/HIDC%20Presentations/Levey,%20Pearl.pdf

CHAPTER 12

Using Teaching and Learning Strategies in the Clinical Setting

Teaching in a clinical setting is one of the most important aspects of your faculty role. The clinical experiences provide the opportunity for the student to (1) use the knowledge, skills, and abilities they have developed in the classroom and apply them to provide evidence-based care for the patient; (2) use critical thinking and clinical judgment processes; (3) develop cultural humility; (4) communicate effectively with patients, colleagues, and the health care team; (5) work with the interdisciplinary and interprofessional health care team; (6) navigate the complexity of the health care system; and (7) develop as a health care professional, leader, and lifelong learner. The purpose of this chapter is to provide information about the various teaching-learning strategies you can use to accomplish these goals in the clinical setting. The chapter concludes with a summary of how you can bring all the components of clinical teaching together to help students have meaningful clinical learning experiences.

While teaching in the clinical setting you will draw on a variety of strategies to assist your students attain professional practice outcomes. You will seek opportunities for the students to attain curriculum competencies, to connect classroom experiences to clinical practice, to perform clinical skills the students have practiced in simulated settings, and to develop the clinical judgment and clinical reasoning expertise to provide safe patient care. You will seek opportunities for students to develop communication, presentation, and interpersonal skills, to use health information technologies, and develop skills for collaboration, working on teams, and interprofessional practice. Students also can set their own goals and reflect on their clinical experiences as they progress to attaining course learning outcomes. Clinical teaching involves maintaining the delicate balance of guiding students as they engage with their patients while assuming responsibility for the patient's safety and encouraging the student to reflect on their patient care experiences with the goal of perfecting the art and science of the discipline.

As is true in the classroom, teaching, learning, and assessment are activities distinct from evaluation and grading (see Part 2), but unlike teaching in the classroom, teaching, learning, and assessment in the clinical setting tend to blur because most clinical experiences do not have a distinct time for evaluation. You must quickly determine if the student is applying theory to practice by providing safe care, and making this determination involves judgment (evaluation) and initiating corrective action.

In this chapter you will learn about evidence-based strategies that are effective in helping students learn to give safe patient care. You will also learn how to integrate assessment activities such as preclinical preparation using simulations or skill practice in a learning resource center or coaching and giving feedback as you are facilitating student learning while they are caring for their patients, and then to clarify for the students when you are evaluating and grading (see Chapter 9).

Strategies to Prepare Students for Clinical Practice

Students must be prepared to implement basic psychomotor (skill performance), cognitive (knowledge and clinical judgment), and affective (professional values, therapeutic and interprofessional communication, team collaboration) skills prior to being assigned to care for patients. You will be responsible for ensuring that students have the necessary preparation to provide safe patient care as they progress toward developing competency at higher levels of each of the three domains of learning.

The development of skills typically occurs in introductory courses that teach psychomotor, communication, and patient assessment skills. These skills may be taught in a learning resources center, in a simulation center using high-fidelity manikins, or by using assigned digital media and virtual reality. Also, you may have responsibilities to teach in these introductory courses, which may be integrated into a part of the clinical learning experience, or when facilitating students' learning as they apply these skills to clinical practice. Students develop and refine skills throughout the curriculum, and some programs have a master skills list that students use to keep a record of skills they have learned, been evaluated as satisfactory, or have performed on an actual patient. Regardless of what course you are teaching, you should be familiar with teaching strategies that are used in all courses in which students have experience with skill demonstration with practice, simulation, standardized patients, and debriefing (see also Part 4).

SKILLS DEMONSTRATION AND PRACTICE

Teaching students to develop proficiency with the skills of their discipline typically occurs in a learning resource center that is designed to replicate a clinical setting, a home, a dental office, an operating/recovery room, or emergency department, which may include patient beds and actual equipment for practicing the skills such as blood pressure monitoring, intravenous (IV) infusion setups, oxygen administration, cardiac monitoring, or physical therapy. Some schools require students to purchase a skills pack, which includes equipment such as dressings, catheters, and tubes used in skill performance. Learning resource centers may also have equipment that students can use to practice a specific skill on task trainers, such as an arm for starting an IV infusion, a bed/stair to learn transfer and ambulation skills, a head/neck model to practice intubation, or a model to teach students to assess a patient's mouth and practice providing oral hygiene. Increasingly, these discipline-specific learning centers are using virtual reality and augmented reality to provide immersive experiences for skill development.

The goal of helping students learn to perform psychomotor skills safely is to develop a level of competency that is refined throughout the curriculum. Skill proficiency is acquired by deliberate practice with continuous feedback (Johnson et al., 2020). The primary approach to helping students learn skills is for students to observe a demonstration of the skill, either by the faculty or by viewing the skill demonstration on a video or other digital media, and then having the student perform the skill. If you are teaching skills in a learning resource center, you will observe the student perform skills according to evidence-based protocols. As the students practice the skill, you will coach and give feedback as the student gains proficiency. Students can also develop and refine their skills when students give each other peer feedback (Kemery & Morell, 2020). Typically there are several safe ways to perform a skill, but students will learn best if they follow a step-by-step approach that is consistent with course materials and evaluation procedures (see Chapter 9). Ultimately students will follow the procedures used at the site where they are having their clinical experience, and you may need to guide students in using best practices as defined at the school and at the clinical site.

As an alternative to learning skills in a resource center, there is a wide range of digital products, virtual and augmented reality software, and simulations that support students' skills learning. You can assign the students to learn specific skills by watching demonstrations presented in the skills package. These products may accompany the students' textbook or can also be easily found by conducting a web search for a specific skill. Digital libraries of patient care skills may also be available on a clinical agency website that students may be able to access. Students and health professionals in practice may find it helpful to have access to information that provides a quick review of how to perform a procedure or information about best clinical practices and standards of care. Because there is a variation in how online resources present ways to perform skills, it is important for you to preview these resources and ensure that the procedures are aligned with the ones that students are learning in their coursework or at the clinical agency.

SIMULATION

Simulation is a replication of authentic clinical situations that provide students an opportunity to practice skills and make clinical judgments in a safe environment that does not involve actual patient care. Simulations can be developed to replicate varying levels of reality and can have low fidelity such as occurs in a role play or case studies, medium fidelity using manikins and models, or as high fidelity using human patient simulators. Recently, screen-based digital clinical experiences involving virtual or augmented reality that more closely simulates patient care experience are available for purchase.

Because simulations replicate a patient encounter, and students can attain the same learning outcomes as they would taking care of an actual patient, many state regulatory bodies have specified that a certain number of clinical practicum hours can be satisfied by using simulations. Part of your clinical teaching responsibilities may therefore include participating in a certain number of simulated clinical experiences. When simulations are used to meet requirements for a clinical practicum experience, the experience must be differentiated from preparation for an actual clinical encounter, which includes a well-developed and tested scenario followed by faculty-led debriefing to ensure the student has attained course learning outcomes like those they would meet if they were taking care of an actual patient.

Your responsibilities may also involve preparing students for clinical practice or providing opportunities for simulated clinical practice experiences when actual clinical experiences are not available due to lack of availability of clinical facilities, weather- or disease-related events that preclude actual clinical assignments, or when a particular learning experience is not available or can be better taught and learned as a simulation. There is a variety of software that simulates a patient care experience in most clinical settings. Links to the software can be embedded in a slide, video, or screen capture presentation or assigned as required viewing. Some textbooks offer digital case studies and web-based virtual worlds that simulate a patient care experience and engage the student in assessing a patient, planning for care, and evaluating the effectiveness of the care. Prior to assigning these learning resources, be sure to preview them, estimate the time commitment required to complete the assignment, and then prepare the students for their use and follow-up afterwards (see Part 4). If the simulated clinical experiences are used as credit for a clinical experience, you should establish similar learning outcomes and then follow up with a clinical postconference debriefing (Box 12.1). (*Resources, products:* Virtual clinical excursions [https://evolve.elsevier.com/education/training/virtual-clinical-excursions/; Digital Clinical Experiences [Shadowhealth.com]; Vsims [https://www.wolterskluwer.com/en/solutions/lippincott-nursing-faculty/vsim-for-nursing])

Developing and implementing a simulation involves writing learning outcomes, designing a scenario, obtaining appropriate resources such as manikins or high-fidelity simulation equipment, preparing the students during a prebrief, facilitating the simulation, and ensuring learning by guiding students through reflection and debriefing (see Box 12.1). Each of these simulation

---

BOX 12.1 ■ Guidelines for Conducting a Debriefing for a Clinical Learning Experience

1. Conduct the debriefing session as soon as possible after the simulated or actual patient encounter.
2. Conduct the debriefing session in an area that is quiet, private, and comfortable.
3. Establish an environment of trust and confidentiality.
4. Begin by giving students 5 to 10 minutes to discuss and reflect about the learning experience. Students' emotions may be heightened by participating in the experience, and faculty should help the students put their feelings into words in a safe environment.
5. Set norms of nonjudgmental participation.

> **BOX 12.1 ■ Guidelines for Conducting a Debriefing for a Clinical Learning Experience** (Continued)
>
> 6. Support students' reflection about the experience.
> 7. Facilitate, guide, and encourage active participation and feedback from students; clarify, but do not correct; ask for alternative strategies.
> 8. Focus on the student's understanding of the clinical encounter established by the learning outcomes and the patient care experience; help students link theory to practice and transfer knowledge gained in the experience.
> 9. Lead discussion about what went well and what could be done differently.
> 10. Focus on the role of the student in the situation. Help students distinguish role of student vs. role of the clinician.
> 11. Use open-ended teaching prompts (see Table 12.1) to guide students' thinking and clinical judgment.
> 12. Talk less so students learn more.
> 13. Summarize (student or faculty can lead this discussion) the key learnings.
> 14. Evaluate the debriefing. Request student anonymous comments; reflect on your role as learning facilitator from the simulation experience.

components require faculty development, training, and expertise, which, unless you have experience or have attended orientation workshops in theses aspects of the simulation strategy, likely will not be part of your responsibilities in teaching in the clinical practicum. You may, however, be asked to participate in the simulation by observing the students conduct the simulation and then leading a debriefing session for your clinical group.

STANDARDIZED PATIENTS

Standardized patients are volunteers or actors who are trained to assume the role of a patient. Faculty may recruit "patients" from the community, or they may be actors from the community or drama schools in the area. These patients may be paid or volunteer their time. As with simulations, the role of the standardized patient is developed to give students an opportunity to practice a variety of skills such as procedures, health assessment, interviewing, communication, and clinical judgment. The learning experience takes place in a learning resource center designed to mimic a clinical setting such as a hospital room, clinic, or home. The "patient" uses a consistent script with each student, and when in teaching-learning mode (as opposed to evaluation mode) can coach the student and give feedback. One of the advantages of using standardized patients is that the student learns to spontaneously interact with the patient in a variety of environments.

Strategies to Develop Critical Thinking, Clinical Reasoning, and Clinical Judgment Skills

The most important aspect of clinical practice courses is to help students develop critical thinking, clinical decision making, and clinical judgment skills. Clinical judgment, clinical decision making, and clinical reasoning are commonly used terms to describe the process by which clinicians make cognitive decisions about collecting information about patients' history, current health and treatment plans, forming hypotheses about the patients' health problems, developing plans to manage the patients' health problems, and establishing standards by which to judge the effectiveness of the plans. Critical thinking is defined as analyzing information to make judgments; it is learned and practiced until the process becomes self-directed and self-monitored by the students. Clinical judgment, often used synonymously with terms such as clinical reasoning or clinical decision making, is defined as the cognitive work of making decisions about patient care.

Various frameworks are used to guide students in developing a systematic approach to making clinical judgments and documenting this critical function of safe clinical practice. These frameworks tend to be discipline specific but have in common a series of cognitive steps that are both sequential and iterative. The information processing model uses six steps: recognize cues, analyze cues, prioritize a hypothesis, generate solutions, take action, and evaluate outcomes (Betts et al., 2019). The SOAP (subjective, objective, assessment, plan) model (Geeky Medics, 2021) is another framework used by health professionals and often as a method of harmonizing the documentation of an interdisciplinary team. Some disciplines use the CHART (complaint, history, assessment, Rx [treatment] and transport) method for thinking through a patient care and documentation process (RC Health Services, 2013). You will be responsible for using the decision-making/clinical judgment framework used in your program and to align activities used in teaching in the clinical practicum with that framework. You should know which framework is being used in the course you are teaching and help students apply it with their patients.

There are a variety of strategies that can be used to help students develop critical thinking and clinical judgment skills. Ideally, the same framework is used throughout the curriculum in both classroom and clinical courses. Before beginning teaching students in the skills lab, simulation lab, or in the clinical setting, you should be familiar with the framework used in the curriculum and understand how much experience the student has with using the framework. Even though you may use a different or hybrid framework to facilitate clinical reasoning in your practice, it is imperative that you help the students apply the model that is used in the program and courses and provide opportunities for students to develop these important judgment skills.

Teaching-learning strategies used to help students develop critical thinking and clinical judgment skills involve using both verbal teaching strategies and written strategies. The goal of both approaches is to help students make their thinking visible, which is the observed outcome of clinical thinking/clinical judgment/clinical reasoning, and provide opportunity for you to coach the students, give feedback, and encourage them to reflect on their thinking processes and judgment skills. Verbal strategies include teaching questions/prompts, coaching, and student presentations. Written strategies include using case studies/unfolding case studies, care plans/care maps, concept maps, and journals/reflection papers.

TEACHING QUESTIONS/PROMPTS

Asking questions is an effective teaching strategy to help the students learn and apply factual and procedural knowledge. Questions in the lower levels of the cognitive domain (understand, know) are useful to determine if the student knows the use or side effect of a drug or has thought through the steps of a procedure. You can also ask questions at higher levels of the domain (apply, create) to prompt students to use the course content in context while using the problem solving/clinical reasoning/clinical judgment model used in the course. Asking questions implies a specific answer. Using questions to teach gives you an opportunity to give feedback as needed. Prompts tend to be more open ended and require the student to generate a variety of answers to which you can give feedback, and prompt for more information as the students' thinking about what they are doing unfolds. Prompts give students an opportunity to make their thinking visible, the observed outcome of making clinical judgments or using clinical reasoning (Hensel & Billings, 2020). Here, you can hold a dialog with students using the clinical judgment/reasoning framework used in the course or in the discipline. Start with asking students about what information/assessment data/cues they have recognized and what conclusion/hypothesis/diagnosis they have formulated. Follow up next by asking about what solutions or plans they have developed and what action they have or will initiate. Conclude with prompting students to indicate how they will know the plan has been successful. You can use these prompts while discussing a patient with students while they are giving care or in a postclinical conference where all students can learn from one example. (Table 12.1 provides examples of teaching questions/prompts.)

TABLE 12.1 ■ Teaching Questions/Prompts

Prompts to elicit the relevant information the student knows about the patient	What from the patient's history was significant? What information did you gather from a health/physical assessment? What laboratory data are significant? What health care provider prescriptions pertain to the patient's health problem? What is the most important issue for the patient at this time?
Prompts to elicit the student's perception of the patient's health problems	What information leads you to identify the patient's health problem/diagnosis? Are there inconsistent findings? Which information about your patient is most concerning?
Prompts to elicit the student's plans and implementation strategies for helping the patient with the health problem(s).	What are your plans for caring for this patient? What are the expected outcomes? What action is needed immediately? Should be done first? What health care team members will be involved in implementing your plan?
Prompts to elicit the student's thinking about evaluating the outcomes of the plan.	Did your plans have the outcome you intended? What findings indicate the plan is successful/not successful? What additional information do you need about the patient care outcomes? What else is needed? What could you have done differently?

COACHING

Coaching is a strategy to help students develop clinical judgement/reasoning skills and clinical competency. After determining what the student knows and the decisions the student is making about giving care, you can enter a dialogue with the student and provide missing information, make suggestions for care, and give feedback as needed. If the care plan involves risk to the patient or if a student is not skilled in performing an aspect of care, you should accompany the student and provide guidance and feedback as the student gives care. Coaching concludes by encouraging the student, asking the student to reflect on what went well, and what could be done differently. Coaching is a teaching-learning strategy, not an evaluation strategy. When coaching, you are not evaluating the student but giving feedback and encouragement. Explain this distinction to your students so they understand you are not grading them and can be more relaxed in giving and receiving information. This strategy is useful throughout the clinical experience to help shape students' behavior toward attaining the course learning outcomes.

CASE STUDIES/UNFOLDING CASE STUDIES

Case studies are representations of actual or contrived clinical situations at one point in time. The cases can be rich with patient information such as health history, lab values, prescriptions, or clinical notes about which the student must make a clinical judgment. Unfolding case studies present a patient situation that occurs over time where the student follows the patient through several phases of a health care encounter. The cases can be presented in written or digital format for the students to work through a clinical judgment process. The cases can also be drawn from an actual patient encounter with a group of students working together to develop a plan of care and giving an oral presentation of the process they used to develop the care plan. Case studies may be included with the course materials, but if you need access to others, cases may be available in a digital product the student is required to purchase as a virtual patient encounter or may be included in the textbook or in ancillary materials that accompany the students' textbook. The case studies provide a link to classroom learning, and your role is to facilitate the students' use of the case to make clinical judgments and decisions centered on evidence-based practices integrated into the patient care plan. Case studies can also be evaluated and graded (see Chapter 9).

CARE PLANS/CARE MAPS

Care plans/care maps are other ways of representing the students' ability to plan and prioritize care for a patient. The format of the care plan is used to guide students' thinking process as they make judgments about data to collect and conclusions to draw from the data to identify and prioritize patient problems, possible actions to resolve the problems, strategies to use to resolve the problem, and evaluation of the outcome of the care. In this sense, the care plan is a linear model of the plan students first develop and then evaluate outcomes of actions taken. The headings of the care plan should correspond with the step of the process students use when planning care and serve as prompts for students' thinking. The care plan also serves as an organizing tool and a worksheet for students. When you use care plans to teach students a care planning process, you can give feedback about the appropriateness of the steps and how they determined what steps to take. Care plans can also be evaluated and graded (see Chapter 9).

CONCEPT MAPS

Concept maps are a visual representation of the students' understanding of a concept and its related parts as it pertains to patient care planning. Concept maps can be represented as graphic organizers, worksheets, tables, process maps, timelines, or infographics. These visual representations of a concept are helpful to students who learn visually to organize care and to understand clinical decision points. Concept maps can be drawn free form by students to show relationships among components of the patient's care. Many faculty use preformed digital concept maps that accompany the textbook into which students enter the concepts and link them to their relationships. As with using care plans, your role is to review the concept map and give feedback. Concept maps can also be used to evaluate students' work (see Chapter 9).

JOURNALS/ REFLECTION PAPERS

These assignments are used to develop metacognitive skills as students write about the decisions/judgments they made and how they connect the experience to evidence and learning outcomes. There should be clear expectations about what the student is to include in these assignments and what evidence of their critical thinking and clinical judgment skills they are to provide. Clear directions will guide the student to better attain the purpose of the assignment. Journals and reflection papers can be evaluated and graded, or you can simply review them and give students feedback (see Chapter 9).

CLINICAL CONFERENCES

Clinical conferences are a hallmark teaching-learning strategy in which the students and faculty anticipate (preconference) or reflect (postconference) on the experience and link theory to practice. The conference is a planned and structured meeting with students that can occur before the clinical or simulated experience (preconference/prebriefing), during the clinical experience (mid-clinical conference), or following the experience (postconference/debriefing). Clinical conferences are held in a quiet and private meeting room and in an environment that ensures patient privacy and observation of Health Insurance Portability and Accountability Act (HIPAA) requirements. Clinical conferences can also be held in an online environment. The conference can be planned and led by a student or faculty. When the conference occurs prior to the clinical experience, the group reviews the learning focus for the day, shares information, asks questions, and discusses plans for patient care. If time permits during the clinical day you can gather available students for a midclinical conference to discuss pertinent care or use an actual or contrived case study that pertains to the clinical focus. During the conference following the clinical experience faculty use a debriefing model (see earlier) to provide students an opportunity to reflect on their experience, discuss clinical judgments, and link their patient experience to evidence for best practice. Your role in these conferences is to facilitate student learning in an empathetic and nonjudgmental manner.

DEBRIEFING

Debriefing is a planned, evidence-based teaching strategy in which students reflect on a simulated or actual clinical experience for the purpose of linking theory to practice. This strategy originated for helping students process the learning from a simulated experience but is also effective to help students think through any patient care experience, whether actual, simulated, or written. Debriefing should occur as soon after the clinical learning experience as possible, and take place in a safe, nonjudgmental environment. While students may be in an observer role while their classmates participate in the simulated, written, or actual patient experience, students who observe their classmates can learn as much as those who participate. You should plan sufficient time for debriefing any actual, written, digital, or simulated clinical experience; for simulations and digital case studies, debriefing time may be twice as long as the simulated experience. Several models have been developed to guide debriefing (e.g., Center for Medical Simulation, n.d.) and, if conducting a debriefing is part of your teaching responsibilities, you should utilize the model used by faculty at your school. Box 12.1 provides general guidelines for debriefing a clinical learning experience.

Strategies to Facilitate Student Development of Oral and Written Communication Skills

Helping students develop effective oral and written communication skills is a significant curriculum competency for which you will seek opportunities for students to develop in the clinical setting. Developing communication skills begins with teaching students how to communicate with their patients and continues as they progress throughout the curriculum and learn how to communicate with other health professionals and interprofessional teams and promote a healthy workplace environmet by communicating concerns for patient safety and confronting incivility. Students also must learn to chart/document patient care and to give professional presentations. You will use a variety of simulated and actual patient care experiences to help students develop these skills.

COMMUNICATING WITH PATIENTS

Prior to participating in any patient care experience, students must learn how to interact with the patient and family members. While this may seem obvious, not all students have the social and professional skills required to introduce themselves to a patient or put the patient at ease. The goal of communicating with patients and families is to reduce their anxiety, provide information about the plan of care, explain the patients' responsibility for learning to manage their care, and indicate the expected outcomes of any diagnostic or therapeutic interventions. Using a framework helps students learn expected communication behaviors. AIDET (*a*cknowledge, *i*ntroduce, *d*uration, *e*xplanation, *t*hank you) is one easy-to-use framework for students (Huron, 2022). At the beginning of every clinical experience, students should first acknowledge the patient by making eye contact and calling the patient by name. Students should then introduce themselves giving their name, their academic affiliation, their experience level, the reason they are assigned to the patient, and who they will be working with (staff, preceptor, faculty). Next students should explain the duration of what will happen during their clinical experience (e.g., what care will be given; if there will be tests, medications, or procedures; and who will be updating the patient on the progress). Students should then give an explanation of what will happen, ask if the patient has questions, and explain what answers the student can provide or will seek others who can. At the end of the experience students should thank the patient for allowing them to provide care. You can teach students to use this or a similar framework with role play or remind students of an approach to communicating with their patients during a preconference.

GIVING A HANDOFF-OF-CARE REPORT TO HEALTH CARE TEAM MEMBERS

A handoff-of-care report is used by health professionals to communicate information about a patient to other health care team members. Using a structured format improves team communications and reduces patient errors (Joy et al., 2011). One such protocol uses the mnemonic SBAR (*s*ituation, *b*ackground, *a*ssessment, *r*ecommendation), in which the health care provider describes the situation and background, gives current assessment data, then recommends an order for medications, lab tests, procedures, or actions to take (Institute for Healthcare Improvement, 2022). Other protocols can be used for interprofessional teams in which information is communicated to all members. Students can learn the technique used at the clinical site, and your role is to seek opportunities for students to develop this communication skill during their clinical learning experience. You can also integrate communication patient information or giving a handoff-of-care report as a role-play activity or written assignments.

COMMUNICATING CONCERNS FOR PATIENT SAFETY

Students also should learn communication strategies to express concern when patient safety is at risk. One strategy is CUS (*c*oncern, *u*ncomfortable, *s*afety), which is used to alert the health care team to a potential or actual problem and to stop their actions (Agency for Healthcare Research and Quality [AHRQ], 2017). When using this strategy, the student will (1) state the concern, (2) state why the student is uncomfortable, and (3) state that this is a safety issue and what alternative action should be taken. Students may have an opportunity to use this strategy during a clinical experience or can reflect on opportunities for its use in their written work.

CONFRONTING INCIVILITY

During clinical experiences students may observe or participate in situations involving uncivil communications. Uncivil behaviors on the part of the student can range from being late to the clinical course, using smartphones for personal communication, rudeness, insults, verbal abuse, sexual harassment, bullying, and aggression (Clark, 2022). Incivility also occurs between faculty and students, students and their classmates, and/or health professionals and colleagues or students. Incivility in the clinical setting disrupts the workplace and puts patient safety at risk. Students can practice effective communication skills to prevent and manage uncivil behavior using role play and reflection (see Part 2). You may be faced with these types of communications and will have the responsibility to deescalate them, and then use the moment as a teaching opportunity for students. Incivility can be managed by serving as a role model, calling out the behavior, and using cognitive rehearsal to manage the incivility. If necessary, refer to the policies in the student syllabus and in the clinical agency to deal with student incivility.

CHARTING/DOCUMENTING PATIENT CARE

When in the clinical setting, students will be required to document the care they give their patients. If your students are allowed access to the charting system at the clinical site, you will be responsible to help the students learn that documentation system. Typically, students learn charting skills in the beginning of the curriculum and may use charting software that simulates the use of an electronic health record (EHR) the program has purchased to use in the learning resource center or can use the training program for the documentation systems used at a specific clinical site (see Part 4). There may be other resources, such as skills videos, that accompanying textbooks. For beginning students it is helpful for them to write what they plan to document, and have you review it before they enter it in a permanent record.

GIVING PROFESSIONAL PRESENTATIONS

Students also need to develop the ability to present information orally and visually. In the clinical setting, students can present a patient case study to their classmates and lead the discussion during a postconference, give a presentation to staff about a topic of interest, or give a shift report. Your role, and that of the classmates, is to be supportive, prompt for information, and contribute to the discussion to ensure key points are shared. You may provide guidelines for these presentations if they are not already included in the course syllabus or course materials. See Chapter 9 for rubrics for grading presentations.

Strategies to Teach the Use of Health Care Technology and Access and Use Information for Patient Care

Increasingly, technology is used to diagnose, manage, and support patients along their continuum of care. Digital health, the convergence of digital information, communication, diagnostic, and learning technologies with health care, is increasingly being incorporated into best practices for health care practitioners. Health care technologies now enable access to health care services via telehealth applications and monitoring devices used in the home. In addition to information online that can be shared with patients, wearable devices such as electrocardiogram monitors, insulin pumps, and dietary intake records enable health care professionals and even the patient or family to perform physical assessments with device attachments such as an otoscope, ophthalmoscope, or heart monitor and transmit data to a health care provider for diagnostic evaluation and management. Robots are being used in the clinical setting to perform surgery, deliver equipment, and perform certain procedures for patients in isolation. Health care technology is increasingly being used in home care settings to remind patients to take medications or perform procedures, to submit electronic data about their health status, and to conduct appointments with their health care providers. If you are teaching in a clinical setting your students will likely be using these technologies and should be familiar with their use. As appropriate, include opportunities to use these technologies when considering patient assignments and require students to integrate their use in written work such as care plans, case studies, or concept maps.

USING TELEHEALTH APPLICATIONS

Telehealth is the use of electronic information and communication technologies, such as secure videoconferencing services, to assess, diagnose, counsel, and evaluate patients and families in their home or a remote health care setting. As state and federal legislation is enacted to support telehealth applications, faculty should include actual and virtual experiences in the curriculum to prepare students for clinical practice in telehealth (Chike-Harris et al., 2021). Competencies for telehealth practice are being developed by professional organizations (Rutledge et al., 2021) and focus on the process and protocols for delivering care by telehealth, use of technology, ethical/legal/privacy considerations, and remote clinical care.

Observational or precepted patient care experiences can be arranged in settings using telehealth. Simulated telehealth experiences can be used in the classroom, learning resource center, or simulation lab.

ACCESSING AND USING INFORMATION TECHNOLOGY FOR PATIENT CARE

In addition to digital health applications, using information technology has become a significant component of working in a health care system, and you will be involved in providing opportunities for students to use these technologies within the constraints of the clinical agency's ability to allow students to use their information systems or mobile devices while in patient care settings. Students should know how to (1) use EHRs, (2) access information from reference materials, (3) access teaching plans for their patients, (4) use electronic formats to develop care plans, and (5) use point-of-care mobile health devices. Introductory courses in most health professions programs include information on how to use library and bibliographic resources to locate evidence for best practices and patient teaching. When possible, you can seek opportunities for students to use these technologies in their clinical experiences.

Strategies for Developing Teamwork, Collaboration, and Interprofessional Practice

Teamwork and interprofessional practice are increasingly integral components of providing safe and high-quality patient care. Your students should be prepared to work in this environment by developing team and interprofessional practice skills.

TEAMWORK

Ensuring patient safety is a primary goal of clinical practice in the health professions. AHRQ has developed tools and guidelines to teach students and practitioners how to work collaboratively and in teams. Using the Team Strategies and Tools to Enhance Performance and Patient Safety (TeamSTEPPS), students and practitioners learn how to promote health care quality using a systematic approach to communications and collaboration. The toolkit presents a framework that has strategies to establish a team structure, use clear communication (see handoff of care, SBAR, and CUS strategies, earlier), develop leadership, monitor results, and give mutual support (AHRQ, 2013). The framework can be used throughout the program to help students develop team skills (Ross et al., 2021). These strategies can be taught using role play, simulation, or case studies (see Part 2).

INTERPROFESSIONAL AND COLLABORATIVE PRACTICE

The program in which you are teaching may provide students experiences with working with other health professions. Designing interprofessional and collaborative practice experiences involves curricular planning with the involved professions, as well as preparation of the students and faculty. The Interprofessional Education Collaborative (2016) has developed a 4-point framework for competencies for collaborative practice (Box 12.2). If you are teaching in a clinical setting where interprofessional practice is an expectation, you may be involved in helping students apply these skills in the clinical setting; be sure you understand the expectations for your role with these experiences

> **BOX 12.2** ■ **Interprofessional Competencies for Collaborative Practice**
>
> - Competency 1: Work with individuals of other professions to maintain a climate of mutual respect and shared values. (Values/Ethics for Interprofessional Practice)
> - Competency 2: Use the knowledge of one's own role and those of other professions to appropriately assess and address the health care needs of patients and to promote and advance the health of populations. (Roles/Responsibilities)
> - Competency 3: Communicate with patients, families, communities, and professionals in health and other fields in a responsive and responsible manner that supports a team approach to the promotion and maintenance of health and the prevention and treatment of disease. (Interprofessional Communication)
> - Competency 4: Apply relationship-building values and the principles of team dynamics to perform effectively in different team roles to plan, deliver, and evaluate patient/population-centered care and population health programs and policies that are safe, timely, efficient, effective, and equitable. (Teams and Teamwork)

INTERDISCIPLINARY/INTERPROFESSIONAL CONFERENCES, PATIENT CARE ROUNDS

Many clinical sites use an interdisciplinary or interprofessional approach to patient care and hold conferences or make rounds that include the patient and family to discuss and plan care for the patient integrating the expertise of all disciplines. As possible, you can encourage students to contribute to or observe these conferences or organize patient care rounds for your students.

Putting It All Together: Planning and Implementing Clinical Experiences

As with teaching in the classroom, when teaching in the clinical setting you will make a lesson plan for each day for and with each student. The plan will start with the course learning outcomes and include an overall focus for each clinical experience. The plan will also include collaborating with students when assigning the types of patients that offer each student an opportunity to identify and attain learning outcomes. Throughout the clinical day you will use the strategies discussed in this chapter to facilitate learning. While each clinical experience is unique for you and for the students, in general, clinical time includes a preconference/prebriefing to set the stage for learning, followed by a patient care experience, and concludes with a postconference/debriefing. You may also use written assignments, such as care plans, reflection papers, or concept maps, to ensure students have obtained the most out of the patient care experience.

COURSE COMPETENCIES AND LEARNING OUTCOMES FOR THE CLINICAL EXPERIENCE

Each clinical experience begins with an intent to provide students an opportunity to meet course learning outcomes. The focus draws on competencies for the clinical course and related didactic course and guides what the student is to learn during this experience. The focus can be specific, such as "conduct a health history," or a broad concept, such as "take care of patients with oxygen deficits." These goals can be attained by all students regardless of the patient assignment, but each patient experience will offer a different example of the skill or knowledge related to the focus. During the postconference, you and students will use the learning focus and the students' patient experience to discuss the variety of examples pertaining to the course learning outcomes.

PATIENT ASSIGNMENTS

Ideally, each student or dyad/triad will have a patient assignment (which can include a team of patients or an observational experience with a particular focus) prior to coming to the clinical experience. The assignment will depend on the focus of the learning experience, the skill and knowledge level of the student, the number of students you supervise, the availability of clinical staff or preceptors working with the students, and suggestions of the agency staff. Depending on the policies at the clinical site, the experience level of the student in the curriculum, and the nature and acuity of the patient, students can choose their patient the day before the clinical experience and prepare for the experience prior to coming to the clinical agency. Another approach is for you to choose the patients and inform the students of the assignment via secure email or within the learning management system (LMS). More realistically, the patient assignments are made on the day of the experience, and all students should be prepared for the focus of the learning experience. Prior to finalizing the patient care assignment, you or the student should seek permission from the patient (and family if appropriate) to care for the patient.

When you are making the assignments for the students, you will need to match their capabilities with the needs of the patient. You will also need to consider how you will manage your time, depending on the student's need for supervision and feedback. Also, you should consult with the nursing staff to obtain their perspective of the assignment, staffing levels and availability to work with a student, and knowledge of the patient's condition or request to not have a student participating in their care. You can also discuss alternative plans with the staff in case a patient will be having a test or surgery. You may find it helpful to develop a worksheet (see Fig. 11.1) to help you organize your day.

THE PRECONFERENCE

The clinical experience should begin with a preconference, which can occur in person (or remotely) with all students; this is a brief meeting with students using a focus sheet, which can be distributed in a LMS or email exchange prior to the experience. During the preconference the student should have a patient assignment and be prepared with a care plan and the knowledge and skills to care for the patient. At this time, you can determine if the student is prepared for providing care and what the student will need from you in terms of assistance, observation, and feedback. This will help you set priorities and timing of working with each student. The preconference is also the time for students to ask questions, clarify their plans, and request your assistance.

THE CLINICAL DAY

You may feel like an air traffic controller as you keep a bird's-eye view on each student, each patient, and many student-staff or student-preceptor interactions! You will plan teaching moments such as prompting for clinical judgment skills, using questioning techniques, or observing a skill performance. You will also coach and give feedback, seek opportunities such as attendance at an interdisciplinary conference or patient care rounds, make alternative learning plans for students as needed, review documentation, and listen to handoff-of-care reports. To accomplish these activities you will need to prioritize super-vision of students to consider when which student (and patient) will need your attention first and when. Depending on the setting, the experience of the student, and the use of a preceptor model, you may be teaching in a situation in which the student is participating in a clinical experience at another clinical site (e.g., in the community, a patient's home, by telehealth, or at other agency), and you will be involved in arranging visits and conferences to occur at a time when you are onsite or meet with the student (and staff or preceptor) via a secure remote connection. Nonetheless, your time with the student/patient/staff will be focused to maximize teaching-learning moments.

Clinical teaching-learning begins when students provide care for their patient(s). Your role is to ensure that each student has an opportunity to maxi-mize learning from the clinical experience. The focus of the experience is learn-ing, not accomplishing tasks; however, there may be occasions when there are gaps in the clinical day such as when the student's patient is discharged, goes to surgery, has a diagnostic test, prefers to sleep, or is talking with visitors. When these situations occur, you will need to make alternative plans to ensure the student still has an opportunity to benefit from the clinical experience. For example, you can assign the student to another patient, ask the student to work with another student or nurse, seek an opportunity for the student to perform a skill, develop a care plan integrating concepts that would have been gained from an actual patient encounter, or use a digital excursion.

During the clinical day you and the students will also interact with staff. You will keep the staff informed of the students' progress in caring for each patient and report concerns and request help as needed. The staff will also keep you informed about the students' and patients' progress, but keep in mind that you are responsible for the teaching and evaluation of the students and use information from the staff to ensure patient safety, as needed. Occasionally there will be situations where staff may take over the care of the patient even when the student is capable, make uncivil remarks, sabotage a student's work, or use poor technique or inappropriate communication with the patient. Use these situations as teaching moments to point out alternative approaches to patient care and communication such as how to state concerns for patient safety or to confront incivility. You may also notice students who are not observing policies for appropriate or academic or clinical practice conduct, and you will need to manage those in the moment as well.

THE POSTCONFERENCE AND FOLLOW-UP ASSIGNMENTS

The clinical experience ends with a postconference. The purpose of the postconference is to help students connect the experience to theory, evidence, and best practices as they relate to the course learning outcomes and clinical focus for the experience. Here you can use strategies such as debriefing, care plans/care maps/concept maps, case studies/clinical scenarios, student presentations, process recordings, and reflection. You may also assign students written work (if noted in the syllabus) that you will read shortly after the clinical experience and to which you may give feedback or a grade.

Ideally, the postclinical conference occurs immediately following the clinical experience at the site of the clinical experience. The advantages of conducting the conference right after the clinical experience include allowing students time to unwind and reflect on their experience, being able to debrief and connect theory to practice, giving immediate feedback, determining if a student has had an upsetting experience, and clarifying misunderstandings. In other situations, it may be necessary to schedule the conference sometime after the experience. While the goal and strategies are the same, the time gap presents a different dynamic as students may have recovered from an upsetting experience, forgotten key aspects of care, or have managed other intervening activities.

The postclinical conference can also be held in an online environment (Petrovic et al., 2020). This may be necessary when the entire clinical experience is held virtually, when the students' experiences are at a variety of locations, or when time or space does not allow for the conference to occur onsite or immediately after the experience. The advantages of a delayed or online postconference include that after long and intense days students are overloaded with information and/or are tired, and the conference can devolve into off-topic discussions and lose the benefit of careful debriefing. When conducting a postconference online, establish norms for respecting student, patient, and agency privacy and confidentiality and a safe space for students to share experiences. You may be the one to lead the conference, but students can do so as well.

Chapter Summary

Teaching in the clinical setting requires you to draw on both your clinical experience and your teaching expertise as you help your students assume the role of a professional. If you are or have been recently working in a clinical setting, you will find that your role will shift from clinician to educator, and you will need to manage your expectations of your students when they are in learning mode. From reading this chapter, you have learned what you might expect in the role of a faculty in a clinical setting and the strategies that will be helpful as you facilitate learning for your students. Here are some key points to keep in mind:

- Clinical experiences connect the theory and evidence for best practices learned in the classroom to care of patients in the clinical setting. If didactic and clinical courses are concurrent and you are only teaching in the clinical setting, be familiar with the content of the didactic course that pairs with the clinical course you are teaching.

■ There are a variety of ways to make patient assignments for students. Students can work in pairs or triads or be paired with a nurse or preceptor. You are responsible for students' learning and evaluation as well as patient safety; the staff retains overall responsibility for the patient. Student-faculty and student-patient ratios are established by state boards of health professions and the clinical stie to ensure patient safety.

■ Effective learning experiences in a clinical setting depend on having positive relationships with the staff. Your time is well spent in learning about agency policies and procedures, explaining course expectations to the staff, and collaborating with staff as you are teaching students.

■ There is a delicate balance between assigning students to care for patients and respecting patient preferences and ensuring patient safety. Understand each student's capabilities and prioritize students who will need supervision and assistance with giving care.

■ There are a variety of teaching-learning strategies that you can use to facilitate students' attainment of course outcomes, including those strategies that might be used in a learning resource center or simulation laboratory that prepare students for clinical care of patients in your course. Common strategies include observing students use psychomotor skills with patients and managing patient care.

■ While much of clinical teaching focuses on seeking opportunities for students to learn the role of care provider, there are also opportunities to help students develop skills in the affective domain such as interpersonal and interprofessional communication skills, leadership and management skills of working with agency staff, and confronting situations in which patient safety is at risk or incivility is disrupting effective patient care.

■ Each clinical experience is structured with a focus on specific learning outcomes. The preconference/prebriefing prepares students to provide safe care. During the patient care experience, you will guide, coach, and give feedback to facilitate student learning. The postclinical conference/debriefing solidifies student learning.

■ Students should have opportunities to care for patients whose age, gender, culture, race, ethnicity is different from theirs. Your role is to guide students as they develop cultural humility, values for diversity and inclusion, and understand the impact of health disparities and the role of health care professionals in ensuring that all patients receive appropriate care.

■ Managing the clinical learning experiences for a group of students (and their patients!) is complex. Plan the learning experience focus with each student, set priorities for where your teaching and supervision will be most needed, and give frequent and meaningful feedback to each student throughout the day.

At the end of each clinical day, take a moment to reflect on your own role in helping students acquire the knowledge, skills, and values of the profession. Know that you are preparing the next generation of caregivers and leaving a legacy.

References

Agency for Healthcare Research and Quality. (2013). *Pocket guide: TeamSTEPPS: Strategies & tools to enhance performance and patient safety.* https://www.ahrq.gov/sites/default/files/wysiwyg/professionals/education/curriculum-tools/teamstepps/instructor/essentials/pocketguide.pdf

Agency for Healthcare Research and Quality. (2017). *CUS tool—improving communication and teamwork in the surgical environment module.* https://www.ahrq.gov/hai/tools/ambulatory-surgery/sections/implementation/training-tools/cus-tool.html

Betts, J., Muntean, W., Kim, D., Jorion, N., & Dickison, P. (2019). Building a method for writing clinical judgment items for entry-level nursing exams. *JATT, 20*(2), S21–S36.

Center for Medical Simulation. (n.d.). *Debriefing assessment for simulation in Healthcare© (DASH).* https://harvardmedsim.org/debriefing-assessment -for-simulation-in-healthcare-dash/

Chike-Harris, K., Garber, K., & Derouin, A. (2021). Telehealth educational resources for graduate nurse faculty. *Nurse Educator, 46*(5), 295–299.

Clark, C. (2022). *Core competencies in civility in nursing & healthcare.* Sigma Theta Tau International.

Geeky Medics. (2021). *How to document a patient assessment (SOAP).* https://geekymedics.com/document-patient-assessment-soap/

Hensel, D., & Billings, D. (2020). Strategies to teach the National Council of State Boards of Nursing Clinical Judgment Model. *Nurse Educator, 45*(3), 128–132.

Huron. (2022). *AIDET patient communication.* https://www.studergroup.com/aidet

Institute for Healthcare Improvement. (2022). *SBAR tool: Situation-background-assessment-recommendation.* http://www.ihi.org/resources/Pages/Tools/SBARToolkit.aspx

Interprofessional Education Collaborative. (2016). Core competencies for interprofessional collaborative practice: 2016 update. Interprofessional Education Collaborative. https://www.ipecollaborative.org/ipec-core-competencies

Johnson, C. E., Kimble, L. P., Gunby, S. S., & Davis, A. H. (2020). Using deliberate practice and simulation for psychomotor skill competency acquisition and retention. *Nurse Educator, 45*(3), 150–154.

Joy, B., Elliott, E., Hardy, C., Sullivan, C., Backer, C., & Kane, J. (2011). Standardized multidisciplinary protocol improves handover of cardiac surgery patients to the intensive care unit. *Pediatric Critical Care Medicine, 12*(3), 304–308. https://doi.org/10.1097/PCC.0b013e3181fe25a1

Kemery, S. R., & Morrell, B. L. (2020). Differences in psychomotor skills teaching and evaluation practices in undergraduate nursing programs. *Nursing Education Perspectives, 41*(2), 83–87.

Petrovic, K., Hack, R., & Perry, B. (2020). Establishing meaningful learning in online nursing postconferences. *Nurse Educator, 46*(5), 283–287.

RC Health Services. (2013). *CHART documentation.* https://instructor.rchealthservices.com/wp-content/uploads/2013/12/CHART-and-SOAP.pdf

Ross, J., Latz, E., Meakim, C., & Mariani, B. (2021). SteamSTEPPS: Curricular-wide Integration, baccalaureate nursing students' knowledge, attitudes, and perceptions. *Nurse Educator, 46*(6), 355–360.

Rutledge, C., O'Rourke, J., Mason, A., Chike-Harris, K., Behnke, L., Melhado, M., Downes, L., & Gustin, T. (2021). Telehealth competencies for nursing education and practice: The four P's of telehealth. *Nurse Educator, 46*(5), 300–305.

CHAPTER 13

Evaluating Teaching and Learning in the Clinical Setting

The last steps of teaching in the clinical setting include assessment, giving feedback while students are learning, and evaluation and subsequent grading of students' attainment of clinical course competencies, which occur after students have had an opportunity to learn and practice. Evaluation is a distinct step in the teaching-learning cycle, but it often becomes blurred in clinical teaching because, unlike teaching in the classroom where evaluation occurs as a regularly scheduled event (e.g., a test, paper, presentation) that is graded and follows opportunities for students to practice and obtain feedback, learning in the clinical setting is ongoing and requires you to distinguish when you are teaching and assessing from when you are evaluating, which will lead to assigning a grade.

This chapter begins with a discussion of how to assess and evaluate students' clinical performance, including identifying who is participating in the evaluation, using course grading criteria, monitoring student progress, recognizing and guiding students whose clinical performance is not satisfactory, and conducting a clinical performance conference with the student. In this chapter you will also learn about the variety of strategies you can use to evaluate students' clinical performance and the instruments you can use to gather and organize the data for evaluating clinical performance and written work associated with students' clinical experience. The chapter concludes by discussing the evaluation of the course, the instruction, and the clinical agency.

Assessment and Evaluation of Student Attainment of Course Learning Outcomes

Assessing and evaluating the progress of the students' development of clinical expertise and attainment of course competencies is an ongoing process throughout the course that culminates in a final evaluation and course grade. The evaluation process is guided by the course learning outcomes and follows the evaluation plan and grading scale posted in the course syllabus, which identifies the relative importance of written, oral, and clinical practice assignments. Information for evaluating students' attainment of course outcomes can come from students' self-evaluation, the students' peers, a preceptor or staff, and your observations of students' written work and clinical performance. While you may receive input from a variety of sources, you are the person who is responsible for judging the students' attainment of the course competencies and assigning the course grade.

USING AN EVALUATION PLAN AND GRADING SCALE

The evaluation plan and grading scale (Fig. 13.1) are developed by faculty to communicate the assignments such as exams, written work, presentations, and clinical performance required to complete the course; the strategies that faculty will use to evaluate the students' completion of the assignments and attainment of course learning outcomes; and the relative weight each assignment will contribute to the course grade. The plan and grading scale are posted in the syllabus and represent a contract with the student. These cannot be changed once the syllabus is distributed to the students. In some clinical courses,

Clinical evaluation in this course is based on submission of 2 care plans by the date due, attaining a minimum of 7 points on a dosage calculation exam, and attainment of clinical course competencies at a satisfactory level or above. The grade in this course will be calculated as follows:

- Care plan #1 (10 Points Possible)
- Care plan #2 (10 Points Possible)
- Dosage calculation exam (10 Points Possible, student must attain 7 points to pass the course)
- Clinical performance evaluation (70 Points Possible)

Total points will be converted to a percentage to determine final grade per the grading scale.

Grading scale

Grade	Percentage
A+	96% to 100%
A	93% to 95.99%
A minus	90% to 92.99%
B+	87% to 89.99%
B	84% to 86.99%
B minus	81% to 83.99%
C+	78% to 80.99%
C	75% to 77.99%
C minus	72% to 74.99%
D+	69% to 71.99%
D	66% to 68.99%
D minus	63% to 65.99%
F	62.99% and below

A grade of "C" is the cut-off for a passing grade in this course.

Fig. 13.1 Evaluation plan and grading scale for a clinical course.

students receive a letter grade based on the extent to which they have attained the course outcomes. In other courses, faculty use a pass/fail approach where it is not necessary to differentiate levels of behavior by letter or numeric grades, but only to note that the student attained (or did not attain) the course outcomes by completing required assignments and clinical experiences. The advantage of this method is that faculty only need to differentiate the students who attained the course outcomes from those who did not. The disadvantage is that students who exceeded expectations and would have received a high letter grade will not have that grade reflected on their transcript. In other grading methods, the grade for the clinical course may be recorded as a separate grade for the course or may be linked to the grade in the didactic course that is a corequisite to the clinical course. In this situation, students must pass the clinical course to receive the grade they attained in the didactic course. Other grading methods blend a percentage of the clinical grade with the course grade to assign one final grade for both courses.

ASSESSING VERSUS EVALUATING STUDENT PROGRESS

During each clinical experience you will have an opportunity to observe the extent to which each student is providing safe and effective care to patients, and you will have opportunities to assess the student's progress and provide feedback as needed. You will provide students with feedback both during and after each clinical experience. In some schools, the students also evaluate their own performance after each clinical experience. You may also use students' written work (care plans, reflection papers) to monitor students' progress. Midway through the course, you may hold in-person midterm evaluation conferences to discuss the students' progress, give feedback, and, as necessary, set learning goals or establish a learning success plan. Toward the end of the clinical experience, you will evaluate student's clinical abilities and collect the necessary data to assign a grade. You will then hold a conference with students individually and give them a report about their grade and, if needed, suggestions for making continuing progress in subsequent courses.

FACILITATING LEARNING FOR A STUDENT WHO IS NOT MAKING SATISFACTORY PROGRESS

If, at midterm, a student is not demonstrating satisfactory performance and progress toward attaining course outcomes, you should discuss with the student which outcomes are not being met and the steps the students should take to attain the outcome. If the student is not progressing, you and the student should make a learning plan (learning contract, clinical performance success plan [Fig. 13.2]) based on course competencies. Both you and the student will sign the plan indicating the agreed upon actions the student will take to improve. The plans can include participating in remedial work for psychomotor skills development, being better prepared to provide care for the assigned patient, connecting theory to clinical practice, or demonstration of

Clinical Learning Success Plan	
Date	
Student Name	
Faculty name	
Course name and number	
Student is not attaining these course expectations and competencies	
To attain course competencies, the student will take the following actions	
Student and faculty will meet on these dates to review student progress	
Satisfactory student progress will be determined by the following measures	
Instructor signature Date :	Student signature Date :

Fig. 13.2   Clinical learning success plan.

professional behavior. The plan should include dates by which improvement will be noted. You will then continue to provide feedback about the student's progress, and if the student is not making progress, meet to discuss the implications of the lack of progress and the possibility of attaining a failing grade. Course failures should not come as a surprise to students, and your documentation of the student's performance must be based on student attainment of course outcomes and shared with the student on an ongoing basis prior to assigning a failing grade.

CONDUCTING THE STUDENT EVALUATION CONFERENCE

Typically the midterm and final course grades are given to each student during a face-to-face (in-person or virtual), private clinical evaluation conference. In this private and confidential meeting with the student, you will discuss the student's strengths and areas for improvement. If students conduct a self-evaluation in your course, or if preceptors provide input to students' grade, you can review this information prior to determining the final grade and share the results with the student during the evaluation conference. Keep in mind that your judgement of the student's attainment of the course outcomes is the most significant factor in determining the final grade, and it is your responsibility to make that judgement. If you have communicated effectively with students throughout the course, they should not be surprised by the final course grade when they come to this conference.

Conducting the Evaluation Conference With a Student Who Will Receive a Failing Grade

Assigning a failing grade is a difficult decision, and you must make the decision based on data and, if necessary, in consultation with the course leader or department chair while at the same time maintaining the student's privacy (unless the student has given permission to disclose the name in these discussions). The judgment to assign a failing grade must be made using the course outcomes and appropriate course, school, campus, and agency policies describing appropriate academic and professional behavior. When making the decision to assign a failing grade, you also need sufficient documentation, have given feedback to the student, and provided an opportunity for the student to improve as described in an agreed upon and signed learning contract. Reasons for not passing the course may include (1) the student gives unsafe care, is unable to perform skills in a safe manner, does not follow agency polices for giving care; (2) the student makes errors in clinical judgment, or cannot prioritize care; (3) the student cannot complete tasks in a timely manner; (4) the student does not attain passing scores on written work (care plans, journals, case studies), which is a component of the course grade; (5) the student demonstrates unprofessional behavior; or (6) the student violates clinical agency or academic misconduct policies (forgery, violations of the Health Insurance Portability and Accountability Act [HIPAA]).

When you are conducting an evaluation conference in which you are assigning a failing grade, you must be prepared to use tact and empathy. Keep the focus of the conference on the student's clinical performance and your objective evaluation. You also must be prepared for the student's reaction, even if the student is anticipating receiving this grade (Frank, 2020). Some students will respond with denial or bargain with you by pleading to receive a passing grade; others may be angry and even violent. It is difficult to predict how a student might respond, and you can, after informing the student, ask a colleague or administrator to be in the room and observe the conference. Students may also bring someone with them, and if they have not asked your permission, you can reschedule the conference and bring your course leader or department chair. At the conclusion of the conference, you can remind students of their options, which may include the right to file an appeal or repeat the course (Jackson et al., 2020). Ultimately, most students accept the decision and can take the next steps in their life.

Evaluation Strategies

After reviewing the syllabus and the evaluation plan for your course, you should familiarize yourself with the evaluation strategies that you will use in your course. Typical evaluation strategies include (1) observation of clinical performance, including during simulation or using standardized patients as an Objective Structured Clinical Exam (OSCE); (2) observing professional and ethical behavior and communication skills; (3) observing students as they make clinical judgments; (4) evaluating/grading oral presentations; and (5) evaluating/grading written work such as care plans, concept maps, and documentation on the electronic health record or patient chart. The evaluation strategy must align with the course learning outcomes and provide information needed to make a judgment about the students' attainment of the course outcomes. Using a variety of evaluation strategies provides students broader opportunities to demonstrate attainment of outcomes.

STRATEGIES TO EVALUATE CLINICAL PERFORMANCE

The most accurate way to evaluate clinical performance is to observe the student when they are giving patient care, communicating with others (the patient, family, staff, health care team), and/or performing a skill. There may be situations in which the student is taking care of an actual patient at a remote setting; in these instances, it is possible to establish virtual site visits using telehealth technology (Harris et al., 2020). You may also evaluate students who are using a simulated patient in a learning resource center. Regardless of the location of the student and patient, be sure you are using the course learning outcomes to guide your observation.

Observing students' clinical performance is a form of sampling, and it is easy to draw conclusions from just one observation. To guard against this, observe students frequently, particularly if they are not attaining course competencies, and look for improvement during the course. Data collection instruments such as checklists, rubrics, and rating scales (see later) help focus the observation. You can also record anecdotal notes to provide more complete descriptions of what you have observed. When you observe students, consider they are likely nervous, and balance your need to evaluate with their need to provide safe care and give feedback. You can use video recordings to capture student performance when it is not possible to observe real-time performance, such as when performing a skill on a manikin, participating in a simulation, or taking an objective structured clinical exam. After making your judgments about students' performance, discuss your findings with individual students. If the observation is for the purpose of assessment (giving feedback), then do so immediately after the event. Throughout the course you will be observing students in the clinical setting and will save and use these evaluations to judge progress toward attainment of course outcomes (formative evaluation), then you will summarize (summative evaluation) the findings as a final evaluation and assign the grade.

STRATEGIES TO EVALUATE CLINICAL JUDGMENT

Students must be able to integrate data, think critically, form hypotheses about their patients' problems, implement a care plan, and evaluate outcomes of their clinical actions. Students' ability to make clinical judgments can be observed by their behavior and by asking students questions or prompting them to talk about how they came to the conclusions they did about the care they have or will give (see Chapter 8). While direct observation and questioning at the time of care will give you the most helpful information to understand how the student is making clinical judgments, you can also evaluate clinical judgment when a student discusses an actual or contrived case study or writes a care plan after giving patient care.

STRATEGIES TO EVALUATE PROFESSIONAL BEHAVIOR AND COMMUNICATION SKILLS

Most clinical courses have an outcome pertaining to professional behavior. Professional behavior is typically defined by state boards of health professions, professional organizations, the college, and the school and included as a course competency in the syllabus. These behaviors include academic integrity, ethical comportment, civility, and course expectations such as participating in all clinical experiences, being on time, and completing course assignments. The course you are teaching may also have outcomes that relate to the students' interpersonal, interprofessional, or professional communication skills with patients, families, staff, the interprofessional team, and classmates (see Chapter 8). You will also evaluate the students' ability to use these skills appropriately. Checklists, anecdotal notes, rating scales, and rubrics are used to collect data about students' professional behavior and communication skills.

STRATEGIES TO EVALUATE MANAGEMENT, DELEGATION, AND PRIORITIZATION SKILLS

You may be evaluating students in courses in which the focus is on managing a group of patients, which requires them to develop team management techniques, delegation skills, and the ability to set priorities. The outcomes for these skills should align with the use of an evaluation instrument because these skills are often difficult to observe as students are using them and may better be evaluated using written papers such as a report, reflection paper, development of an organizational chart, or a written plan for priority patient needs, in which students describe how they will/did manage a group of patients, set priorities, and to whom they will/did delegate tasks.

STRATEGIES TO EVALUATE ORAL PRESENTATIONS

If your course evaluation plan and grading scale include evaluating students as they make a presentation such as presenting their patient during clinical rounds, teaching a group of patients or staff, or making a presentation to classmates or at a professional conference (see Chapter 8), you will need to evaluate the student according to the course outcomes for this activity. Instruments to gather data when students are being evaluated when they make a presentation include video recording, rubrics, rating scales, and checklists.

STRATEGIES TO EVALUATE WRITTEN WORK

Most clinical courses use teaching strategies that include written work such as care plans, concept maps, papers, charting/documentation, or memos (see Chapter 8). The most effective and efficient way to evaluate written work is to use rubrics that clearly describe what is to be included in the written work and the level (grade) the work is to be completed to earn the highest grade.

Evaluation Instruments

Evaluation instruments are designed to collect information that will be used to evaluate students' attainment of learning outcomes and professional behavior. Observation, rating scales, rubrics, and checklists are the most common types of instruments used to evaluate students' clinical performance and assign a grade.

The evaluation instrument used to gather the data should be valid and reliable. The validity of the instruments used to evaluate student's clinical performance can be established by ensuring the instrument is gathering information relevant to clinical practice. The instrument should also be practical, easy to use, and clearly understood by the student and faculty. The reliability of the instrument is noted when it provides predictable and consistent information.

In courses in which there are several sections of the clinical component of the course that use the same syllabus, evaluation strategies, and instruments as well as the same grading scale, there are likely several faculty who are involved in evaluating the students in their section of the course. In these situations it is easy to have a variety of ideas about how to evaluate and grade students, and students soon learn who is considered the "easy" grader and who is "strict." To avoid the inevitable unevenness in grading the students across the entire course, it is helpful for all faculty to have a consensus about how to evaluate and grade students' clinical performance. As you are first learning to evaluate students, it is helpful to discuss how you are evaluating students with a mentor or course leader. It is also possible for the course faculty to establish interrater reliability by constructing a case scenario or using a videotape of student clinical performance and asking each faculty to rate/grade the students' performance using the same grading criteria/rubric. The ratings can then be averaged to determine a percentage of agreement among the evaluators. When agreement is less than 60% to 70%, faculty should discuss how to harmonize the grading for the course.

ANECDOTAL NOTES AND VIDEO RECORDINGS

When observing students' clinical performance (performing skills, giving patient care, and communicating with the patient, staff and interprofessional teams) in real time, anecdotal notes and video recordings can be helpful instruments. Observations of students' clinical performance can be annotated by making a written record of the observation as an anecdotal note (Fig. 13.3), which can be written soon after the observation or recorded electronically using the note or recording function of an electronic device and shared with students as a digital attachment if permitted by the school and agreed upon by

Example of an Anecdotal Note Format	
Date	
Student	
Setting	
Course Competency	
Observation	
Suggestions for improvement	
Instructor Signature & Date	
Student signature & Date	

Fig. 13.3   Example of an anecdotal note format.

the students. Observations recorded in an anecdotal note describe an example of how well students attained course competencies as well as an observation that requires students to improve.

The anecdotal note should include the date, setting, clinical focus or competency, and a detailed description of the observation. You should sign the note and share it with students; if needed you can ask students to sign that they have read the note and add their comments. Using digital formats, if permitted and agreed upon by students and faculty, can expedite sharing of information. Anecdotal notes can be used as an assessment or feedback (formative evaluation), and then saved for a cumulative record for a final evaluation and assigning a grade (summative evaluation). It is easy to become biased when using anecdotal notes as an evaluation instrument. To avoid bias, be sure that your observations relate to course competencies and professional behavior.

Video recordings are another way of gathering data for formative and summative evaluation when you are not able to be present at the time. Video recordings are often used when the student is conducting a health assessment, performing a skill, giving a presentation, or participating in a simulation or OSCE. The recording provides a record of the event that you (and the student) can use to evaluate the clinical performance. When making video recordings of students taking care of standardized or actual patients, be sure to obtain permission from the student and the patient according to school and clinical setting policies.

CHECKLIST

A checklist is used to determine if the student correctly performed a skill or followed a protocol or procedure. The checklist includes a column for the skill/behavior/step of a process and a column(s) for noting how the student performed the skill with gradations of two (yes/no) or three (satisfactory, needs improvement, unsatisfactory or alone, with assistance, did not perform). Checklists primarily are used in learning resource centers as the student is developing psychomotor skills or in simulated clinical experiences for which the behavior can be observed and quantified. If your course uses a checklist, review this instrument before you use it with your students.

RATING SCALES AND RUBRICS

Rating scales and rubrics are used to differentiate levels of the behavior being evaluated. Rating scales are similar to a checklist but describe in more detail the extent of the behavior and the quality of the behavior on a numeric point scale (typically with 3–7 points along a continuum) Scales distinguish the differences of expectations and relate the behavior to a judgment or grade. Rating scales can also be developed to reflect the consistency with which the student demonstrates the behavior by using words such as *always*, *sometimes*, or *never*.

Rubrics are descriptions of behavior that are leveled to describe what constitutes behavior ranging from satisfactory to unsatisfactory or from the top letter grade or percentage to the lowest grade, or from pass to fail. Rubrics can be used to evaluate written work, oral presentations (e.g., Columbia Gorge Community College, n.d.), and clinical performance. Using rubrics is particularly helpful to both you and the student because the expected behavior at each grade level is clearly described. Rubrics, unlike checklists and rating scales, provide rich descriptions of the behavior to be evaluated and describe the behavior in three to five levels, corresponding to the grade. Rubrics developed as a clinical performance evaluation instrument use course competencies as the behavior with descriptions of student behaviors for attaining the learning outcome with three to five levels of behavior.

CLINICAL PERFORMANCE EVALUATION INSTRUMENTS

Each clinical course has a clinical performance instrument that faculty use to assign clinical grades. The instrument is aligned with the course learning outcomes and may take the form of a checklist, rating scale, or rubric. Review the instrument used in the course you will be teaching before you use it. Examples of clinical performance evaluation instruments can be located online (e.g., University of Houston, 2012).

Student and Faculty Evaluation of the Course, Instruction, and Clinical Setting

At the completion of the course, you and the students will evaluate all aspects of the course, including the course structure and clinical experience, teaching effectiveness, and appropriateness of the clinical setting. You or someone at the school or campus will initiate the evaluation process by providing the link to the evaluation form.

The evaluation of the course and instruction asks students to respond to questions about the opportunity to meet course outcomes, the availability of resources, and the effectiveness of the instructor (i.e., you!). Your school may also obtain information about the suitability of the clinical setting, and if involved in the instruction of students, the preceptor or staff. This evaluation obtains information about the ability of the clinical site to support the students' learning needs as well as how well the site fulfilled expectations of the contract with the school. Evaluation of the clinical site may also include obtaining information about the physical facilities (e.g., classrooms, locker, and location), the suitability and availability of patients to meet the course competencies, and the clinical staff support and ability to serve as role models for the students. Both you and the students will participate in this evaluation. Findings from this evaluation can be used to determine future use of the clinical setting or to improve the school's relationship with the setting. Before you teach the course, review the evaluation instruments your school uses to gather data about the course, instruction, and clinical agency.

Regardless of how the course evaluation takes place, you will receive the results. At this time you will review the findings and determine if changes need to be made to the course design, the course instruction, and the use of the clinical site. Likely, you will receive a variety of responses; some responses will be very complimentary, some that may have helpful suggestions, and others that represent students' frustration with the experience. While it is normal to focus on the uncomplimentary remarks, step back and find a balance. Decide which comments are helpful and ones that you can or should do something about and put the others in perspective. Findings from course evaluations are essential for quality improvement of the course, the instruction, the curriculum, and the academic program. The findings can be used for faculty performance review and provide data for promotion and tenure decisions. Data that are aggregated from all clinical courses can be used to make decisions about the use of a clinical agency, to provide information for program review, and may be submitted as a part of an accreditation report.

Faculty (i.e., you!) will also have an opportunity to evaluate the course and your role in teaching and evaluating the students. Typically, you will write this evaluation as a reflection that includes information about what went well and what, if any, changes you will make in your teaching or use of the clinical agency the next time you teach the course. Make a folder to compile the student's evaluation and yours for discussion with the course leader or department chair in an annual performance review. You can include this written reflection with other data you provide during a faculty performance review.

Chapter Summary

When assessing and evaluating students' attainment of course competencies and learning outcomes in the clinical setting your role will be to give feedback and coach students while they are learning to provide safe patient care, and at the same time you will ultimately evaluate the students' attainment of course outcomes and assign a grade. From reading this chapter you have learned that an evidence-based evaluation process uses a variety of evaluation strategies and instruments to guide you in making judgments about the students' clinical performance. At the end of the course, you and the students will also evaluate the effectiveness of the course, the instruction, and the clinical experience. Here are key points to keep in mind:

- The clinical practicum provides an opportunity for students to apply what they have learned in didactic courses, and therefore evaluation strategies used in clinical courses must align with teaching-learning strategies and experiences in corequisite courses
- Evaluating students' clinical performance is linked to teaching and assessment. The clinical experience is a time for learning as well as for assessment and evaluation.
- Assessment (feedback, coaching) facilitates student progress in the clinical course.
- Early in the course, identify students who are not making progress and develop a learning plan/contract with them to define the expectations for improvement.
- Depending on the course, clinical evaluation focuses on students' skill performance, clinical judgment abilities, professional behavior; communication skills; management, delegation, and team skills; and oral and written work.
- There are a variety of strategies to determine students' attainment of course goals; the strategies are specified as part of the course evaluation plan in the course syllabus and linked to teaching strategies used in the clinical and/or didactic courses.
- Evaluation instruments guide the collection of data used to make judgments about students' attainment of course outcomes. Instruments must be valid, reliable, and easy to use. If you are teaching a section of a course that has other sections and other faculty using the same syllabus, evaluation strategies, evaluation instruments, and grading criteria, be sure your judgments are aligned with all faculty teaching in the course. At the same time, be sure you are applying evaluation and grading criteria equitably and fairly among the students in your course.
- Align your expectations of student behavior with the level of the students in the curriculum, the course outcomes, and the amount of clinical experience students have. Expectations of the clinical abilities of students in the first semester of the program will be different from those you could have of students at the end of the program.
- Assigning a failing grade is a difficult decision. Prior to making the decision, provide opportunities for students to improve and offer remedial assistance as needed; document your observations of the students' performance and validate with them; initiate a learning contract as needed; and discuss the students' progress with your course leader/administrator and seek assistance in coming to a decision to assign the failing grade. Discuss the grade in private with each student; have an administrator present if

needed; advise students of the grade appeal process and allow them time to process the situation and determine their next steps.

- Evaluation of the course, instruction, and clinical site provide information for improving the course and instruction and for determining the effectiveness of the clinical facilities to offer learning experiences to support course outcomes.

Evaluating students' clinical performance and attainment of course outcomes is one of the most important activities of a faculty member. You now have the information you need to use evaluation strategies and instruments, and along with your clinical expertise and wisdom, you are prepared to assign grades that are thoughtful, fair, and based on evidence.

References

Columbia Gorge Community College. (n.d.). *Oral communication rubric.* https://www.cgcc.edu/sites/default/files/accreditation/Evidence-2020/Core%20Learning%20Outcome%20Rubrics.pdf#:~:text=Framing%20Language%20Oral%20communication%20takes%20many%20forms.%20This,is%20recommended%20that%20each%20speaker%20be%20evaluated%20separately

Frank, N. J. (2020). Dealing with the aftermath of student failure: Strategies for nurse educators. *Journal of Professional Nursing, 36*(6), 514–519. https://doi.org/10.1016/j.profnurs.2020.04.009

Harris, M., Rhoads, S. J., Rooker, J. S., Kelly, M. A., Lefler, L., Lubin, S., Martel, I. L., Beverly, C. J. (2020). Using virtual site visits in the clinical evaluation of nurse practitioner students, student and faculty perspectives. *Nurse Educator, 45*(1), 17–20.

Jackson, D. C., Hoffman, J., & Schaller, F. (2020). How to successfully navigate a nursing student academic/grade grievance. *Journal of Professional Nursing, 37*(1), 149–154. https://doi.org/10.1016/j.profnurs.2020.06.004

University of Houston. (2012). *Rubrics for evaluating the competency of students in field practicum IV: Clinical.* https://www.uh.edu/socialwork/_docs/field/forms/2016%20Rubric%20for%20FP%20IV-CLINICAL.pdf

Using Technology in Teaching and Learning

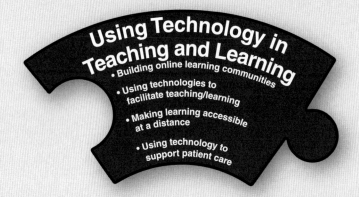

Using Technology in Teaching and Learning
- Building online learning communities
- Using technologies to facilitate teaching/learning
- Making learning accessible at a distance
- Using technology to support patient care

Technology is an essential teaching and learning tool that all faculty are expected to incorporate into their practice as educators. The purpose of Part 4 is to provide hands-on information designed to prepare you to effectively use the technology that you will encounter in your faculty role. In Chapter 14, you are introduced to the faculty role and responsibilities associated with using technology, as well as the competencies you will need to acquire to integrate technology into your teaching practice. Chapter 15 provides information you will need to get started with using technology in the classroom, clinical and online educational settings, including understanding the policies that guide the use of technology in your institution and program, and accessing resources available to assist you, such as instructional designers, distance education specialists, and instructional technology staff. Chapter 16 introduces a variety of software programs and the hardware that you will likely use in your classroom courses. Chapter 17 discusses the technologies you will encounter when teaching in a clinical setting. Chapter 18 focuses on facilitating distance learning in both synchronous and asynchronous settings. In Chapter 19 you will learn how to use technology to evaluate the effectiveness of teaching, course, curriculum, and academic programs. Appendix D lists documents, policies, and procedures you should review as you are getting started using technology to facilitate your teaching and support your students' learning.

CHAPTER 14

Introduction to Using Learning Technology

As you get started teaching in the health professions you will be using a variety of technologies to support your teaching and the students' learning in the classroom, the clinical setting and in the simulation center or learning resources center (Bonnel, Smith & Hobbs, 2022; Burke & Weill, 2022). In the classroom you will use projection systems and presentation software, digital multimedia, and testing software and you may use administrative support systems to enter student grades or access student advisement records. Likely, you will also use aspects of a learning management system (LMS) to manage course activities such as posting grades, engaging students in discussion, distributing course materials and course evaluations, and assessing student learning. Increasingly, simulations using high-fidelity manikins are used to prepare students for clinical practice and you may have responsibilities to teach in settings where these complex technologies are used to facilitate learning. In clinical settings, you will assist students use of technology to access patient records, record progress notes, and teach patients about their care plan. Use the self-assessment checklist at the end of this chapter to determine your readiness to integrate these learning technologies into your teaching practice and the need for additional orientation you may need to use the technologies available in your school.

Faculty Role and Responsibilities Related to Using Learning Technology

Your role as a faculty member will invariably involve using a variety of technologies. While you may be responsible for entering and retrieving data from information systems such as the registrar's office to post grades, or the human resources office to apply for faculty benefits, your most important role will be to use learning technologies in the classroom and clinical environment. In the classroom and learning resources center or simulated learning settings you will use presentation software, interactive games, digital video, virtual and augmented reality, and testing software. The courses you teach may be offered in a fully or partially online format and you will need to know how to navigate the LMS and use its many functions that connect you and your students. Additionally, much of teaching now is situated in, or supported by, learning technologies such as simulations and virtual and augmented reality. Also, you will prepare your students for using digital health applications such as charting using an electronic health record, mobile health applications such as wearable devices for managing patients' health and wellness, tracking patient progress using data retrieved from diagnostic devices, and the use of telehealth to provide patient care. Consider the following competencies as you prepare to use technology in your faculty role.

Educator Competencies for Using Learning Technology

USING TECHNOLOGY IN THE CLASSROOM AND STUDENT SUPPORT SERVICES

Teaching in the classroom relies heavily on the use of learning technology. You will use technology to assist you in the delivery of your lesson plan and to engage students with the content through active learning strategies. Students experience their first encounter with technology as they apply for admission, register for classes, apply for financial aid, and track their transcript in preparation for graduation. They may also encounter the use of technology in the academic advising process. Students will need to use basic word processing, presentation, and spreadsheet applications to complete assignments. In your courses, students will use learning technologies such as e-textbooks, videos of skills demonstrations, and interactive case studies. Box 14.1 lists competencies you will need to develop as you teach in the classroom.

BOX 14.1 ■ **Competencies Related to Using Learning Technology in the Classroom**

- Use technology to support the teaching-learning process.
- Make and use digital video.
- Use online interactive teaching-learning tools.
- Use technology to support assessment and evaluation in the classroom such as test administration and proctoring software, electronic gradebooks.
- Make and use presentations using slides and screen capture recordings.
- Use classroom projection systems.
- Review media, multimedia, digital media for applicability to learning and lesson plan.
- Use, assign, and critique e-books, test banks, and ancillaries that accompany textbooks.
- Use polling and audience response systems embedded in learning management and teleconferencing systems.
- Access library resources; conduct literature searches.

USING LEARNING TECHNOLOGY IN STRUCTURED, SIMULATED, AND CLINICAL SETTINGS

When teaching in a skills or simulation center and when you are in the clinical environment with students, you will use a variety of technologies to support learning such as patient care simulations using high-fidelity manikins, simulated health records, and virtual reality case studies. Because you are preparing students for patient care that increasingly involves digital health applications such as remote health assessment and monitoring, home health care delivery, and patient teaching for wellness promotion and health maintenance, you will also need to be

---

BOX 14.2 ■ Competencies Related to Using Technology in Structured, Simulated, and Clinical Settings

- Use technology to support patient care.
- Use electronic health records.
- Use technology to access patient teaching and health information resources.
- Use technology to access library and evidence-based practice guidelines.
- Use technology to support assessment and evaluation in the clinical environment.
- Use mobile health technologies in clinical setting.
- Use simulations and high-fidelity manikins to develop clinical scenarios and conduct prebrief and debriefing sessions with students.
- Use telehealth systems.
- Use mobile devices for health monitoring, tracking teaching, maintenance.

---

familiar with the digital health practices used in the clinical agency. Box 14.2 lists competencies you should develop as you teach in the clinical setting.

USING TECHNOLOGY TO SUPPORT ON-CAMPUS AND DISTANCE-DELIVERED COURSES

Whether you teach online or in the classroom, you will be expected to learn how to use technology to deliver course content to students. Two common forms of technology used to deliver course content are LMSs and videoconferencing platform systems. One challenge to delivering content through a technology-mediated environment is knowing how to create a supportive and engaging learning environment for your students. LMSs are sophisticated software programs that provide a learning platform containing all the instructional information that students need to support achievement of student learning outcomes. Course materials, links to online resources and e-textbooks, discussion forums, test administration, grading, assignment submission, email and course announcements, and integrated videoconferencing links are some examples of the learning resources LMSs can provide to support student learning. Videoconferencing platforms allow for real-time, web-based (synchronous) interactions. Videoconferencing platforms have exploded in use in education as recent pandemic health care concerns limited in-person classroom interactions. They are likely to remain a valuable tool in reaching distant student populations.

The use of a LMS is not confined to online and hybrid (blended) courses. Increasingly, courses that meet in the classroom use LMS platforms to provide supplemental learning resources for students and support faculty-student and student-student communication outside of the classroom. Given the prevalent use of LMSs most higher education institutions provide significant development resources for faculty and students to learn how to effectively use the campus-supported LMS in their teaching and learning activities. Box 14.3 llists competencies that you will need to develop to successfully implement LMS and videoconferencing technology into your courses.

BOX 14.3 ■ Competencies Related to Using Technology to Support On-Campus and Distance-Delivered Courses

- Use learning management systems.
- Use videoconferencing systems.
- Engage students in online courses; create social presence.
- Develop content modules that support achievement of course outcomes.
- Develop active learning strategies that foster interaction.
- Observe legal/ethical aspects of using technology and teaching in an online environment.

USING TECHNOLOGY TO SUPPORT PROGRAM AND CURRICULUM EVALUATION PROCESSES

Technology is very useful in supporting the many evaluation processes associated with program and curriculum implementation. For example, a variety of technologies are used to support the collection of learning analytics data to improve the student learning experience. Curriculum and course evaluation processes can be greatly enhanced using information systems that support the tracking and curriculum mapping of concepts, outcomes, and competencies as integrated across the curriculum, as well as student achievement of expected student outcomes in clinical and classroom settings. Technology is also used to help aggregate data and detect program trends that support faculty decision making related to program improvement and help with preparing reports for regulatory and accreditation agencies.

Technology is also used to support course and faculty evaluation. Most course evaluations are administered using electronic surveys and retrieval of stored data. Course evaluations for individual courses and faculty may be complied as aggregated data that compare the results of student surveys of faculty teaching effectiveness tracked over time for an individual faculty and to compare individual faculty teaching effectiveness with other faculty in the school or university. Box 14.4 lists competencies you will need to be familiar with as you collect and interpret data about your course, curriculum, and the academic progress of your students.

To increase one's skill with using technology, you will find it helpful to conduct a self-assessment of your competence in using technology to support

---

BOX 14.4 ■ Competencies Related to Using Technology to Support Program, Curriculum, and Course Evaluation and Accreditation and Other Reports

- Use online survey tools to track student learning outcomes.
- Assess course and program quality indicators, including distance education.
- Use tracking systems to manage curriculum mapping, clinical placements, student compliance, program evaluation, accreditation reports.
- Understand use of information management systems used to manage student records for admission, progression, graduation.

teaching, learning, and patient care. Table 14.1 provides a listing of technology competencies for novice educators. Take the time to evaluate your experience level with each competency, review your self-assessment, and create a plan to increase your competence in the various areas. It may be helpful to consult with a mentor or your supervisor to better understand the areas in need of improvement and prioritize the self-improvement activities that will be most beneficial. With focused effort on improving your skill set, you will find you enjoy integrating technology into your teaching practices in the classroom and clinical settings.

TABLE 14.1 ■ Self-Assessment of Competencies Related to Using Learning Technology

Consider to what extent you feel comfortable performing the following competencies, then check the appropriate box. After you complete the checklist, develop a plan to gain skill in the competencies in which you have less experience. Share your plan with your mentor for additional feedback.

Educator Competency	I Have No Experience	I Have Some Experience	I Have Much Experience
Make and use digital video			
Use test administration and proctoring software, electronic gradebooks			
Make and use presentations using slides and narrations			
Use classroom projection systems			
Review media, multimedia, digital media for applicability to learning and lesson plan			
Use/assign/critique e-books, test banks, and ancillaries that accompany textbooks			
Use polling and audience response systems			
Use technology to support patient care			
Use electronic charting systems			
Use technology to access patient teaching and health information resources			
Use technology to access library and evidence-based practice guidelines			
Use technology to support assessment and evaluation in the clinical environment			
Use mobile health technologies			
Use technology to support assessment and evaluation in the clinical environment			
Use learning management systems			
Use videoconferencing systems			

Continued on following page

TABLE 14.1 ■ **Self-Assessment of Competencies Related to Using Learning Technology** (Continued)

Educator Competency	I Have No Experience	I Have Some Experience	I Have Much Experience
Engage students in online courses; establish social presence			
Observe legal/ethical aspects of using technology and teaching in an online environment			
Use technology for faculty, course, and curriculum evaluation			
Use technology to gather and report information for accreditation and other reports			
Use curriculum tracking systems			

Chapter Summary

In this chapter you have read about the competencies you will need as you are getting started using a variety of technologies to support student learning. Here are key points for you to consider as you begin your journey:

- Understand the pedagogic value of each technology and integrate its use into your course and lesson plan appropriately.
- Each school, academic program, and clinical setting uses specific technology applications to support their work; familiarize yourself with the specifics of each application you will use with your students.
- Learning technologies are an integral component of in-person and distance-delivered courses; understand how to use them appropriately for each instructional setting.

References

Bonnel, W., Smith, K., & Hober, C. (2022). *Teaching with technologies in nursing and the health professions: Strategies for engagement, quality, and safety* (2nd ed.). Springer Publishing.

Burke, L., & Weill, B. (2022). *Information technology for the health professions*. Pearson.

CHAPTER 15

Getting Started Using Learning Technology in the Educator Role

Using technology is an integral aspect of your faculty role (Bates, 2022; Cornelius & Wilson, 2022; Harnish et al., 2018). While you will be expected to know how to use the institution's information and administrative technologies and the clinical agency client-based information systems when teaching in the clinical environment, most of the time you will be involved in using technology to facilitate student learning. After reading this chapter you will know how to get started using the various technologies you will encounter in your faculty role.

Introduction to Using Technology

Before you start your course, you will need to (1) obtain access to the technology services provided at the institution and/or clinical agency, (2) learn to use the technologies that students use in your courses, (3) ensure students have access to the technology and know how to use it, (4) meet the technology support personnel and know who to contact for assistance, and (5) understand policies that guide faculty and student responsibility pertaining to the use of information and learning technologies at your school.

ACCESS TO TECHNOLOGY SERVICES

Before you begin teaching, one of the first things you will do is obtain access to the technology services used at your school and, if needed, the clinical agency. This typically requires establishing a user identification and password, email account, access to library resources, access to the learning management system (LMS), and learning how to use software used by your students. This information may be included in an orientation session before the semester begins or from the course leader or the person to whom you report, or IT support personnel may assist you in obtaining the technology access you need for your course.

TECHNOLOGIES IN THE CLASSROOM AND CLINICAL AGENCY

If you are teaching in the campus classroom or at a clinical agency, you will need to know how to use technology equipment such as computer and projection systems, videoconferencing systems if delivering content to students at remote sites, microphone and audio systems in the classroom, presentation software such as PowerPoint, and how to access the internet for yourself and students. This information may be provided in an orientation program taught by faculty or technology service support staff at the school or institution or by the course leader. You will find it helpful to conduct a test run with the technology before you use it with students.

EXPECTATIONS FOR STUDENT USE OF TECHNOLOGY

You will also need to understand what technology the students are required to use and know how to use the programs in your course. For example, will the students need to have access to high-speed internet at the university? In their home or place of study? Will students use a digital device (laptop, tablet, or phone) in your classroom; if so, will they be oriented to the ethical and appropriate use of the technology in your course? Are students required to purchase the software used in the course such as e-books, course packs, content review books, or digital case studies? Will tests be administered in your course in an online environment such as a LMS? If so, do students need access to testing and proctoring software? Will students need to practice taking technology-administered tests before they take a test in your course? Does the institution or school provide the LMS, or does the student need to purchase access?

In clinical courses, will students be required to be oriented to clinical information systems such as electronic health records or using telehealth or patient teaching and monitoring software or apps? If so, who will communicate these expectations to the student? If information about the use of technology is not explained elsewhere, you will need to be informed and prepared to do so.

There may be other components of your course or corequisite courses that use technology. For example, your students may learn skills and practice in a learning resource center, skills laboratory, or simulation center, and you will need to ensure that the students are oriented to the appropriate technology to participate in these learning experiences.

PEOPLE TO KNOW: THE TECHNOLOGY SUPPORT STAFF

Most colleges and many professional schools have a technology support service that includes technical staff to assist you and your students with accessing the campus technology. Such technology includes the internet, computer security programs, email and word processing, the library and literature search software, LMS, and the technology Help desk. The technology support staff is essential to your successful experience using technology, and if introduction to the support team is not included in an orientation program then be sure to arrange to meet them and know how to contact them. Establishing contact with the librarian support staff is also an important step as they will be invaluable to you as you identify library resources to use in your courses.

POLICIES ADDRESSING TECHNOLOGY USE

The use of technology in the classroom, online courses, and clinical agencies is guided by policies related to ethical use, fair use, and protection of student and patient privacy. The policies may be developed by the library, student services, or technology services. Policies may also describe what information can be abstracted from textbooks or journals and used in course packs that faculty develop for student use. Appendix D provides examples of policies that are used to regulate technology access and use in educational settings and clinical agency environments. Before you use or assign students to use any technology, familiarize yourself with the following policies:

- *College use policies.* Prior to having access to college-supported technologies, students and faculty must agree to the institution's technology policies for using technology on campus, online, and with mobile devices. These policies typically include protection of privacy, appropriate academic use, fraud, harassment, and limits on political activities. Review the technology user polices at your institution; students and faculty may be required to sign an agreement to observe the policies.
- *Clinical agency use policies.* If you and your students are having learning experiences in the clinical environment, you will need to be familiar with agency use policies. Some agencies do not allow students, and in some cases faculty, to have access to clinical information systems and may restrict any internet access to public spaces. As appropriate, familiarize yourself with the policies at clinical agencies where you will be supervising students. Students will also be expected to observe patient confidentiality when using technology-supported electronic health records or when discussing patient situations in an online course or on social media.
- *Intellectual honesty, student academic conduct, and policies pertaining to using technologies.* Universities and schools have policies pertaining to academic conduct for both faculty and students, and these policies may indicate that the technology can be used only for academic use; users must communicate civilly and observe privacy laws and policies. Review these policies and ensure students have read and signed their agreement to observe them.
- *Copyright laws.* Copyright laws protect original works of authorship. These works include music, publications, and videos, among others. The Fair Use section of the copyright laws specifies situations in which copyrighted material can be used with and without permission. Check with your library or technology services office to determine if your proposed use is permissible.
- *Common Creative Attributions License.* This license indicates that faculty can use or share work with attribution to the owner of the content. Check with your library or technology services if you need additional information.
- *Technology, Education and Copyright Harmonization Act of 2002* (TEACH Act, 2002). This act is designed to provide broader access to materials that are used in distance education courses offered by accredited, nonprofit institutions. Check with your library or technology services office if your proposed use is permissible.

Integrating Technology Into the Course and Lesson Plan

As you become more familiar with the course, student learning needs, and available resources you may decide to change or add additional learning resources. Digital learning resources come with most textbooks or course packages, and the student may be required to purchase these. In addition to reading the textbook, you should review any digital learning resources that are provided, or if you are choosing software for your courses. See Boxes 15.1 and 15.2 to learn how to preview software and use it with students. This

---

BOX 15.1 ■ Considerations for Previewing Digital Instructional Software for Use in Course or Lesson Plan

- Does the digital instructional software align with the course and lesson learning outcomes?
- Review the entire product. Follow all paths that a student might take, particularly those that are not correct.
- Does the product provide instructional support, coaching, and feedback throughout the program?
- Does the product show procedures, thinking processes, and clinical judgment processes that follow those taught in your class and curriculum?
- Are the visuals and animations suitable for your students? Is their diversity represented in the people and patients in the program? Does the content and activities in the digital instructional software represent reality?
- Consider the time it will take the student to use the product. Does the time spent justify the learning benefit? Is this the best way to help the student learn and apply this content?
- Consider the hardware requirements. Will all students have access to the device on which the digital resource is best used? Do all students have online access and high-speed internet if needed?
- Plan to develop pre- and postlearning activities for the product. What information will students need to have before they use the product? How will the students know they have attained intended learning outcomes after they use the product?
- Determine if the cost of the product is justified. Is the school purchasing a user license or do students purchase their own product?

BOX 15.2 ■ How to Integrate Digital Instructional Software Into a Course or Lesson Plan

- Determine expected learning outcome(s) for the course and verify how the selected digital instructional software will help student attain them.
- Orient students to both technical and instructional use.
- Determine if the assignment of the software is required and supports the main instruction or is optional and used to enhance learning or appeal to students' preferred learning style. Can the software be used by groups of students learning together? Will there be test questions embedded in the program? If so, are they used for grading or assessment? Inform the students about your expectations for the use of the assignment and how to get the most out of it.
- Consider using a study guide, summary of key points, or practice test questions to help students achieve expected learning outcomes.
- Follow up with students about the effectiveness of the digital instructional software and its contribution to their learning.

involves both previewing the digital instructional software and considering its benefit and alignment with expected student learning outcomes, preparing yourself and students to use it, and evaluating its effectiveness after use. Assigning instructional technology programs is only part of the learning activity; you will need to prepare the students before they use the program and then follow up after they have used the program to ensure the students have attained the learning outcomes.

Preparing to Use a Learning Management System

Course management software, also known as a LMS, is increasingly used in both asynchronous and synchronous learning environments. You will likely find yourself using a LMS to also support courses that meet in person. Because of the expenses associated with the use of a LMS and the instructional personnel required to support widespread implementation of the platforms, most institutions adopt one commercial LMS product that is deployed throughout the institution for use by all academic departments. You will want to familiarize yourself with the learning platform utilized by your institution and explore the technology support resources that are available to help you orient yourself to the use of the software. Seek out faculty development resources at both the institutional level (often located in teaching and learning centers) and within your program. Find out what instructional design and technology support is available to help you develop your courses for online delivery within the LMS and who you should contact if technology issues arise during the teaching of your course. Be sure to give yourself adequate time to orient to the use of the LMS software prior to teaching your first class.

Regardless of which LMS vendor your institution subscribes to, all have similar capabilities. The prime advantage to using an LMS, even in courses that meet in person, is that the LMS provides a secure, convenient environment for all class communications, dissemination of course materials, assignment submissions, and links to course resources. Box 15.3 lists more common course management functions that you can expect to find in an LMS.

BOX 15.3 ■ Course Management Functions of a Learning Management System

- Delivery of course content (syllabus, course calendar, learning units, modules)
- Submission of course assignments
- Provide feedback on student assignments
- Administration of quizzes and tests
- Support of course communication (emails, course announcements)
- Facilitation of asynchronous student-student and student-faculty interaction through discussion forums
- Maintain record of student grades
- Integration of links to learning resources (library, databases, synchronous communication, multimedia)
- Maintain record of student attendance/participation
- Track student achievement of course competencies and outcomes

One of your first decisions will be to determine which of the LMS course management functions you will use in your course and to seek instructional design guidance on how best to utilize those functions. In some cases, the faculty in your program may have made collective decisions about the template to be used by all faculty for courses that are delivered using an LMS. A consistent LMS template is often recommended to be used within a program to maintain consistency in course design for students. As students enroll in multiple courses that have an LMS presence, providing consistency in course design will help minimize the amount of time students spend on learning how to navigate the various courses and allow them to focus more on course content and achieving learning outcomes. Additionally, certain student resources (links to library resources and electronic databases, academic policies, etc.) may be automatically included as standard links in all courses for the convenience of students and faculty. Once you understand any design parameters that have been set by your program you will be ready to design your course within the LMS.

Chapter Summary

In this chapter you have read about the knowledge and skills you will need as you are getting started using information and learning technologies. Here are key points to consider:

- Know how to use all hardware and digital instructional software programs that will be used in your course. Know who and how to contact them for assistance.
- Understand expectations for student use of technology in your course. Ensure all students have access to the internet and know how to use any required devices such as mobile phones, computers, or special equipment.
- Understand policies that pertain to using technology at the university or clinical agency such as appropriate use, ethical use, and legal aspects of using course materials from external sources.
- Learning management systems are used in both in-person and distance learning courses and provide you with many resources by which to organize your course and interact with your students. Meet with instructional design personnel and utilize your institution's center for teaching and learning excellence to orient yourself to the LMS platform used by your institution and how to use it most effectively in your courses.

References

Bates, A. W. (2022). *Teaching in a digital age, guidelines for designing teaching and learning.* BC Campus. https://opentextbc.ca/teachinginadigitalage/

Cornelius, F., & Wilson, L. (2022). Educational technology. In Whitman-Price, R. A., Godshall, M., & Wilson, L., *Certified nurse educator review.* Springer Publishing Company.

Harnish, R. J., Bridges, K. R., Sattler, D. N., Signorella, M. L., & Munson, M. (Eds.). (2018). *The use of technology in teaching and learning.* Society for the Teaching of Psychology. http://teachpsych.org/ebooks/

Technology, Education and Copyright Harmonization (TEACH) Act. (2002). https://www.congress.gov/bill/107th-congress/senate-bill/487

CHAPTER 16

Using Learning Technology in the Classroom

Technologies that support teaching, learning, assessment, and evaluation have become an essential adjunct to student learning in the classroom. Students likely have as much access to mobile devices such as smartphones, computers, and tablets as they do to a pencil, and there is increasing availability of digital resources, software programs, and apps to establish an interactive environment within your classroom. Your role is to determine how using technology-assisted learning activities will support student achievement of course learning outcomes and integrate its use into your lesson plan.

The use of technology in the classroom is most effective when it meets teaching-learning goals to (1) provide opportunities to apply course content, (2) decrease reliance on linear types of learning tools (books, handouts, Power-Points), (3) link course content to patient care, (4) develop clinical judgment skills, (5) promote active learning, (6) appeal to students' particular learning style, (7) facilitate accommodations for students with disabilities, (8) support needs of students for whom English is an additional language, and (9) promote collaboration (Gallegos & Nakashima, 2021).

There are a variety of ways you can integrate learning technologies into the classroom setting. Learning technologies can be used in the classroom as (1) a stand alone learning experience, (2) preparation for participating in a class session or clinical learning experience, (3) an optional learning experience, and (4) remediation. In this chapter you will learn about the variety of ways you can use technology to facilitate learning outcomes and meet students' specific learning needs.

Technology to Provide Course Content

One of the most important aspects of your role as an educator is to facilitate students' learning, not only so they know and understand the foundation of the content and concepts of your course, but also so they can apply and synthesize the information to make effective clinical judgments and evaluate patient care outcomes. There are a variety of technologies that you can effectively use within your courses to help facilitate student learning. E-books, course packs, presentation software, screen capture recordings, and technology-supported student presentations are some examples of such technologies and are described further in this section.

E-BOOKS AND COURSE PACKS

Textbooks and related materials are the foundational sources of content in most courses. While students may purchase a hard copy of course materials, some schools require students to purchase e-books and other digitally supported course materials. These may be bundled in a course pack, the purchase of which is included in the students' course fees. You will need to obtain instructor access to these materials. As an instructor, you may also have access to ancillary textbook instructional materials such as PowerPoints, content outlines, and test banks with a variety of questions that may or may not relate to your learning outcomes and course content. While these instructor resources are readily available, you must evaluate them for relevance to your learning outcomes, curriculum philosophy, and student learning needs.

PRESENTATION SOFTWARE

Faculty and students have become accustomed to teaching and learning with the use of presentation software such as PowerPoint or Prezi. These presentations can be useful in the classroom and in online courses to (1) help organize information, (2) provide structure for complex concepts, (3) provide documents for students to review important information before and after class, (4) help students (and faculty!) maintain focus on the topic, and (5) guide students in the application of the content to clinical practice.

Using presentation software, while helping the students learn and understand the content, is generally considered a low-level cognitive domain learning activity. To encourage students to apply, synthesize, and evaluate the content, you can embed learning activities such as case studies or practice test questions in the presentation, or follow the presentation with activities in which the students are expected to apply the information to patient care. Box 16.1 provides information about effective design and use of presentation software.

BOX 16.1 ■ How to Design and Use Presentation Software

- Organize the presentation to facilitate students' attainment of the outcome.
- Use Calibri font with titles of font size of 36 to 54 and the body of the slide at 24- to 28-point font size.
- Design for focus and clarity: avoid distracting templates, clip art, transitions, sound effects.
- Use visuals to focus key words, concepts, and application to clinical practice.
- Use color and bold font to emphasize key points.
- Use bullet points or graphics to explain steps of a process.
- Keep one idea per slide.
- Plan on a maximum 35 to 40 slides per 60-minute session.
- Insert video clips, as appropriate, to provide illustrate examples of concepts.
- Embed interaction into the presentation such as polling questions, case studies, calculations, pause-think-write an application of concept.
- Conclude with summary of key points and an assessment activity (reflection, practice test questions, case study).
- Rehearse using the classroom presentation system; when displaying in the classroom, ensure all students can see the slides.

SCREEN CAPTURE RECORDINGS

Screen capture recording is another form of presentation software that adds narration to visual images allowing you to combine audio and visual presentations of the content. You can assign these recordings as preparation for participating in active learning strategies in class, or they may be used as a follow-up or resource for students who wish to review the content more than once. These recordings can also be helpful to students for whom English is an additional language or for those who have difficulty hearing. Using screen capture recordings to deliver content can better facilitate meeting the diverse learning needs of students. Because you are narrating and explaining what is seen on the screen, you can convey excitement and caring and amplify the content with examples. By adding the voiceover to the presentation, students tend to feel more connected to the faculty and each other (Toulouse, 2020). You can use screen capture recordings for course orientation, syllabus and course expectations, feedback, and to provide content and amplify assigned readings (e.g., Prezi Present [www.Prezi.com], Pechakucha [www.pechakucha.org], FlipGrid [https://info.flipgrid.com/]).

If you plan to create your own screen capture recordings, first find out what resources are available for your use and then request technical support well in advance of the time you plan to use it. You will need to allow time to learn the technical skills and to design the learning activity.

Students can also make their own screen capture recordings as an assignment or for a presentation to their classmates. As in the classroom when presenting content alone or as a member of a panel, you can assign students to be the ones to contribute content through presentations using presentation software, short videos, or screen capture software. For example, students (individually or in teams) can use graphic design platforms to (1) make infographics to use integrated text and images to convey information, (2) make documents or posters to demonstrate application of course content, and (3) share their work with peers or with patients in patient education sessions (e.g., Canva [http://canva.com], FlipGrid [https://info.flipgrid.com/]).

Technology to Facilitate Engagement in Learning

Students learn best when they are actively engaged in learning. Obtaining the students' attention, increasing their motivation, and providing opportunities for collaboration are features of games, game-based learning (gamification), and digital whiteboards. Prior to use, be sure students understand what learning outcomes they are to attain and how to use the program. Following the learning activity, debrief with the students about the experience and how they achieved their learning goals through participation in the activity.

GAMES

Online games are a fun and easy way to engage students in an activity that helps them learn or assess their basic knowledge. Often called frame games, the game is played by filling in a two-dimensional grid or frame that organizes content by category and increasing levels of difficulty. You or the students can design these games or use an online product (e.g., Kahoot [http://www.kahoot.com; Nearpad [http://www.nearpad.com]).

GAME-BASED LEARNING

Game-based learning, or gamification, is the use of game-based features in non-game situations. Gamification also involves interactive digital learning using a scenario-based learning approach, which requires the users to follow rules and compete (with self or others). Playing games requires application of knowledge, promotes engagement in learning, and can teach students how to make clinical judgements. Other benefits of gamification include increased motivation to learn and apply knowledge, improve ability to receive feedback, facilitate development of affective skills, distinguish between relevant and irrelevant clinical data, learn to work within time constraints, and receive tangible rewards such as a certificate or badge. Emerging evidence suggests that gamification is a strategy that assists students in attaining learning outcomes (Dahlke et al., 2020) and leads to increased knowledge, improved clinical decision making, and student satisfaction (Malicki et al., 2020; Reed, 2020). Game-based learning can take place in the virtual learning environment as well as the physical classroom environment such as using board games and simulations (e.g., 3D Game Lab, Saturday Night in the ER).

DIGITAL WHITEBOARDS

Students often learn more when they are working with others. There are a variety of technology tools available to facilitate student collaboration or working in teams in both synchronous and asynchronous learning environments. Digital whiteboards (e.g., Jamboard [www.http//:jamboard.com], Padlett [http://www.padlett.com], Kaptivo [http://www.kaptivo.com]) are an example of such technology. Digital whiteboards are stand alone or added components to a learning management system (LMS) and group conferencing systems. Students may use these tools to brainstorm ideas, collaborate on group projects, use sticky notes, make a concept map to categorize or visualize information, use decision-making processes to solve a case study, and summarize and reflect after participating in a learning activity.

When using teamwork as a strategy it is important to have clear learning outcomes established and clearly communicated directions for what students are to brainstorm, solve, produce, or submit. You will also need to ensure that students know how to access and use the technology. If needed, orient students to the expectations for group process, state privacy expectations, and allow sufficient time to accomplish the goal of the experience.

Technology to Access Information

One outcome of health profession education is for students to learn how to access information and evaluate it for accuracy, relevance to their professional development, and usefulness for clinical practice. The course you are teaching likely requires students to search the professional literature for information and evidence-based findings pertaining to clinical care best practices. As you prepare to teach your course(s), be sure you understand the program's expectations for students to develop search skills and use bibliographic software as well as the librarian and library resources at the institution. Students can also access information from a variety of sources online, and your role is to help students evaluate the accuracy and quality of the information found. Students should also be instructed in how to observe ethical use policies of information accessed and referenced.

Technology to Assess and Evaluate Student Learning

Instructional technology plays an important role when you are assessing and evaluating student learning and attainment of course competencies (Frith, 2022). Being able to assess students as they are learning provides the student a gauge for knowing what they have learned and gives you a sense of where additional instruction might be needed. Digital products can also be used for administering tests in the classroom and in online courses to evaluate student learning. There are a variety of technology tools designed to assess and evaluate student learning (e.g., test authoring and grading software in your LMS; Nearpad [http://www.nearpad.com]). The following sections further describe these technology tools.

CLASSROOM RESPONSE SYSTEMS FOR ASSESSMENT AND EVALUATION

Classroom response systems, often referred to as clickers, allow you to easily create questions that can be displayed in the classroom or posted to the students' computer or device during an on-campus course or in an online synchronous course for students' response. Students submit their response, and the anonymous responses are aggregated and then displayed to the class to foster discussion. Additionally, polls or surveys can also be used to create multiple-choice questions that can be embedded in presentation or videoconferencing software. Such questions can be used as a pretest to gain students' attention, as a practice test during the class session, or as a graded quiz. Polling questions or surveys can also be used to obtain information about student demographics, values, or opinions and the results used to stimulate reflection or discussion (e.g., polling function in your LMS; Zoom [http://www.zoom.com], Turningpoint [https://www.turningtechnologies.com/turningpoint/], polling questions in videoconferencing programs, classroom response systems).

DIGITAL VIDEO

With the advent of mobile devices and portable digital cameras, videos can be used to assess and evaluate learning. The use of digital video is particularly useful in assessing and evaluating skill performance, student presentations, communication skills, role play, simulation, and preparation for students' job interviews. Students can make their own video of their performance using their mobile device and submit it as a digital file for feedback and grading.

Videos are a component of high-end simulation labs, and if you have access to these systems you can use the video that captures the students' performance to encourage them to review, reflect, and identify areas for improvement; you can also use these videos for evaluation and grading of student performance. If you are integrating the use of digital video into your evaluation plan, ensure that all students have access to the technology and understand how to use it. You will also want to develop rubrics when using the video as a guide for evaluation.

ADMINISTERING TESTS FOR ASSESSMENT AND EVALUATION

Instructional technology can be used when administering tests that are used for assessment or evaluation of student learning. Most learning management and videoconferencing systems, and stand alone test administration and item analysis products, as well as classroom presentation software and classroom response systems (clickers), have capabilities for administering test questions in assessment or evaluation modes. In assessment mode, questions are deployed within the LMS, videoconferencing system, or classroom response systems, and settings are used to allow the students to practice and review their scores without recording the score as a grade. Settings can also be used in evaluation mode, and the results can be forwarded to the gradebook.

As usual, you will need to let the students know if the questions are being used for assessment or evaluation purposes. If the questions are being used for evaluation with an assigned grade, it will be important to document how the questions fit within the course evaluation plan. Various products, including tools in a LMS and stand alone products, provide exam statistics, including scores, mean, standard deviation, and item analysis (see Part 2). Examples of resources and products for the LMS include: Canvas, Blackboard, Desire to Learn; for videoconferencing systems: Zoom, Microsoft Teams, WebEx; for classroom presentation systems: PowerPoint, Prezi; for classroom response systems/digital response systems/electronic voting: EZ vote; and for exam administration and item analysis products: ExamSoft.com.

Technology to Ensure Academic Integrity

Technology can also be used to monitor students' academic integrity. Opportunities to cheat on exams, overlook copyright laws, plagiarize, violate classmate and patient privacy, and disregard student and faculty codes of conduct are abundant whether the learning environment is in person or remote. Technology tools such as those described in the following sections can help establish a safe learning environment and ensure students are observing appropriate academic practices.

ESTABLISHING A CULTURE OF ACADEMIC INTEGRITY

Technology, with all its positive uses, also offers an environment in which students can easily access resources and papers online on any assigned topic, find answers to test questions, plagiarize, and spread untruths. The first steps to establishing a culture of academic integrity in your courses is to establish course norms, have students read and agree to institution and program policies related to academic integrity and incidents of academic misconduct, provide access to online orientation programs that explain academic integrity, and invoke consequences as noted in academic integrity policies (see Appendix D).

REMOTE PROCTORING

While live, onsite proctoring is the gold standard for proctoring exams, using remote proctoring programs and services is a viable option for monitoring students while they are taking exams outside of a proctored classroom (Furby, 2020). These systems use cameras and audio on the students' computer for live streaming and recording of the students' actions while taking the exam. The remote proctor has a view of all students while they are taking the test and can record actions, submit a red flag when they observe inappropriate behavior, or terminate the test-taking session. One proctor can observe 10 to 15 students at one time. Remote monitoring of simulated clinical experiences can be accomplished by using telepresence robots operated from an i-Pad with video and audio capabilities (Mudd et al., 2020).

While remote proctoring can be used on demand and allows students flexibility for scheduling exams, it also poses risk for academic misconduct. As it is an accreditation requirement that institutions and programs be able to validate student identity in the case of distance or remote learning to ensure the student enrolled in the course is the person doing the coursework, it is increasingly common for institutions and programs to establish proctoring policies for online or distance learning courses. Institutions may choose to enter a contract with vendors who provide proctoring services for all academic programs, or programs may select their own proctoring services. Check with your course leader or program chair to determine if your program uses proctoring services and what your responsibility is for accessing the services (e.g., Learning with Integrity [Canvas/proctoring software/proctoring services/your school's LMS toolkit], your school's technology support services).

PLAGIARISM DETECTION

If your assignments require students to submit original written work, there is a possibility that students are (1) submitting papers that can be purchased or are available at no cost online, (2) unintentionally using all or parts of works of others without citation, (3) intentionally using without citation all or parts of published works, or (4) asking or paying someone to complete the assignment for them. If you have reason to doubt that students are submitting their own work, you can use plagiarism software to scan the paper and compare it to a vast library of published work to verify that the student is submitting original or appropriately cited work. You can also encourage students to use this software before they submit the paper to help them understand when to cite others' work. Most institutions provide access to plagiarism checking software through the LMS. Plagiarism detection software may be available online at no cost, but the features may not be robust (e.g., Turnititin [turnitin.com], Grammarly [www.grammarly.com]), and test proctoring software is available (e.g., Examity [www.examity.com], Exam Soft [www.examsoft.com]).

Putting It All Together in the Classroom

Because of the wide availability of mobile devices and software to support classroom activities, it is likely that the course you are teaching will integrate a variety of technology-supported learning activities. Learning technologies are continually evolving, and you will want to remain alert to new technology that will be appropriate to incorporate into your courses. Box 16.2 offers guidelines for you to consider as you make decisions about integrating new or additional learning technologies into your course.

BOX 16.2 ■ Integrating Technology to Support Classroom Teaching-Learning, Assessment, and Evaluation Activities

- Review course and lesson learning outcomes and determine if the technology application facilitates students' attainment of the expected learning outcome.
- Consider overall course requirements and time allocation for the technology-supported learning activity. Technology should facilitate learning without adding unnecessary time requirements for its use. Be mindful of the technology to time ratio!
- Make sure students have access to the required technology (such as mobile devices) and know how to use the software application if there is a technology-supported requirement in your courses. Some schools may provide a mobile device with preloaded software for use throughout the program.
- Determine what preparation students need prior to participating in the technology-supported learning activity and what follow-up (e.g., writing a paper, taking a test, making a presentation) will ensure students have attained the expected learning outcome.
- Determine if the technology-supported learning activity will be used by each individual student, or if the students will be participating in a group or using a think-pair-share approach to the activity.

Chapter Summary

In this chapter you have learned about technologies that support teaching, learning, assessment, and evaluation in the classroom. Here are some key points to remember as you consider how best to incorporate the use of technology into your classroom teaching:

- Use technology to support pedagogy and student learning needs. Consider the course outcomes and lesson learning outcomes and how technology can best be used to support student attainment of these expected outcomes. How can the chosen technology be used to effectively assess and evaluate student learning?
- Using technology in the classroom will help you assist students to attain learning outcomes, encourage active learning, and offer content in a variety of ways that meet the diverse learning needs and preferences of students.
- Consider how you can use technology to facilitate the linkage of course concepts to the application of patient care, to increase the clinical decision-making skills of your students.
- Ensure you know how to use any technology that you choose to incorporate into your courses. Request an orientation to the technology, attend faculty development opportunities, and seek out technology support as needed.
- Review all institution and program policies that pertain to the ethical use of technology and established guidelines for ensuring appropriate academic integrity behaviors.
- Before using any type of technology, be sure all students have access to the required technology and know how to use it to support their learning.
- When using technology to present course concepts, include active learning strategies to ensure students can apply the concepts and associated content to patient care scenarios.
- Preview every technology-assisted learning experience you assign to students such as e-books, digital videos, and clinical excursions to validate that the chosen experience will help facilitate achievement of learning outcomes in a time-effective manner.
- When recommending the purchase of hardware or software, or the integration of specific technology into a program or course, always consider the cost-benefit ratio associated with its use. Does the benefit to learners justify the cost to the institution, program, or student?
- Learn how to access clinical information and evidence for best practices, teaching students to do the same.
- Use technology to give students an opportunity for deliberate practice through such active learning strategies as the use of gaming, practice questions, polling and surveys, technology-supported group learning, and assessment of their ability to apply the course content.
- Technology can be used to effectively administer and grade exams. Faculty and students are responsible for knowing the institution and program academic integrity policies, following academic guidelines for ethical use, and demonstrating academic integrity when using these products. Proctoring services are increasingly in use to validate student identity in online and distance testing situations; validate the policies in use at your institution and program.

References

Dahlke, S., Hunter, K., & Amoudu, O. (2020). Innovation in education with acute care nurses. *The Journal of Continuing Education in Nursing, 51*(9), 420–424.

Frith, K. (2022). How technology can aid in competency-based nursing education. *Nursing Education Perspectives, 43*(1), 66–67.

Furby, L. (2020). Are you implementing a remote proctor solution this fall? Recommendations from NLN Testing Services. *Nursing Education Perspectives, 41*(4), 269–270.

Gallegos, C., & Nakashima, H. (2021). Mobile devices: A distraction, or a useful tool to engage nursing students. *Journal of Nursing Education, 57*(3), 170–173.

Malicki, G., Vergara, F., Van de Castle, B., Goyeneche, P., Mann, S., Schoot, M., Seiler, J., Meneses, Z., & Whalen, M. (2020). Gamification in nursing education: An integrative literature review. *The Journal of Continuing Education in Nursing, 51*(11), 509–515.

Mudd, S. S., Mclitrot, K. S., & Brown, Kristen, M. (2020). Utilizing telepresence robots for multiple patient scenarios in an online nurse practitioner program. *Nursing Education Perspectives, 41*(4), 260–262.

Reed, J. M. (2020). Gaming in nursing education: Recent trends and future paths. *Journal of Nursing Education, 59*(7), 37–38.

Toulouse, C. (2020). Screen capture recordings enhance connectedness among students, course content, and faculty. *Journal of Nursing Education, 59*(9), 531–535.

CHAPTER 17

Using Learning Technology in Simulated and Clinical Learning Settings

The overarching goals of using technology to support clinical learning in simulated and actual clinical learning environments are to (1) prepare students for clinical practice and (2) orient students to technologies they will experience with their patients in the clinical setting. Technology can be used to support the development of clinical decision-making skills in simulated learning resource settings that are designed to replicate the clinical practice environment. Such clinical learning resource centers also provide students with access to instructional materials that support the acquisition of clinical psychomotor skills through practice and demonstration. The instructional materials may include hands-on access with medical supplies, models, and equipment; digital media; and the use of high-fidelity manikins to simulate clinical cases. Such simulated clinical learning scenarios provide students with the opportunity to first practice patient care in a safe, controlled environment before transferring their learning to the care of actual patients. Alternative simulated clinical learning methods can also be useful when actual clinical settings are not available for student learning or do not provide clinical experiences with particular types of patients as needed to meet curriculum expectations.

In this chapter you will learn about digital media that simulate patient care experiences to provide review and practice for developing clinical decision-making and psychomotor skills. You will also learn about using simulated clinical information systems and electronic health records (EHR) to provide students with the opportunity to learn documentation skills and how technology is increasingly used to monitor patients' health data. As you begin teaching your clinical courses, familiarize yourself with the availability of technologies that support students' preparation for clinical practice at your school.

Technology to Simulate Patient Care Experiences

There are a variety of clinically focused technologies that can be used to help students attain the required clinical competencies of their discipline. Clinical teaching in many health care environments can be chaotic and unpredictable and will not always provide the learning experiences that students need to hone their clinical skills. For safety reasons, clinical agencies may also restrict the numbers of students allowed in their facility and the types of clinical skills they are allowed to perform on patients. One advantage to simulating patient care experiences is that faculty can ensure all students can consistently provide patient care in predetermined clinical scenarios where they can safely practice their psychomotor and clinical decision-making skills without harm to patients. Simulated learning environments can also provide for student remediation as needed, and as demonstrated in recent years they can be beneficial to health professions programs when clinical sites are unavailable for student learning. This section outlines the use of technology in high-fidelity simulations and digitally simulated clinical practice.

HIGH-FIDELITY SIMULATIONS

Many schools and clinical agencies have dedicated simulation centers where students and staff can practice clinical skills, evaluate the effectiveness of their clinical judgments, simulate care of patients when it is not possible to have an actual clinical experience, and work with interdisciplinary and interprofessional teams (Jeffries, 2022; Lioce et al., 2018). The centers can be designed to mimic an actual patient experience in many different clinical environments. For example, clinical scenarios may be created for an operating room, recovery room, triage center, labor and delivery rooms, telehealth and remote patient care in rural community hospitals, and the monitoring of patients in their homes and assisted living facilities. To effectively use this technology faculty and staff who work in these simulation centers must have completed training in helping students learn in these environments and understanding how to work with the technical staff who manage the manikins. Unless you have received some training and orientation on how to use simulation to facilitate student learning, you should not be asked to assume these responsibilities in a simulation center. However, it is important that you familiarize yourself with the types of experiences your students have there and be prepared to follow up with what they have learned during their experiences. While it is beyond the scope of this book to expand upon how to prepare to teach in a simulated learning environment, there are several simulated learning resource facilities that offer faculty development opportunities in simulation technology to prepare students to work in clinical environments in which interprofessional practice is a model for patient care. If this is an area of teaching that appeals to you, you may wish to investigate these training and development programs as part of your own career development goals.

DIGITAL SIMULATED CLINICAL PRACTICE PROGRAMS

There is a variety of software that simulates a patient care experience (Aebersold & Dunbar, 2021). This software may be used in the classroom, in a preclinical conference, as a substitute for clinical experiences when none are available, or to supplement their learning experiences when students have time during their clinical practice. Some textbooks offer digital case studies and web-based virtual worlds that simulate a patient care experience and engage the student in assessing a patient, planning for care, and evaluating the effectiveness of the care. Prior to assigning these learning resources, be sure to preview them, estimate the time commitment required to complete the assignment, and then prepare students for their use and follow-up afterwards. If the simulated clinical experiences are used as credit for a clinical experience, you should establish similar learning outcomes, and then follow up with a clinical postconference debriefing or some other means by which to evaluate student achievement of the learning outcomes of the assignment (e.g., virtual clinical excursions [https://evolve.elsevier.com/education/training/virtual-clinical-excursions/], Vsims [https://www.wolterskluwer.com/en/solutions/lippincott-nursing-faculty/vsim-for-nursing]).

Technology to Facilitate Development of Psychomotor Clinical Skills

If you are teaching in a clinical course or there is a component of your course that requires students to learn psychomotor clinical skills in a learning laboratory or resource center, there is a wide range of digital video products, virtual and augmented reality software, and simulations that support students' psychomotor skills learning. You may be integrating these products into lesson plans in your clinical course or expecting students to independently use these products to practice or review a skill prior to performing it in the clinical setting.

These products may accompany the student's textbook and can be easily found by conducting a web search for a specific skill. Digital libraries of patient care skills may also be available on a clinical agency website that students may be able to access. As an example of use, students and health professionals in practice may find it helpful to have a quick review of how to perform a procedure or locate information about administering a pharmacologic agent.

When selecting learning technologies and products to help facilitate the acquisition of psychomotor clinical skills, there are several factors for you to consider. Because there is a variation in how online resources illustrate how clinical skills can be performed, it is important for you to carefully preview these resources and ensure that the procedures are relatively aligned with the ones that students are learning in their coursework or in the clinical agencies. While it may not be possible to find resources that are in complete alignment with your curriculum or clinical agencies, you should be aware of any differences and be prepared to discuss those practice differences with your students.

In addition, these resources can be costly with budgetary implications, and they often have potential application across several courses or even health care programs. It is rare that you would be deciding to purchase software on your own without consulting with your faculty colleagues and validating the program has the resources to purchase the product. It can be beneficial to see these programs in use prior to purchase by either asking the vendors to demonstrate the products or viewing them on display in exhibits at health professions conferences. You may also benefit from contacting other programs who are using the products to determine their level of satisfaction before committing to a purchase.

Using Technology to Manage and Monitor Patient Care in the Clinical Environment

Increasingly technology is being used to document, manage, and support patient care. Regardless of the health professions discipline, your students will be expected to use patient care and health information technology safely, effectively, and with attention to privacy and confidentiality when delivering care to their assigned patients. Health care technology also requires a strong component of understanding interprofessional teamwork and collaboration. This section provides an overview of the types of patient care and health information technology that your students will be exposed to and that you will need to incorporate into your teaching to ensure students can begin developing competencies associated with technology in health care.

USING TECHNOLOGY TO DOCUMENT PATIENT CARE

Most clinical agencies have transitioned to the use of technology to support patient care planning, charting, and documentation. The use of the EHR has greatly impacted how patient care is documented, requiring faculty and students to develop and maintain competencies needed to accurately document the care given by students when in the clinical agency. Gaining access to the clinical agency's EHR requires significant advance planning and coordination with the agency. If you are teaching a clinical course, you can anticipate that you will be required to undergo training on the appropriate EHR before being able to access it in the clinical setting.

To help facilitate their students' learning, some programs arrange to simulate the use of an EHR, which may be provided by a vendor, or in some settings the training program for documentation systems used at a specific clinical agency may be available to students in the program's health professions learning resource center or at the clinical agency. To facilitate your students' learning of EHR, you will want to allow enough time for you to be oriented to not only the program's functional uses but also the policies and procedures that the clinical agency has adopted to guide the implementation of the system (e.g., skills videos accompanying textbooks; skills videos available online from clinical agencies, schools of nursing, and commercial vendors; charting software such as DocuCare [https://www.wolterskluwer.com/en/solutions/lippincott-nursing-faculty/lippincott-docucare] or EHRtutor [EHRtutor.com]).

USING TECHNOLOGY FOR PATIENT MONITORING AND PATIENT TEACHING

Health care technologies now enable access to health care via telehealth applications and to home care by monitoring devices used to promote safety and health maintenance in the home. In addition to online information that can be shared with patients, devices are now available to enable health care professionals and even the patient or family to perform physical assessments with device attachments (e.g., otoscope, ophthalmoscope, heart monitor) and send data for diagnostic evaluation. Robots are being used in the clinical setting to perform surgery, deliver equipment, and perform certain procedures for patients in isolation. Health care technology is increasingly being used in home care settings to remind patients to take medications or perform procedures, to submit electronic data about their health status via the telephone, and to conduct appointments with their health care providers. Patients also use wearable technology such as cardiac monitoring devices, insulin pumps, or exercise trackers.

If you are teaching in a clinical setting your students will likely be using these technologies, and if you are teaching in the classroom your students should understand the use of health care technology and mobile health. Beyond the use of the technology itself, health professions students should understand privacy, confidentiality, and ethical issues that are related to the use of health information technology in various health care environments.

Be alert to various initiatives that address the use of health information technology and how it will continue to impact health care. For example, the Agency for Healthcare Research and Quality (AHRQ) has a Health Care Information Technology Integration initiative in primary care (https://www.ahrq.gov/ncepcr/tools/health-it/index.html). The nursing profession has long participated in the Technology Informatics Guiding Education Reform (TIGER) initiative (https://www.himss.org/what-we-do-initiatives/technology-informatics-guiding-education-reform-tiger), which is a product of the Healthcare Information and Management Systems Society (HIMSS). TIGER is an interprofessional initiative and over the years has identified competencies for nurses and other health care professionals. These resources and others can be useful to you and your program as decisions are made about how to incorporate patient care technology into your curriculum.

USING TECHNOLOGY TO OBTAIN PATIENT CARE INFORMATION AND RESOURCES

Students should know how to search relevant literature and product databases that can be used for patient care. These databases provide clinical guidelines, information about drugs, treatments, and procedures, as well as information for developing a teaching plan. Faculty should include time in their courses to teach students how to critique the information for accuracy and applicability to patient care. Students may also have access to the internet during a clinical experience, and faculty should teach students about trusted resources for information about drugs, procedures, patient teaching plans, and evidence for best practices used at the clinical agency.

USING TECHNOLOGY TO CONNECT PATIENTS TO CARE PROVIDERS: TELEHEALTH

Telehealth is the use of electronic information and communications technologies, such as secure videoconferencing programs, to assess, diagnose, counsel, and evaluate patients and families in their home or remote health care setting. Learning experiences can be designed to simulate a patient encounter via telehealth experiences and can be used in the classroom, learning resource center, or simulation lab. Your students may also have a clinical experience with an actual patient using telehealth. When students are learning to use their clinical skills in telehealth patient encounters, be mindful of the need to include information about patient privacy and ethical use of telehealth in your lesson plans.

Putting it All Together

Technology is increasingly becoming an integral component of patient care, and your role is to prepare students for this future of clinical practice. Fortunately there are many resources to assist students prepare for providing safe patient care. Box 17.1 includes guidelines for integrating technology-supported learning activities into your clinical courses and lesson plans.

BOX 17.1 ■ Integrating Technology-Supported Learning Activities into Clinical Courses and Lesson Plans

- Review clinical course and lesson learning outcomes to determine how technology can most effectively contribute to students developing their psychomotor and clinical decision-making skills.
- Technology can be used to foster development of students' clinical skills through independent study or group work, through review and repetition of skills to be mastered prior to application in the actual clinical settings, and through use for remediation purposes. Consider the various ways you intend to use the technology when evaluating its applicability for your clinical courses and lesson plans.
- When selecting digital media or designing simulated learning experiences to supplement or replace actual patient clinical learning experiences, review the selected media and simulated learning experiences to ensure there are clearly established learning outcomes that align with the intent of the clinical experience and facilitate student achievement of the expected learning outcomes.
- Ensure students are oriented to the use of the selected technology.
- Develop lesson plans to include preparation and follow-up for each technology-supported learning activity. Consider the use of anticipatory set activities to help students understand the intent of the learning activity and debriefing activities following the conclusion of the activity.
- Evaluate use, application to development of clinical decision-making skills, attainment of student learning outcomes, and student satisfaction after implementing a technology-supported clinical learning activity.

Chapter Summary

In this chapter you have learned about technologies that are used to support learning in structured simulated clinical environments such as learning resource or simulation centers or in the actual clinical environment. Here are key points for you to consider when integrating these technologies into your simulated or clinical practice environments:

- A variety of technologies are available to facilitate learning as students prepare to care for patients in a clinical environment. These include multimedia to teach and reinforce learning for clinical skills and virtual case studies to help students develop assessment, communication, and clinical judgment skills, and chart and document care.
- The clinical practice environment is increasingly dependent on the use of technology to manage digital health applications. Students will be actively engaged in using these technologies to assess and diagnose patients' health status, monitor patients' health, and develop teaching plans.
- Students should know how to access and critique online information to locate evidence-based practices, seek information on medications, and find appropriate patient education materials for their patients.
- Knowing how to use telehealth technologies to reach patients in their homes and at health care facilities in rural and remote areas is becoming an essential skill for health care professionals and should be integrated into students' clinical experiences.
- Your role is to thoughtfully and intentionally use technology to facilitate student learning in the clinical environment.

References

Aebersold, M., & Dunbar, D. M. (2021). Virtual and augmented realities in nursing education: State of the science. In T. A. Schneidereith (Ed.), *Annual review of nursing research: Healthcare simulation* (pp. 225–242). Springer Publishing. https://doi.org/10.1891/9780826166340

Jeffries, P. (2022). *Simulation in nursing education: From conceptualization to evaluation* (2nd ed.). Lippincott Williams & Wilkins.

Lioce, L., Graham, L., & Young, H. M. (2018). Developing the team: Simulation educators, technical, and support personnel in simulation. In C. Foisy-Doll & K. Leighton (Eds.), *Simulation champions: Fostering courage, caring, and connection* (pp. 429–444). Wolters Kluwer.

CHAPTER 18

Using Learning Technology to Facilitate Distance Learning

Distance education is playing an increasingly important role in higher education and the education of health professions students. Whether students are enrolled as traditional students on campus or from a distance, an increasing number of college students will likely take at least one course via distance technology during their education. In 2019 the National Center for Educational Statistics (NCES, 2019) reported that over 3.4 million students were enrolled in exclusively distance education courses, while another 3.8 million were enrolled in at least one distance education course, representing a total of 37% of all students enrolled in postsecondary education. With the onset of the global pandemic, this number has dramatically increased as higher education institutions rapidly shifted to the use of synchronous and asynchronous distance education to safely maintain campus operations (Jeffries et al., 2022). Many faculty suddenly found themselves teaching online courses with minimal lead time for preparation. Because of this recent widespread immersion into distance education, faculty in higher education programs will likely continue to learn how to most effectively utilize technology to facilitate learning, and the use of distance technologies will expand.

Health professions faculty have often been leaders in the implementation of distance education on their campuses. As an educator in the health professions, there is every likelihood that you will be asked to teach a distance education course at some point in your teaching career. Teaching a distance education course requires you to invest much time into planning and organizing the course and determining how best to design learning activities that will foster student engagement and achievement of course outcomes, and the ability to effectively evaluate student learning. This chapter addresses the use of distance education technology, how it impacts your teaching role, and how to most effectively create distance learning environments that facilitate the achievement of student learning outcomes.

The Distance Education Environment

Distance education is not a new phenomenon in higher education. It has been successfully used for decades to extend educational opportunities to those students who live at a distance from campus. Additionally, distance education has often been used to facilitate the educational goals of working adults whose work schedule and responsibilities do not allow them to regularly attend in-person classes. This has been particularly beneficial for health care professionals, such as nurses, who return to school to further their education while working. There is a rich database of evidence-based literature that has studied the effectiveness of distance learning in facilitating the achievement of student learning outcomes (Pei & Wu, 2019). You can start your preparation for teaching from a distance by conducting a literature search on the use of distance education in your discipline and gain an understanding of evidence-based best practices to help you plan your own development as a distance education teacher.

The distance education environment is generally described as being one of three types: asynchronous, synchronous, and hybrid or blended. An asynchronous distance education environment is one in which courses are taught entirely online with no real-time interactions. Students can access the course at any time or place that is convenient for them. All student-faculty interactions are mediated using integrated learning management systems (LMS), which are sophisticated course management software platforms that contain all course materials, discussion forums, assignment submissions, and testing functions. In this learning environment and with the use of a computer connected to the internet, students have a single point of access (the LMS) to attend class and access all the course materials needed to facilitate their achievement of expected learning outcomes.

The synchronous distance education learning environment is one in which students and faculty have real-time interactions mediated across the miles through technology. Synchronous distance education requires students to attend class sessions at a set time. In the recent past, the technology used in synchronous distance courses consisted primarily of videoconferencing systems supported by the institution or in some cases regional or statewide education partnerships. Such videoconferencing systems can link multiple sites together at the same time with the use of cameras capable of autofocusing on the speaker, thus allowing students from all sites to participate and see each other as they interact. These systems require a significant amount of resource investment, both in terms of equipment and personnel, to maintain. More contemporary versions of videoconferencing are supported by web-conferencing software companies that provide software platforms to support audio video interactions between participants. This area of technology is currently enjoying a rapid expansion in growth because of the global pandemic, both in corporate and educational uses. Common commercially available platforms include Zoom, GoToMeeting, WebEx, and it is likely this market will continue to evolve. Participants must have access to a computer or other device equipped with a web-camera and microphone and stable broadband access to the internet to log on to the platforms.

A hybrid or blended distance education environment is one that combines both asynchronous and synchronous learning to facilitate student learning. This model of distance education allows students to have the convenience of learning in their own time, with periodic sessions of real-time interactions with

---

BOX 18.1 ■ Competencies for Creating Effective Distance Education Learning Environments

- Using distance education technology effectively
- Creating a learning community to foster interaction
- Fostering student engagement and active learning
- Evaluating student learning in a distance education environment

---

their peers and faculty. The synchronous interactions can occur in person, or student cohorts who are geographically dispersed can use videoconferencing technology. LMS may integrate links to web-based conferencing platforms within the system to easily facilitate synchronous interactions from a distance within hybrid courses. With the use of LMS and web-based videoconferencing, it is becoming increasingly easy to combine asynchronous and synchronous learning activities in your course.

In your teaching role, you may be asked to teach in all three types of distance education environments as it is not uncommon for programs to use both asynchronous and synchronous courses, as well as hybrid courses, in the delivery of the curriculum. Regardless of whether the courses you teach are asynchronous, synchronous, or hybrid, you will need to develop competence in several areas to be an effective teacher in the distance education environment (Box 18.1).

Using Distance Education Technology

A first step toward teaching a distance education course is to familiarize yourself with the technology that you will use to deliver the course. When teaching a distance education course, you will want to ensure that you are using the technology to facilitate learning, not creating barriers to learning. You can only do that if you understand how best to leverage the technology to create a supportive learning environment. The most common forms of technology used to deliver distance education courses to students are, as noted, learning management systems, institutional videoconferencing systems, and web-based videoconferencing platforms. Additional multimedia, such as podcasts and vodcasts, may also be utilized in conjunction with these common forms of technology to deliver content to students (Friesth, 2020).

LEARNING MANAGEMENT SYSTEMS

One of the most common technologies used to deliver distance education is the LMS. If you are teaching an asynchronous online course, the LMS will be used to hold and manage all your course materials, facilitate course discussion, submit assignments, administer tests, and post grades. You may also use the LMS to send course announcements, email your students, and post links to external learning resources. Links to web-based conferencing (e.g., Zoom) can also be embedded in the LMS to conveniently set up synchronous interactions as needed. When effectively designed, the LMS supports student learning by creating easy access to course materials and allows the students to navigate the course site with minimal difficulty. It is a comprehensive course organization tool for faculty and students alike.

If you are teaching a synchronous or blended course, the LMS is still a valuable course management tool. You can select the LMS functions that you wish to use to support the delivery of your course. For further description of the functions that the LMS can perform, see Chapter 15.

INSTITUTIONAL VIDEOCONFERENCING SYSTEMS

Institutional videoconferencing systems are used to synchronously connect students and faculty from various remote classroom sites. The use of such technology requires students to be present at a preset time and at a specific geographic location so that they can sign on to the class and participate in class discussions. The requirement to be present at a specific location may be a disadvantage to some students who are juggling work, family, and school responsibilities. As faculty, you will need to understand what your role will be in the operation of the videoconferencing system and how to access technical support as needed to facilitate use of the equipment by faculty and students who are remotely located. The use of such systems requires coordination of scheduling and support personnel contacts at remote sites to ensure that students have access to the room and equipment during the scheduled class time.

You will want to allow time for your own orientation to the equipment prior to using it to teach your course. Students will need to be made aware of who to contact at the remote location if they encounter difficulties with accessing the classroom or using the equipment. One of your teaching challenges when using this technology is to not rely on lecturing during class time, but to consider how to foster student interaction and active engagement with the course content.

WEB-BASED CONFERENCING SYSTEMS

With the use of web-based conferencing systems increasing in higher education during the global pandemic, it is becoming more likely that you will conduct synchronous class sessions using a web-based conferencing platform, rather than an institutional videoconferencing system. The main advantage to web-based conferencing for students is that participants can sign on wherever they are located if they have access to the internet with enough bandwidth to support the transmission of audio and video. Additional advantages for the institution are that web-based conferencing does not require extensive investment in specialized videoconferencing equipment and requires fewer personnel to support synchronous course delivery. The institution does need to purchase a license to deliver courses using the conferencing platform. A disadvantage to using web-based conferencing is the quality of audio and video can be disrupted if the internet connection is not stable or does not operate with sufficient bandwidth.

As a teacher you will face the same challenges as with institutional video-conferencing related to engaging students with the content and interacting with each other. There is a temptation to solely rely on lecture as a teaching strategy, which is not conducive to active learning. However, one advantage with web-based conferencing is that you can create individual "rooms" within the conferencing platform to allow for student interaction and group work.

Creating a Learning Community in a Distance Learning Environment

When developing a course to be taught in a distance learning environment, your primary goal is to create an environment that will enable students to successfully demonstrate and achieve the course's expected learning outcomes. Technology, if not utilized effectively, can erect barriers within the learning environment and cause students to feel isolated from their classmates and teacher and disempowered from being responsible for their own learning (Regmi & Jones, 2020). This is true of both asynchronous and synchronous distance learning. There are several steps that you can take as a faculty when designing your distance learning course that will help establish a student-centered learning community that fosters student engagement and active learning.

Garrison et al. (2000) developed the Community of Inquiry framework, which outlines a process by which online learning can be designed to effectively facilitate student learning. They created the term "community of inquiry" to refer to those who are participants in the learning process; the community of inquiry consists of students and teachers, thus a learning community is formed. The Community of Inquiry model describes three elements in the design of online learning experiences that are believed to be necessary to build a sense of community among learners, foster higher-order thinking, and enable achievement of student learning outcomes. Those three elements are cognitive presence, social presence, and teaching presence (Garrison et al., 2000). An important concept of the model is that the three elements of presence must interrelate for the purposes of creating a community of inquiry that encourages meaningful interactions leading to achievement of learning outcomes (Garrison & Cleveland-Innes, 2005). The Community of Inquiry framework has been extensively researched over the past 2 decades, and you will be able to find much evidence-based literature that addresses its utility as a framework for designing online education.

While the Community of Inquiry framework was developed for asynchronous online learning, the concepts related to social, cognitive, and teaching presence also have applicability to the design of other technology-mediated distance education models, including blended courses and those taught solely through videoconferencing. As you design your course for distance learning, consider the following tips to help you develop a course that fosters cognitive, social, and teaching presence, facilitating higher-order thinking and achievement of student learning outcomes.

CREATING COGNITIVE PRESENCE

Garrison et al. (2000) considered cognitive presence to be the element of the Community of Inquiry framework that was most critical to student success. Cognitive presence as defined by the authors means "the extent to which the participants in any particular configuration of a community of inquiry are able to construct meaning through sustained communication" (Garrison et al., 2000, p. 89).

In the health professions, the cognitive domain is focused on students being able to critically think (engage in higher-order learning), connect theory to practice, and apply knowledge learned to clinical decision making and patient care. Using the definition of cognitive presence, as put forth by Garrison et al. (2000), your role as teacher is to create learning experiences that allow students to construct meaning and develop the cognitive, psychomotor, and affective competencies necessary for the provision of safe patient care. You will want to leverage the use of the technology to facilitate the acquisition of competencies, minimizing any technology barriers. The importance of creating learning activities that foster transparent and clear communication of course concepts is paramount as you consider teaching and learning strategies that will engage students in the learning process and encourage them to connect their newly acquired theoretical knowledge to application to real-life situations.

Box 18.2 provides examples of teaching-learning strategies that can help you create cognitive presence in both synchronous and asynchronous learning environments. With attention to your course design and by implementing a variety of strategies, you will be most likely to appeal to your students' various learning styles and learning needs, leading to the acquisition of expected learning outcomes.

BOX 18.2 ■ Creating Cognitive Presence in Distance Learning Environments

- Contemplate the knowledge foundation students will need to construct in the cognitive, psychomotor, affective learning domains to successfully demonstrate course outcomes.
- Develop learning modules that will serve as knowledge foundation building blocks, organizing course content into logical units of study and identifying the learning module topic, related student learning outcomes, reading assignments, learning activities and due dates for associated assignments.
- Consider teaching-learning strategies and activities that will encourage students to apply theoretical knowledge to their clinical practice and demonstrate their decision-making skills. As examples, such strategies can include problem-based learning scenarios, case studies, virtual reality scenarios, and simulations.
- Design learning activities that require students to engage in inquiry, critique, analysis, and synthesis of course concepts. Such strategies can include written assignments, debates, concept maps, literature reviews/reports, and presentations.
- Create opportunities for students to engage in self-assessment and self-directed learning based on their identified learning needs. As examples, such strategies can include debriefing sessions, journaling, portfolio development, and 1-minute papers.
- Seek out the guidance and feedback of your institution's teaching and learning centers, and instructional design experts to learn how to best leverage technology to promote higher-order learning.

CREATING SOCIAL PRESENCE

Social presence was the first presence identified as having importance for online learning and has been the most researched presence in the Community of Inquiry model (Swan et al., 2009). Social presence was defined by Garrison et al. (2000) as "the ability of participants in the Community of Inquiry to project their personal characteristics into the community, thereby presenting themselves to the other participants as real people" (p. 89). Social presence is thought to play a role in supporting cognitive presence and helping learners achieve higher-order thinking. A lack of social presence in your course can lead students to feel isolated in the learning process without a supportive learning environment that enables them to do their best work. A feeling of isolation eventually can lead to a lack of student satisfaction, failure to achieve learning outcomes, and withdrawal from the course.

Fostering social presence has been thought to be particularly important to promoting learning in the affective domain, as well as promoting cognitive learning (Garrison et al., 2000). In the health professions, addressing the affective learning domain is an essential component to providing safe, compassionate patient care. There are many learning opportunities in which health professions students are asked to explore professional beliefs, values, emotions, and ethical dilemmas related to the care of clients. Students are most likely to feel free to express those feelings if they can do so in a risk-free, safe environment, in which the dialogue is constructive and supportive.

While students can engage in self-reflection, it is also important that they learn to collaborate and work in teams to achieve their learning goals. Creating a social presence, one in which they believe themselves to be members of a supportive learning community, will encourage them to share their thoughts and engage with others. In fact, the online learning environment can provide students, especially those who are more reticent with sharing, with increased opportunities to provide thoughtful, reflective comments in group learning settings. For example, online environments have been successfully combined with in-person clinical learning experiences to promote reflection in online postconference learning situations, generating more thoughtful discussion than in postconferences that are held in person immediately following the clinical setting (Petrovic et al., 2020).

Designing a course that utilizes a blended design with both asynchronous and synchronous learning is one means by which you can facilitate social presence. However, just encouraging student interaction is not sufficient. You will want to design learning activities that encourage students to engage in meaningful dialogue that remains on point and promotes in-depth discussion of course concepts. It is also possible to promote social presence in asynchronous learning environments especially through collaboration and group activities. Box 18.3 provides examples of teaching-learning strategies designed to promote social presence in your distance learning course.

BOX 18.3 ■ Creating Social Presence in Distance Learning Environments

- Have students collectively identify and share teaching and learning behaviors that best support their learning in distance environments.
- Ask students to create course interaction guidelines for course communications that will demonstrate respectful interactions and civility, whether they be asynchronous or synchronous; post the guidelines where they will be readily accessible by all.
- Encourage students to post introductions in a shared discussion forum to create a sense of community; create a discussion forum where students can go to interact as desired outside of required course activities.
- Create learning circles in courses that have a high enrollment so that students can come together to discuss course concepts in smaller, more intimate teams of learners.
- Be intentional in designing learning activities that require communication with peers and faculty.
- Respond in a timely manner to student inquiries.
- Create a discussion forum where students can post course questions that can be answered by anyone who knows the answer, student or faculty.
- Design learning activities that promote collaboration, require students to provide peer feedback, student discussion, or groupwork.
- Use technology to provide office hours online, via teleconference, web-based conferencing.
- Provide prompt feedback on assignments.

CREATING TEACHING PRESENCE

The third element of the Community of Inquiry framework is teaching presence. There are two roles typically associated with creating teaching presence within your course: designing the educational experience and facilitating discussion and learning (Garrison et al., 2000). Anderson et al. (2001) defined teaching presence to be "the design, facilitation, and direction of cognitive and social processes for the purpose of realizing personally meaningful and educationally worthwhile learning outcomes" (p. 5). They further elaborated that creating teaching presence encompasses the activities the teacher engages in to design the course, plan learning activities, facilitate course discussion, and provide instruction to students as needed.

The importance of teaching presence in your course cannot be overstated; research has indicated that teaching presence can lead to increased student satisfaction and perceived learning (Swan et al., 2009). Creating a teaching presence in your course contributes to the extent that social presence and cognitive presence will also be evident. Box 18.4 provides examples of actions you can take to create teacher presence as you design your course and facilitate course discussion. The next section of this chapter focuses on how to foster student engagement and active learning in the activities that you design for your distance education course, in both asynchronous and synchronous learning environments.

Fostering Student Engagement and Active Learning

Fostering student engagement and active learning in your course can help facilitate students' achievement of expected learning outcomes. Active learning

---

BOX 18.4 ■ Creating Teaching Presence in Distance Learning Environments

- Create clear statements of course outcomes and expected student learning outcomes, emphasizing their importance to students.
- Organize course content into learning units or modules that promote logical learning progression, creating a learning "roadmap" for students to follow.
- Establish clear expectations for student participation in the class.
- Provide students with an opportunity to share their expectations of you as their teacher (i.e., what behaviors will help promote their learning in the distance learning environment).
- Use teacher-directed instruction as necessary to promote understanding of complex concepts (e.g., brief lectures, podcasts, narrated PowerPoints).
- Design learning activities to support achievement of course outcomes, with accompanying rubrics to be used to guide evaluation of student assignments.
- Provide clear instructions and due dates for all assignments.
- Focus student discussions and reinforce student contributions as needed; provide constructive feedback and correct misunderstandings of content.
- Encourage student participation as needed, reaching out to students who are not meeting course participation expectations.
- Pose questions to clarify and prompt deeper understanding of content.

---

strategies are more likely to increase higher-order thinking and the decision-making skills of learners. Good practices in education that lead to higher-order thinking include (1) encouraging student-faculty contact, (2) developing student reciprocity and cooperation, (3) using active learning strategies, (4) giving students prompt feedback, (5) emphasizing time on task, (6) communicating high expectations, and (7) respecting diverse ways of learning (Chickering & Gamson, 1987). While developed in 1987 for undergraduate education, these seminal teaching principles are still relevant and can be applied to the design of distance education courses. Keeping such practices in mind as you create your distance learning course can help ensure that your students are engaged in the learning process.

If you have access, an instructional designer will be able to help you design your course to incorporate a variety of teaching-learning strategies to meet diverse student learning needs and promote active learning. You will want to avoid posting your lectures online as that will only lead to passive learning. While selected snippets of teacher-provided lectures in the form of podcasts, narrated PowerPoints, among others, can have their appropriate place in the design of online courses, they should be short (10–15 minutes at most) and limited with a goal of providing clarification of selected and usually more complex concepts. This is also true for synchronous videoconferencing: Resist the temptation to simply lecture to your geographically dispersed students. Instead, consider ways that you can invite their participation in the course, allowing them to continue to hold responsibility for meeting their own learning needs. To get started with your course design, make an appointment with your instructional design support personnel to determine how you can best convert your face-to-face course to distance learning, or if you are initially developing the course, integrate active learning experiences throughout the course. Table 18.1

TABLE 18.1 ■ Fostering Student Engagement and Promoting Active Learning

Principle	Tip
Encouraging student-faculty contact	• Establish office hours via technology • Share preferred means of contact • Be available to respond to course questions in a timely manner (discussion forums, web-based conferencing, telephone)
Developing student reciprocity and cooperation	• Promote student discussion via use of technology, including LMS discussion forums • Provide opportunities for students to provide peer feedback • Design group/teamwork, collaborative learning assignments • Create learning circles to promote facilitate smaller discussion groups
Using active learning strategies	• Case studies, problem-based learning, team-based learning • Application exercises • Debates, pro/con discussions • Reflection, writing assignments • Portfolio development • Use of technology (videos, podcasts, vlogs)
Giving students prompt feedback	• Set timelines by which students can expect to receive graded assignments • Use formative evaluation strategies • Use student peers to provide initial feedback on assignments
Emphasizing time on task	• Communicate due dates for all course work • Allow adequate time for students to complete assignments • Employ consistent course template design for all modules • Minimize technology barriers and maximize ease of course navigation
Communicating high expectations	• Clear communication of course outcomes and expectations for student participation • Encourage self-directed learning • Reach out to students who may be falling behind as evidenced by minimal participation, late assignment submissions • Empower students to identify and pursue own learning needs
Respecting diverse ways of learning	• Incorporate a variety of teaching/learning strategies • Provide learning activity "options" for students to select from when feasible • Encourage respect for diverse opinions • Allow student to select topics for further/deeper study for select learning assignments • Create a balance of collaborative work and self-reflection activities

provides tips based on Chickering and Gamson's (1987) seven principles of good practices that you can use to foster student engagement and promote active learning in both asynchronous and synchronous distance learning environments.

Evaluating Student Learning in the Distance Learning Environment

As with face-to-face courses, evaluating student learning in the distance learning environment requires careful forethought. The evaluation strategies that you implement need to demonstrate the same level of rigor as your face-to-face courses and be designed to measure student attainment of the expected course outcomes. Ideally, you should utilize both formative and summative evaluation strategies so that you can best monitor and understand your students' ability to acquire and demonstrate understanding of the expected course outcomes.

Formative evaluation strategies are those that assess student learning as they are engaged in learning the concepts being taught and applying them to practice. By using formative evaluation strategies you will have a chance to assess student understanding and modify your teaching plans as needed to best meet their learning needs. Formative teaching strategies can include administering pretests before beginning a new learning module and a posttest following the learning module to gauge the improvement of students' knowledge about the concepts being taught. When using formative evaluation strategies you are not assigning a grade to the activity; rather, you are using the formative evaluation to assess whether the lesson plan and activities have been successful in facilitating student engagement and learning.

Classroom assessment techniques, such as those designed by Angelo and Cross (1993), can be readily adapted to the distance learning environment. For example, you can use the discussion forum to ask students to post short comments about the concepts they are having trouble understanding and need further clarification about (muddiest points). You can also do a round-robin exercise in which your students can respond with a short reply to a question you pose to them, either in a synchronous class session or in an online discussion forum. The 1-minute paper can also be assigned to quickly gather data about the students' understanding of a specific concept, in which you pose a question for them to respond to in a short paragraph. Formative evaluation is a quick way to gauge how your learners are doing with the course material, and you can be creative in designing the formative learning strategies that you want to use.

You will conduct summative evaluation when you are ready to measure the students' achievement of the expected course outcomes. Even though it is a distance education environment, you will be expected to measure the course outcomes at the equivalent level as expected in a face-to-face class. As such, it is important to understand the purpose of the evaluation and carefully select the evaluation strategy that is appropriate for the learning domain that you are measuring. Using a variety of evaluation strategies is usually most appropriate to comprehensively measure student achievement. For example, this may be a test that consists of multiple-choice questions, a written paper assignment, development of a presentation, or a portfolio process. In health professions courses, it could also be a simulated experience using a learning laboratory facility with standardized patients or high-fidelity mannikins where students come to demonstrate their acquired clinical skills.

Whichever evaluation strategy you select, you will need to investigate how to best implement those strategies in a distance environment, whether they are asynchronous or synchronous. Administering tests will likely require you to arrange for proctors or use other security measures to minimize academic dishonesty. Hands-on demonstration of clinical skills will require having access to learning laboratory facilities and personnel. Again, proactively accessing the

---

BOX 18.5 ■ Getting Started: Evaluating Student Learning in Distance Learning Environments

- Establish clear course outcomes and expected student learning outcomes.
- Identify the competencies that students will need to demonstrate to successfully meet course outcomes.
- Select a variety of evaluation strategies that will effectively evaluate the learning domains (cognitive, psychomotor, affective) associated with the identified competencies.
- Develop clear instructions and grading rubrics for each evaluation strategy to share with students at the beginning of the course.
- Provide prompt and frequent feedback on student performance throughout the length of the course.
- Integrate the use of formative evaluation strategies in the course to assess students' ability to grasp course concepts.
- Address academic integrity and student identity validation policies as they pertain to your selected evaluation strategies, adhering to institutional and program policies.
- Identify the resources needed to implement your chosen evaluation
- Strategies (e.g., test banks, proctors, plagiarism detection software, computer-assisted instruction, simulation facilities).

---

expertise of an instructional designer is a good place to get started with designing your evaluation strategies for your distance education courses. Box 18.5 provides you with some planning strategies to help create evaluation measures that will be reliable and valid for use in your course.

Chapter Summary

In this chapter you were introduced to the design of distance learning courses and how to prepare yourself to teach in asynchronous, synchronous, or blended distance learning environments. Here are some key points to consider to get you started in the design and implementation of your distance education courses:

- Distance learning in higher education has increased significantly in recent years. Health professions programs have often been leaders in using distance education technology on their college campuses. Be sure to tap into the expertise of your faculty colleagues as you begin developing your distance learning courses.
- There are three main types of distance learning course models typically used in higher education: asynchronous, synchronous, and blended (hybrid) courses.
- Use the expertise of instructional designers and your institution's center for teaching and learning excellence resources, if available, to help you create a course design that will facilitate achievement of student learning outcomes.
- Common forms of distance education technology for you to familiarize yourself with are course management software (learning management systems), institutional videoconferencing systems, and web-based conferencing systems.

- Your primary goal as a teacher of a distance learning course will be to create a learning environment that supports the development of a learning community that supports student achievement of expected learning outcomes.
- The Community of Inquiry framework outlines a process by which online learning can be designed to facilitate student learning. The three elements necessary to build community among learners are cognitive presence, social presence, and teaching presence. While designed for online courses, this framework also has applicability to synchronous and blended distance learning courses. As you design your distance learning course, you will want to incorporate teaching-learning strategies that support the creation of cognitive presence, social presence, and teaching presence in your course.
- Fostering student engagement and active learning in your distance learning courses are more likely to increase the higher-order thinking of your students.
- Utilize formative and summative evaluation strategies to assess and evaluate student learning in distance education courses.
- Evaluation strategies for distance learning courses need to measure the same course outcomes and demonstrate the equivalent rigor of courses that are taught in person.
- Distance learning courses are not easier or inferior to face-to-face courses. Teaching a distance learning course requires much planning and organization, a keen understanding of curriculum and how to design learning activities that will foster student engagement and achievement of course outcomes, and the ability to reliably evaluate student learning.

References

Anderson, T., Rourke, L., Garrison, D. R., & Archer, W. (2001). Assessing teaching presence in a computer conferencing context. *Journal of Asynchronous Learning Networks, 5*(2), 1–17.

Angelo, T. A., & Cross, K. A. (1993). *Classroom assessment techniques. A handbook for college teachers.* Jossey-Bass.

Chickering, A., & Gamson, Z. (1987, March). Seven principles for good practice in undergraduate education. *American Association for Higher Education Bulletin*, 3–7.

Friesth, B. (2020). Teaching and learning at a distance. In D. Billings & J. Halstead (Eds.), *Teaching in nursing: A guide for faculty* (6th ed., pp. 392–408). Elsevier.

Garrison, D. R., Anderson, T., & Archer, W. (2000). Critical inquiry in a text-based environment: Computer conferencing in higher education. *The Internet and Higher Education, 2*(2-3), 87–105.

Garrison, D. R., & Cleveland-Innes, M. (2005). Facilitating cognitive presence in online learning: Interaction is not enough. *The American Journal of Distance Education, 19*(3), 133–148.

Jeffries, P., Bushardt, R., DuBose-Morris, R., Hood, C., Kardong-Edgren, S., Pintz, C., Posey, L., & Sikka, N. (2022). The role of technology in health professions education during the COVID-19 pandemic. *Academic Medicine, 97*(35), S104–S109. https://doi.org/10.1097/ACM.0000000000004523

National Center for Educational Statistics (2019). IPEDS Data Explorer 2019-2020. https://nces.ed.gov/ipeds/search/ViewTable?tableId=28442

Pei, L., & Wu, H. (2019). Does online learning work better than offline learning in undergraduate medical education? A systematic review and meta-analysis. *Medical Education Online, 24*(1). https://doi.org/10.1080/10872981.2019.1666538

Petrovic, K. A., Hack, R., & Perry, B. (2020). Establishing meaningful learning in online nursing postconferences: A literature review. *Nurse Educator, 45*(5), 283–287. https://doi.org/10.1097/NNE.0000000000000762

Regmi, K., & Jones, L. (2020). A systematic review of the factors—enablers and barriers—affecting e-learning in health sciences education. *BMC Medical Education, 91*, 1–18. https://doi.org/10.1186/s12909-020-02007-6

Swan, K., Garrison, D. R., & Richardson, J. C. (2009). A constructivist approach to online learning: the Community of Inquiry framework. In C. R. Payne (Ed.), *Information technology and constructivism in higher education: Progressive learning frameworks* (pp. 43–57). IGI Global.

CHAPTER 19

Evaluating the Use of Learning Technology

Because the use of technology is increasingly integral to support teaching, learning, and patient care, you will be involved in evaluating its effectiveness to facilitate student learning, design the course, and use the technology itself. When evaluating student use of technology, it will be important to evaluate the technology before assigning it for student use (availability of technology, usability of hardware and software, student readiness to use the technology), while the students are using the technology (formative evaluation), and after students have used the technology (summative evaluation). In this chapter you will learn how to evaluate the pedagogic value of technology, use a rubric to determine the effectiveness of an online course, and use best practice standards for evaluation and accreditation of distance-delivered programs.

Evaluating the Use of Learning Technologies

As you begin to use various learning technologies in your courses, you will find yourself making judgments about its ease of use and value to student learning. Frith (2020a; 2020b) recommends evaluating the technology, both hardware and software, for accessibility, ease of use, cost, and impact on student and faculty productivity. You can also evaluate the technology you are using for compliance with Americans with Disabilities Act (ADA) guidelines and universal design for learning principles. Your experiences in using various types of learning technology and noting these factors will help you understand the benefit the technology has for your students. Once you have gathered evaluation data on these factors, consider changes that will improve the use of the learning technologies in your courses.

ACCESSIBILITY OF REQUIRED TECHNOLOGY

When considering the use of technology that requires access to high-speed internet outside of the classroom, you must ensure that all students have internet access and a device that can connect to the internet. Your first step before selecting technology is to determine the digital literacy of your students and any technology access issues that exist within your student population. The digital divide that exists in higher education in the United States accompanied by educational inequities that exist among students who are low-income, first-generation college attendees or minority learners continues to potentially impact students' ability to be successful in college (Buzzetto-Hollywood et al., 2018). Institutions have a responsibility for assessing and evaluating students' technology learning needs to address any barriers that may exist. If it is a program expectation that students will have access to the internet and a computer with certain specifications, it is important for the program to set forth these expectations when students enroll in the program.

Access to instructional materials implies that students have ready access to a computer; however, some students may be accessing materials from a mobile phone and thus dealing with slow download times. While some campuses offer hotspot internet access for students, having to come to campus to access the internet puts students who are working remotely at a disadvantage. Before choosing any technology for use outside the on-campus setting, you will want to verify if your institution or program has any policies that address computer and digital literacy requirements for all students, as well as the level of digital literacy and access to computers and broadband infrastructure your students possess. If you are teaching in a clinical facility, you should also evaluate the accessibility of internet access for students who are searching clinical information and evidence-based practices for patient care or if they will be able to access digital course materials during their clinical experiences.

COMPLIANCE WITH ADA GUIDELINES

The ADA (2007) provides guidelines for ensuring that materials to be accessed online meet the needs of students with disabilities such as low vision or difficulty hearing. These guidelines provide strategies such as adding text to images for students with low vision and specifying color and font size and use of html or rich text format for documents posted on the website. For assistance with compliance, check with your technology support service or instructional designers as they will be the most knowledgeable about the design of any digital learning materials that will be accessible to all students

UNIVERSAL DESIGN FOR LEARNING

Universal design was first developed in the field of architecture with a goal of designing environments and products that are accessible to all, regardless of age or ability (Anderson et al., 2019). As applied to learning, universal design recognizes that individuals have variable learning needs and provides a process by which curriculum is designed to systematically address the learning differences that exist among all learners (Anderson et al., 2019). Universal design goes beyond assuring accessibility to those who have a disability. The use of the universal design process ensures all learners can access the learning environment and have access to the resources they need to be successful. The focus is on providing an inclusive learning environment with multiple and flexible learning opportunities for all students. Levey (2018) conducted an integrative review to address the use of universal design in nursing education. While this study was focused on nursing education, the findings have implications for other health professions educators as well. Levey's (2018) study indicated that many nurse educators did not understand universal design, and this was a major barrier to its use in classroom and clinical settings. Instructional designers are a good source of information for how to ensure your courses use technology that follows universal design principles. Seek out resources within your institution and search your discipline's literature to expand your knowledge of universal design, and include questions about the use of universal design principles in the technology evaluation plan.

EASE OF USE

Technology must also be easy for the least tech-savvy student in your class to use. Usability testing is a process for evaluating hardware and software programs with all levels of students before requiring its use. While most of the hardware and software used in the courses you will be teaching have likely undergone usability testing, you will want to provide students with an orientation to the hardware or software along with clear explanations of your expectations of how they are to use the technology to achieve the expected learning outcomes. For example, if you are using a LMS to make course materials available to students, provide students with clear directions on how to navigate the system to locate course resources such as learning modules, where to find instructions for how to complete and post assignments, how to use the communication tools to interact with peers and faculty, and how to access and take online tests.

COST AND EDUCATIONAL VALUE FOR LEARNING

Hardware and software, as well as technology fees charged by the institution, add substantially to the cost of attending classes. If you are the one recommending purchase decisions, be mindful of assigning expensive programs, understand the value the student will obtain from them, and identify who will be bearing the cost. Is it the school or program in the institution or the student? When possible, identify multiple ways the technology can be used to benefit students' learning experience. Can the technology be used across numerous courses or programs to help justify the cost investment? Additionally, if you anticipate that the students will bear the cost of implementing the technology, be mindful of your institution's policy regarding charging additional student fees. Many institutions require central administration approval when additional student fees are being proposed, which will require advance planning to obtain prior to purchase and implementation.

Along with cost, you will want to determine not only to what extent the use of technology devices and assigned software contribute to student learning but also the time involved for the student to use the program. You should conduct a trial use of the entire program you are assigning to know how productive the learning time is. Is the use of the technology the most effective and efficient means by which to achieve the desired learning outcomes? Does the technology support the diverse learning needs of your students? How quickly will the technology and content become outdated and require further investment for updates? (See Chapter 15 for further considerations.)

STUDENT SATISFACTION

When using any type of technology you should also understand how satisfied students are with the technology and the content. You can seek student input in a variety of ways using both formative and summative evaluation strategies. When using learning technologies, especially for the first time, it is important to gather feedback from students about their experiences with the technology and how it is affecting their learning before the end of the course. Seeking student input midcourse provides you with an opportunity to make any adjustments that may be needed to improve the students' learning experience. You can gather summative evaluation data by including questions on the course evaluation and asking the students directly for feedback after completing a technology-assisted learning activity.

Evaluating Design and Use of Online Courses

Course evaluation is an essential responsibility of faculty to ensure curriculum quality and determine if the course is achieving its intended goals for student learning. While the evaluation of online courses encompasses the usual course evaluation elements of student learning outcomes, faculty and student satisfaction, and effectiveness of student learning activities, there is also a need to evaluate additional elements related to the online learning experiences of students and faculty. These additional elements include an evaluation of the course design, ease of access and navigation of the course, and the degree of interaction fostered within the online environment.

If you are new to online teaching, you will want to seek assistance with designing and evaluating your course. Instructional designers can help you design a course in which course concepts are organized into learning modules, active learning strategies are developed to encourage student engagement, and the navigation of the course is user friendly. They can also help you develop a plan for evaluating the effectiveness of the overall course design. Depending upon the scope of resources available at your institution, you may have access to instructional designers at both the institution and program levels. Many institutions have centers for teaching and learning that provide faculty support and development in teaching and evaluating online courses. See Chapter 18 for further information about designing online courses.

Designing the evaluation plan for your online course will require you to access a variety of resources, including the feedback of your peers. Arranging to have peers evaluate your course and provide feedback can be a very useful strategy. Proactively planning on how you will evaluate your online course as you design it will yield the most beneficial feedback from all stakeholders.

There are also several online resources available that are specifically designed to help faculty develop, teach, and evaluate quality online courses. Two of the most prominent online resources devoted to facilitating quality in online learning are the Online Learning Consortium (OLC) and Quality Matters. The OLC was founded in 1999 as the Sloan Consortium (Sloan-C) and has evolved over the years into a global consortium. The OLC (2022) offers best practices focused on five pillars of online learning: learning effectiveness, faculty satisfaction, student satisfaction, scale (enrollment capacity), and access (academic, administrative, technical). Quality Matters began with the Maryland Online consortium that received federal funding to launch a nonprofit organization focused on measuring quality in online education. Quality Matters provides training and certification opportunities to higher education personnel who are responsible for implementing online education for their campuses. Quality Matters (2022) has developed standards and rubrics that can be used to evaluate online courses and other resources. The course design rubrics and standards are made available to members addressing the following areas: course overview/introduction, learning objectives, assessment and measurement, instructional materials, learning activities and learner interaction, course technology, learner support and accountability, and usability.

Both organizations offer institutional membership that allows faculty who are employed by member institutions access to all resources. Both organizations also offer individual membership options. You will want to ascertain if your institution is a member of either. While some of the resources are available free, the complete robust collection of tools, standards, and rubrics is only available to members. Workshops and webinars, as well as repositories of evidence-based literature related to online learning, are also available.

Evaluating Distance Learning Programs

Evaluating your distance learning programs and courses requires you to evaluate the usual program and course components. Institutional and programmatic accreditation bodies and regulatory agencies typically have specific criteria related to distance learning programs (asynchronous, hybrid, and synchronous), and it is important that you be aware of the criteria stipulated for your health professions discipline. Box 19.1 lists distance learning elements that accrediting

---

BOX 19.1 ■ Distance Education Program Evaluation Elements

- Student identity verification
- Test integrity
- Technology resources
- Faculty development
- Rigor of courses
- Credit hour/workload hour alignment
- Achievement of expected student learning outcomes
- Student resources

agencies typically evaluate and the collection of specific evaluation data. These areas are expanded upon next.

STUDENT IDENTITY VERIFICATION

When you teach in a distance education program or course, it is an expectation that the institution and program will have processes in place that allow you to verify and authenticate the identity of the students who have registered for the course. This is an expectation of the federal government, as promulgated by the 2008 Higher Education Opportunity Act (HEOA), Public Law 110-315, Section 602.17, subsection G, which sets forth accreditation criteria for institutions and programs that offer distance education programming and receive Title IV funds for student financial aid. The criteria state that institutions are required to use methods such as the following to verify student identity: (1) secure logins and passcodes to access course content, (2) proctored examinations, and (3) any new or other technologies that can effectively verify student identity. Institutions are also required by law to protect student privacy and notify students at the time of registration or enrollment of any additional fees that are being charged to verify student identity. Because of these accreditation regulations, you can expect your discipline's accreditation agency to seek evidence that your institution and program are adhering to the criteria. The institution and program will have to provide documentation that outlines the processes and means being used to verify student identity and protect student privacy.

As you can see, it is important that you ascertain, to the best of your ability, that the students enrolled in your distance education course are the individuals doing the coursework. The technology used to deliver distance education instruction needs to be secure and accessible only by students who are registered in the institution and enrolled in the course.

Your role as a teacher of a distance education course is to understand the policies and processes in place to comply with these federal regulatory expectations. Failure to adhere to the criteria can jeopardize your institution's and program's accreditation status and access to student financial aid. Your first step is to review your institution's policies related to student identity verification and clarify any questions you may have. You will need to ensure that your course adheres to the policy. You will also want to understand any institutional procedures in place to protect student privacy.

The use of a course LMS, in which only registered and enrolled students who have had their identity verified by the institution are allowed access to the course, provides some measure of security. This is one reason why it is beneficial to conduct all course-related work within the LMS. Proctoring examinations is another way to validate the identity of the student taking the test. Plagiarizing detection software can be used to help determine if written assignments contain original work.

Students also have the responsibility to keep their student identification (ID) numbers and passcodes secure. Institutions typically have stringent policies in place that address the students' responsibility for protecting their unique student ID and passcodes and the consequences of sharing the information with others. Sharing the institution's and program's academic honor code with your students is another important step in creating an environment that discourages academic fraud and supports academic integrity.

TEST AND WRITTEN WORK INTEGRITY

In the health professions, evaluating a student's clinical decision-making competence and achievement of expected student learning outcomes as measured by valid and reliable tests is of critical importance. Addressing test integrity in a distance education environment is an important consideration for faculty, and (as previously discussed) is a requirement of accrediting agencies. Faculty will want to take steps to ensure that the enrolled student is the individual who is taking the test and that they are doing so without cheating. These same concerns can be extended to other graded assignments that the student submits as coursework.

Proctoring examinations is one strategy used to ensure test integrity. Students can be required to go to a secure location such as a testing center that has in-person proctoring or they can be proctored remotely using technology. There are several commercial vendors that specialize in providing proctoring services to educational institutions. Determine your institution's policies regarding test proctoring and if the institution has an established contract with a commercial proctoring service.

Ensuring that written work is original to the enrolled student is another challenge requiring faculty to consider strategies to discourage academic dishonesty. Such challenges are not unique to distance education, as students in the traditional classroom setting can also submit written assignments that are not their own work. The use of plagiarizing detection software can help minimize the likelihood of plagiarism. Many institutions and programs have policies about the use of such software, notifying students in writing that all written assignments will be submitted for review to detect plagiarized material.

TECHNOLOGY RESOURCES

Accrediting agencies will want to see evidence of adequate technology resources to support teaching and learning in distance education programs (e.g., Accreditation Council for Occupational Therapy Education, 2022). Technology resources include the hardware and equipment needed to deliver the courses either via the internet or via teleconferencing systems, software to support course delivery (e.g., LMS, instructional design tools, plagiarism detection), classrooms equipped for teleconferencing if using synchronous telecommunication delivery, and electronic learning resources such as library databases. It is expected that faculty will be oriented to the use of the equipment. It is also an expectation that students will be informed of the technology requirements of the distance education program and courses prior to their enrollment.

In addition to adequate hardware and software it be necessary to demonstrate that you have access to adequate support personnel to assist you in the design and delivery of your course. Do you have access to instructional designers and other instructional technology support personnel to help you prepare your course for distance delivery? Such support may be at the institutional or program level. Is there Help desk support for both faculty and students that can be used to report problems and request assistance? If so, how much support is provided—is it available 24/7 or more limited?

Other distance education technology support resources typically expected by accreditation agencies are technology orientation sessions, designed to help faculty and students to learn how to use the technology to support teaching and learning. Such support may include in-person training as well as access to online resources.

FACULTY DEVELOPMENT

An important evaluation criterion for the delivery of quality distance education is for the institution and program to offer a robust faculty development program to prepare faculty for teaching in a distance learning environment. For you to be successful in teaching from a distance it will be important for you to develop competency in doing so; it is not simply a case of transferring your teaching from an in-classroom presence to the distance education environment. It will be important for you to invest time into preparing yourself to be an effective teacher in a technology-mediated environment, as will be evaluated on your teaching effectiveness in the distance education environment and held to the same level of performance expected of you in the face-to-face classroom. Chapter 18 further describes the competencies required to develop a teaching presence in a distance education environment that is conducive to fostering student learning.

There is an expectation by institution and program accreditors that distance education courses will demonstrate the same level of rigor that exists in courses that are taught in person in the classroom. You will need to demonstrate that the course objectives, expected student outcomes, and evaluation processes of your distance education courses are held to the equivalent level of achievement as they would be if taught in the classroom. Grading scales and policies are expected to be the same as well. This is an important consideration as you develop courses for distance delivery. How can you achieve the same learning outcomes in the distance learning environment? This will be your creative teaching challenge as you design your distance education course, developing learning experiences that enable students to demonstrate the course's expected learning outcomes. Seek out faculty development opportunities to help you master these competencies.

ACHIEVEMENT OF EXPECTED STUDENT LEARNING OUTCOMES

Students who are enrolled in distance education programs must be able to demonstrate the expected competencies and outcomes as set forth in the curriculum and by the discipline's standards. You will be responsible for determining how to measure student learning outcomes in your course, and (as discussed previously) students must be held to the same level of rigor as in-person courses. Of special significance in health professions programs is how best to connect theory and practice, and to measure your students' clinical competence in a distance learning environment. Clearly identified course outcomes, learning activities and evaluation rubrics, grading policies, and transparency about the evaluation process (which incorporates both formative and summative evaluation feedback into the course) are necessary elements to facilitating student achievement of expected learning outcomes. Faculty are also expected to ensure that the workload required of students to achieve the expected student learning outcomes is aligned with the credit hours that are assigned to the course.

Distance education courses are also expected to provide students with ample opportunities to engage in peer-peer and student-faculty interactions throughout the course. As you develop your course, you will want to consider how you will foster such interactions so that a supportive learning environment is created in which students can demonstrate success in achieving learning outcomes.

STUDENT SUPPORT RESOURCES

Accreditors expect that students who are enrolled in distance learning programs will have the equivalent access to student support services as students who attend on-campus classes. This includes, for example, access to academic advising, various academic support services, tutoring, accommodations as needed for disabilities, financial aid, and registration. Extending these services to distance enrolled students requires institutional resources and coordination of student support services across multiple departments. You will want to ensure that you understand how students in your distance education courses access the student services necessary to support their academic success.

Chapter Summary

In this chapter you have learned how to evaluate the use of a variety of learning technologies in the classroom, online, and distance learning environments. Here are key points for you to consider:

- Before making assignments in your courses that require students to use technology to achieve their learning outcomes, ensure that all students have access and the digital competencies to use the learning technologies assigned.
- Prior to using technology, determine that students have been oriented to the purpose of the use of the technology and what learning outcomes they are to attain.
- When developing evaluation plans for the use of learning technology, you will want to consider the following factors: accessibility, ADA compliance

and universal design principles, cost and educational value, ease of use, and student satisfaction.

■ Use formative and summative evaluation strategies to evaluate student satisfaction with the use of learning technologies.

■ Useful resources for evaluating the design, instruction, usability, and effectiveness of online courses include the Online Learning Consortium (OLC) and Quality Matters.

■ In addition to the usual course evaluation elements, you will want to evaluate distance-delivered courses (asynchronous, hybrid, and synchronous) for their design and ability to foster student achievement of expected learning outcomes.

References

Accreditation Council for Occupational Therapy Education. (2022). *ACOTE standards and interpretive guide.* https://acoteonline.org/accreditation-explained/standards/

Americans with Disabilities Act. (2007). *Website accessibility under Title II of the ADA, ADA best practice tool kit for state and local governments (chap. 5).* https://www.ada.gov/pcatoolkit/ch5_toolkit.pdf

Anderson, K. M., Davis, D., & McLaughlin, M. K. (2019). Implementing universal design instruction in Doctor of Nursing Practice education. *Nurse Educator, 44*(5), 245–249. https://doi.org/10.1097/NNE.0000000000000642

Buzzetto-Hollywood, N., Wang, H. C., & Elobaid, M. (2018). Addressing information literacy and the digital divide in higher education. *Interdisciplinary Journal of E-skills and Lifelong Learning, 14,* 77–92.

Frith, K. (2020a). Assessment of online education: Part 1. *Nursing Education Perspectives, 41*(5), 320–321.

Frith, K. (2020b). Assessment of online education: Part 2. *Nursing Education Perspectives, 41*(6), 386–387.

Levey, J. A. (2018). Universal design for instruction in nursing education: An integrative review. *Nursing Education Perspectives, 39*(3), 156–161. https://doi.org/10.1097/01.NEP.0000000000000249

Online Learning Consortium. (2022). *Five pillars of online learning.* www.onlinelearningconsortium.org/

Quality Matters. (2022). www.qualitymatters.org

PART 5

Participating in Program Evaluation Processes

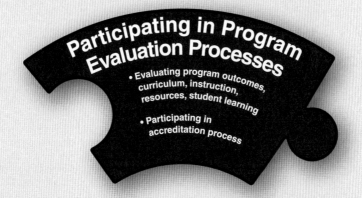

Participating in Program Evaluation Processes
- Evaluating program outcomes, curriculum, instruction, resources, student learning
- Participating in accreditation process

Health professions education programs are accountable to their stakeholders for achieving program outcomes and providing quality educational experiences to their students. Having a robust program evaluation plan that systematically measures how effectively a program is meeting these two goals is part of the continuous quality improvement process. Accreditation is a closely related program evaluation process that publicly attests to a program's quality. As faculty, you are a stakeholder in the process, and being a knowledgeable participant in program evaluation activities is one of your faculty responsibilities. Part 5 provides you with a foundation in program evaluation and accreditation processes. Chapter 20 introduces you to concepts related to program evaluation. Chapter 21 highlights the faculty role in program evaluation. Chapter 22 addresses the development of a systematic evaluation plan and describes the various program elements that are typically evaluated. Chapter 23 addresses accreditation and how to prepare yourself to participate in the accreditation process. In Chapter 24, common issues associated with program evaluation are discussed along with strategies for avoiding pitfalls associated with them. Chapter 25 discusses how to review the effectiveness of your program's evaluation plan.

At the back of the book you will find Appendix E, which contains a listing of documents to gather and review as part of your teaching responsibilities related to participating in curriculum development. Appendix F contains a listing of health professions accrediting agencies.

CHAPTER 20

Introduction to Program Evaluation and Accreditation

As a new health professions educator, most of your time and energy will understandably be devoted to gaining comfort with your role as a teacher and designing learning experiences for your courses that will help students demonstrate the expected learning outcomes. The courses you teach must fit seamlessly within the larger context of the program's curriculum ensuring that students progress in a timely fashion to achieve the end-of-the program outcomes and successfully graduate with the competencies required for safe practice. For the curriculum to produce quality graduates, all faculty must work together toward the common goal of implementing the curriculum as planned to meet program outcomes. At the same time you are responsible for teaching your assigned courses, you are also responsible for understanding how your courses and teaching practices mesh with your faculty colleagues' efforts to contribute to the greater good of meeting the program's mission.

Health professions education is complex, and the programs within which our students learn have many elements that must be constantly and systematically monitored for quality. Program evaluation is a key component to the success of any health professions program. In your role as an individual faculty member, you are a stakeholder in the program evaluation process and expected to be an informed, collaborative participant. A successful program evaluation process will help you in your teaching role by providing you and your colleagues with reliable and valid data that can be used to inform program decision making.

Program evaluation has both internal and external aspects to it. The institution and program faculty are responsible for designing internal evaluation processes that are implemented with the purpose of monitoring quality and improving outcomes of academic programs. Most institutions of higher education have entire departments dedicated to gathering and analyzing data related to institutional effectiveness. Many health professions programs also have access to personnel dedicated to collecting data to monitor program effectiveness. In addition to these internal evaluation processes are external evaluation processes that institutions and programs are subjected to as well. These external evaluation processes are carried out by regulatory agencies (such as licensing and certification boards) and accrediting agencies that accredit health professions programs and institutions of higher education.

The purpose of this handbook is to provide you with an overall understanding of the purposes of program evaluation and your role as a faculty in the program evaluation process. The accreditation process for health professions programs and how accreditation provides a valuable source of external program evaluation will also be discussed. The purpose of this chapter is to introduce you to the concepts of continuous quality improvement (CQI), systematic program evaluation (SPE), and accreditation with a focus on how these processes work together to ensure educational quality in health professions programs.

Purposes of Program Evaluation

Health professions education programs are accountable to society for the quality of the graduates they produce. The faculty and administration of those programs hold responsibility for ensuring that the program has the curriculum and resources it requires to consistently meet the learning needs of students. To maintain program quality it is essential to have an evaluation process in place that calls for the systematic collection and analysis of data for all elements of the program. Box 20.1 lists program elements that require regular and ongoing monitoring and evaluation. Faculty are expected to play an integral role in carrying out the evaluation process as designed, usually documented in the form of a systematic evaluation plan (SEP). It will be important for you to understand what your role in the evaluation plan is expected to be so that you can be prepared to participate as needed.

As noted in Box 20.2, program evaluation serves several purposes (Ellis, 2020). First and foremost, program evaluation is used to determine how effectively and

---

BOX 20.1 ■ Evaluated Program Elements

- Governance structure
- Mission, goals, values, vision
- Curriculum
- Policies and publications
- Resources (e.g., facilities, technology, fiscal, supplies, equipment)
- Faculty
- Student support services
- Record of student complaints
- Successful student achievement:
  - Completion and graduation rates
  - Employment rates
  - Licensure/certification pass rates

From Ellis, P. (2020). Systematic program evaluation. In D. Billings & J. Halstead (Eds.), *Teaching in nursing: A guide for faculty* (7th ed., pp. 514–559). Elsevier; Halstead, J. (2017). The accreditation process in nursing education. In M. Oermann (Ed.), *A systematic approach to assessment and evaluation of nursing programs* (pp. 79–91). National League for Nursing.

BOX 20.2 ■ Purposes of Program Evaluation

- Determine overall program effectiveness in achieving outcomes
- Establish to what extent program mission and goals are being met
- Assess how various program elements interface and impact program effectiveness
- Identify the extent to which the program is being implemented as planned
- Provide faculty with data to guide program decision making
- Determine adequacy of resources to maintain or improve program quality

---

From Ellis, P. (2020). Systematic program evaluation. In D. Billings & J. Halstead (Eds.), *Teaching in nursing: A guide for faculty* (7th ed., pp. 514–559). Elsevier.

---

to what extent the program is meeting its stated mission, goals, and expected program outcomes. Expected program outcomes encompass all outcomes and benchmark measures established by faculty for the program elements listed in Box 20.1.

A second purpose of evaluation is to determine if all elements of the program are being implemented as administration, faculty, and staff envisioned. Program elements can interact with each other to influence whether outcomes can be achieved as desired. For example, faculty may have set a goal to increase scholarship productivity among the faculty by 10%; however, lack of resources to support faculty scholarship efforts may prove to be a hindrance to meeting this expected goal. In another example, faculty may be concerned about trending lower student pass rates on licensure examinations. The root cause(s) of this student performance decline could lie in any number of program elements: faculty preparation, student quality, curriculum, or student support services. Only a comprehensive review and evaluation of multiple program elements will reveal possible areas that would benefit from an improvement plan and improve the pass rate scores.

A third purpose of evaluation is to provide faculty with the data reports they need to make informed, evidence-based decisions about changes to improve program performance. Additionally, evaluation data can help faculty decide how to deploy scarce program resources most effectively to improve program quality or in what areas they need to acquire additional funding.

As you can see, program evaluation is a pervasive activity that you will be engaged in to some extent throughout your career as an educator. Some faculty emerge as leaders on their campus in the use of evaluation data to improve education quality, building a program of research on outcome evaluation, while others are content to remain informed participants of the process and consumers of the data produced. There is a need for all faculty to have knowledge of the evaluation process, understand how to use data effectively to make program decisions, and improve program performance. Faculty can most effectively engage in program evaluation when they promote a culture of CQI within their program.

Continuous Quality Improvement in Health Professions Education

The program evaluation process is most successful in institutions and programs that intentionally cultivate among faculty and staff an organizational culture that promotes CQI. Historically, health professions programs have embraced CQI as a means of maintaining program quality and are often campus leaders in ways to effectively engage in CQI efforts and conduct program evaluation activities. The National League for Nursing (NLN), in its *Hallmarks of Excellence Nursing Model,* advocates for programs to develop a culture of CQI (Adams & Valiga, 2022). In this model, CQI is defined as "a comprehensive, sustained, and integrative approach to assessment and evaluation that aims toward continual improvement and renewal of an individual and/or a total system" (p. 182).

While the NLN *Hallmark* model was developed for implementation in nursing education programs, the concepts are universal for quality education and can be extended beyond nursing to other health professions disciplines. Besides developing a culture of CQI, the NLN advocates that for programs to achieve excellence, faculty should strive to incorporate these core elements to ensure quality program outcomes: innovative curricula, evidence-based strategies to promote learning, engaged students, well-prepared faculty, adequate resources to meet goals, commitment to the scholarship of teaching and learning, and effective leadership at institutional and professional levels (NLN, 2020). These core elements are commonly referenced and expanded upon in the accreditation standards of health professions education programs and are the foundation upon which SPE processes are developed. We will next discuss both of these processes—the process of program evaluation that is systematic in nature and the accreditation process—and how these processes influence program evaluation.

Continuous Quality Improvement and Systematic Program Evaluation

To effectively ensure ongoing program quality, the CQI process must be consistently applied to the evaluation of academic programs using a systematic, ongoing approach that yields valid and reliable assessment data. Sporadic or serendipitous attempts at measuring program effectiveness will not provide the data faculty need to make informed program decisions. To effectively conduct program evaluation activities, program faculty need to have a SPE process in place to determine if the program is consistently meeting expected program outcomes. Without such a plan, program stakeholders will remain uninformed about program outcomes, program quality will undoubtedly be compromised, and student learning will be negatively impacted.

Developing a process for SPE allows faculty to assess and evaluate all elements of the program with the intention of measuring and improving outcome achievement. Box 20.3 identifies the steps that faculty must take to begin the SPE process (Halstead, 2022). These steps are typically documented in what becomes the program's written SEP. The SPE process is described in further detail in Chapter 22.

BOX 20.3 ■ Process of Systematic Program Evaluation

- Consider needs of program's stakeholders (students, faculty, clinical partners, etc.)
- Develop well-defined program outcomes and goals
- Establish benchmarks as indicators of program success
- Develop means for collecting, analyzing, and using data to support program decision making

---

From Halstead, J. (2022). Culture of continuous quality improvement. In M. H. Adams & T. M. Valiga (Eds.), *Achieving distinction in nursing education* (pp. 49–59). National League for Nursing.

Continuous Quality Improvement and the Accreditation Process

Accreditation is another important CQI process closely associated with demonstrating program quality. Guided by a set of discipline-specific standards, program accreditation is a form of external peer review attesting to the program's compliance with the standards and the program's quality. Most health professions programs are accredited by their discipline's accrediting body. The accreditation process involves an evaluation of the program's compliance with accreditation standards that have been established by the discipline. Chapter 23 addresses the accreditation process in more depth and how you might expect to participate in the process.

The purposes of CQI, SPE, and accreditation are closely related with the ultimate goal of maintaining and improving program quality (Halstead, 2022). SPE is an internal CQI process that the program administration and faculty undertake. Accreditation is an external CQI process that involves the faculty's self-review of the program, as well as an external review by others who are expert in the discipline and higher education. Both processes help the program achieve the goals of demonstrating quality, highlighting program effectiveness with achieving outcomes, and identifying areas for improvement. The two processes of SPE and accreditation are somewhat interdependent as well. Without a strong plan for SPE, programs will find it difficult to successfully achieve and maintain program accreditation, as having a systematic approach to evaluating program outcome achievement is usually a key accreditation standard that programs are expected to meet.

Self-Assessment of Competencies Related to Program Evaluation

Now that you are familiar with the processes of CQI, SPE, and accreditation, let's consider the competencies that are needed to be an informed participant in program evaluation in your faculty role. Box 20.4 identifies educator competencies associated with program evaluation and accreditation. Table 20.1 provides you with an opportunity to do a self-assessment of your current readiness to participate in program evaluation and accreditation activities.

BOX 20.4 ■ Competencies Related to Program Evaluation and Accreditation

- Assess and evaluate achievement of expected program outcomes.
- Participate in continuous quality improvement efforts at the program level.
- Design and use tools to measure program effectiveness.
- Collect and interpret data related to program effectiveness.
- Participate in continuous quality improvement efforts at the course level.
- Design and use tools to measure course effectiveness.
- Collect and interpret data related to course effectiveness.
- Implement discipline-specific program assessment models designed to gather aggregate student data related to achievement of end-of-program curriculum outcomes.
- Possess familiarity with discipline-specific accreditation process and standards.
- Participate in the accreditation process, including site visit.
- Write accreditation self-study report.
- Develop and implement SEP to evaluate program elements.
- Establish benchmarks by which to measure program success at achieving outcomes.
- Participate in faculty discussions using data to make decisions about program changes.

TABLE 20.1 ■ Self-Assessment of Competencies Related to Program Evaluation and Accreditation

Consider to what extent you feel comfortable performing the following competencies and check the appropriate box. After you complete the checklist, develop a plan that will help you develop skill in the competencies in which you have less experience. Share your plan with your mentor for additional feedback.

Educator Competency	I Have No Experience	I Have Some Experience	I Have Much Experience
Assess and evaluate achievement of expected program outcomes			
Participate in continuous quality improvement efforts at the program level			
Design and use tools to measure program effectiveness			
Collect and interpret data related to program effectiveness			
Participate in continuous quality improvement efforts at the course level			
Design and use tools to measure course effectiveness			
Collect and interpret data related to course effectiveness			
Implement discipline-specific program assessment models designed to gather aggregate student data related to achievement of end-of-program curriculum outcomes			
Possess familiarity with discipline-specific accreditation process and standards			
Participate in the accreditation process, including site visit			
Write accreditation self-study report			
Develop and implement systematic evaluation plan to evaluate program elements			
Establish benchmarks by which to measure program success at achieving outcomes			
Participate in faculty discussions using data to make decisions about program changes			

Chapter Summary

In this chapter you were introduced to the purposes of program evaluation and the processes of CQI, SPE, and accreditation. Here are some key points about how these processes influence program quality:

- The program evaluation process is key to documenting and maintaining program quality.
- There is a common set of program elements that all health professions programs evaluate for quality (see Box 20.1).
- The institution and program faculty are responsible for designing internal evaluation processes that are implemented with the purpose of monitoring quality and improving outcomes of academic programs.
- External program evaluation processes are carried out by regulatory agencies (such as licensing and certification boards) and accrediting agencies that accredit health professions programs and institutions of higher education.
- Faculty can most effectively engage in program evaluation when they promote a culture of CQI within their program.
- Developing a process for SPE allows faculty to assess and evaluate all elements of the program with the intention of measuring and improving outcome achievement (see Box 20.3).
- The purposes of CQI, SPE, and accreditation are closely related.
- Without a strong plan for SPE, programs will find it difficult to successfully achieve and maintain program accreditation.

References

Adams, M. H., & Valiga, T. M. (Eds.). (2022). *Achieving distinction in nursing education*. National League for Nursing.

Ellis, P. (2020). Systematic program evaluation. In D. Billings & J. Halstead (Eds.), *Teaching in nursing: A guide for faculty* (7th ed., pp. 514–559). Elsevier.

Halstead, J. (2017). The accreditation process in nursing education. In M. Oermann (Ed.), *A systematic approach to assessment and evaluation of nursing programs* (pp. 79–91). National League for Nursing.

Halstead, J. (2022). Culture of continuous quality improvement. In M. H. Adams & T. M. Valiga (Eds.), *Achieving distinction in nursing education* (pp. 49–59). National League for Nursing.

National League for Nursing. (2020). *The hallmarks for excellence in nursing education model*. https://www.nln.org/education/teaching-resources/professional-development-programsteaching-resources/hallmarks-of-excellence-%C2%A9-dffbb05c-7836-6c70-9642-ff00005f0421#:~:text=Innovative%2C%20Evidence%2DBased%20Approaches%20to,Effective%20Institutional%20and%20Professional%20Leadership

CHAPTER 21

Getting Started With Program Evaluation

In Chapter 20 you learned the purposes of program evaluation and the concepts of continuous quality improvement and systematic program evaluation as applied in higher education. The importance of the regular and ongoing monitoring of program elements that affect the quality of program outcomes were also addressed. These same program elements are most commonly evaluated by all health professions accrediting agencies, thus you can expect to find those elements represented in any systematic evaluation plan (SEP) that is adopted for your health professions program.

If you completed the self-assessment of your competencies related to program evaluation, you have a good idea of your current readiness to participate in program evaluation and accreditation activities, and the areas in which you may wish to strengthen your knowledge. But how does all this information relate to your faculty role especially as a new educator? The purpose of this chapter is to help you apply this information to your faculty role as you gain an understanding of the program evaluation process and how your actions as a faculty member can help your program effectively evaluate its outcomes.

Understanding the Faculty Role in Program Evaluation

As a member of the faculty, you play a vital role in the success of how your program's evaluation plan is conducted. It can be common for faculty to hold the general belief that program evaluation is primarily the responsibility of administration, and if not administration then maybe the curriculum committee or some other such centralized entity. However, program evaluation is an essential shared responsibility of everyone associated with the program (Frye & Hemmer, 2012), including administrators, faculty, and staff. You can expect to be involved in the evaluation of the aspects of the program for which you have direct responsibility (e.g., your courses and individual faculty accomplishments) and to contribute to the evaluation of other program elements that impact how you implement your faculty responsibilities (e.g., instructional resources, curriculum, faculty support). Appendix E contains a listing of documents and policies to gather and review as part of your teaching responsibilities related to program evaluation.

Preparing to Participate in Program Evaluation

In addition to reviewing documents and policies related to the evaluation process used by your institution and program, there are several action steps you can take to inform yourself about the approach your institution and program take to evaluating academic programs. These steps include understanding the evaluation process used by your institution and program, and the accompanying policies; knowing the key players who lead the evaluation process; and being familiar with your program's SEP.

UNDERSTANDING THE PROGRAM EVALUATION PROCESS

In most institutions of higher education, the evaluation of academic programs takes place at two levels: the institution level and the program level within academic units. While the focus here is on program-level evaluation, it is important for you to understand how the evaluation process in your health professions program is coordinated with the institution's evaluation process, as you will likely be expected to participate in the evaluation data collection process at the institutional level.

Institutions collect and report aggregate data on their academic programs for multiple reasons. One of the most important reasons is to be compliant with the expectations of the institution's accrediting agency. Other major reasons include fulfilling reporting requirements related to receiving federal financial aid for students, applying for external grant funding, and sharing outcome data with community partners and potential donors. Additionally, institutions collect data to evaluate the effectiveness and success of specific institutional initiatives such as those related to distance education; civic engagement; and campus diversity, equity, and inclusiveness, to cite a few examples. Enrollment data, student demographics, and graduation rates are representative of the types of data that institutions collect and report to various constituents.

Institutions also play a role in evaluating curriculum. Universities and colleges regularly evaluate the outcomes of the general education core curriculum and conduct reviews of individual academic programs. Most have a centralized course evaluation process that is administered at the institutional level with course evaluation data being collected and the results being disseminated back to faculty. Institutions also collect data to evaluate the effectiveness of university services that support faculty teaching and student learning efforts, such as instructional support and student support services.

In your faculty role you may be asked by the institution to provide data for any of these reasons. Depending on the organizational structure, institutions often have departments responsible for institutional research and assessment that oversee the collection and analysis of institutional data. There are also likely to be institutional general education curriculum committees or academic review committees composed of faculty representatives from the various academic units. You will want to seek out information regarding the department and committee structures in place at your institution and develop an understanding of their responsibilities with the evaluation process.

Overseeing the institution's academic policies is usually the responsibility of the provost's or academic affairs office. Your institution will possibly have academic policies that direct the evaluation processes related to faculty teaching, courses, academic programs, and the general education curriculum. Familiarizing yourself with those policies will help you understand the data you will be required to collect for your faculty teaching and course evaluations, as well as data for other evaluation efforts led by the institution.

Within your program, evaluation processes may be managed by an administrative office or a faculty evaluation committee. While evaluation policies need to be congruent with policies at the institutional level, it is usually the responsibility of the program faculty to determine the policies and process that are used to evaluate faculty teaching, courses, and other program elements. The schedule for evaluation is determined by a written SEP that all faculty have input into developing. Chapter 22 explains the process of developing and implementing the SEP.

KNOWING THE KEY PLAYERS IN THE EVALUATION PROCESS

As you review the evaluation materials that you have gathered (from Appendix E), you will also want to take note of who has lead responsibility for the evaluation processes within your program. The processes may be managed by an administrative office, or it could be the responsibility of a faculty evaluation committee.

Your immediate supervisor can also be very helpful in providing information about what will be expected of you in the evaluation process, especially regarding the evaluation of your courses and teaching. You will want to be sure that you have access to the correct evaluation tools that are expected to be administered to students enrolled in your courses as there may be several surveys that are used to gather data. You will also need to understand the timeline used to administer the tools.

Frequently the course and teaching evaluation instruments are administered electronically by the institution and deployed directly to the students enrolled in your courses. You may also have additional program-level evaluation surveys to administer. For example, if you teach a clinical course, you can anticipate asking students to evaluate the clinical agency setting and preceptors or staff involved in your students' learning.

When reviewing the results of the evaluation process, mentors can be valuable in helping you to process and make sense of evaluation feedback that you receive from students and other sources. It is also helpful to know who represents your program or school on any institutional-level evaluation committees. Your representatives can be a source of information regarding what evaluation data the institution asks faculty to report on regular basis, as can the directors of centralized institutional departments that provide assessment and evaluation assistance. In your first year or so of teaching you will be primarily focused on the evaluation process as it applies to your immediate teaching assignments. As you grow in your role and expand your responsibilities in your program, you will come to appreciate that evaluation is a key element of any professional initiative that you are likely to undertake, whether it be related to your teaching, scholarship, service, or practice. Being alert to opportunities from evaluation experts to develop and expand your knowledge about assessment and evaluation strategies will be beneficial to your professional development as faculty.

BECOMING FAMILIAR WITH THE PROGRAM'S SYSTEMATIC EVALUATION PLAN

When you start your new teaching position, you should receive a copy of your program's SEP. If you do not receive it and cannot locate it, you should make a point of requesting a copy. While all aspects of the SEP are important, you will want to initially focus your SEP review on the evaluation components that are related to your teaching role, making note of the evaluation calendar and the methods used to evaluate your courses and teaching role. A full discussion of the SEP can be found in Chapter 22.

Chapter Summary

In this chapter you were introduced to steps you can take in your first year of teaching to prepare yourself for participating in the program evaluation process. Here are some key points to consider as you prepare yourself to be a participant in your program's evaluation processes:

- Program evaluation is a shared responsibility of all who are associated with the program (faculty, staff, and administrators).
- Program evaluation activities are conducted at the institutional level and program level; you may be asked to participate in evaluation efforts at both levels.
- To prepare yourself to be a knowledgeable participant of your program's evaluation plan, you will want to gather and review documents and policies that will assist you in understanding the process (see Appendix E).
- Be proactive in seeking out information related to the evaluation of your courses and your teaching performance; ensure that you have the correct evaluation tools and timelines.
- Request a copy of your program's SEP so that you can reference the areas for which you are responsible.
- Seek opportunities within your institution and professional organizations to expand your knowledge about program assessment and evaluation strategies.

Reference

Frye, A. W., & Hemmer, P. A. (2012). Program evaluation models and related theories: AMEE guide 67. *Medical Teacher*, 34(5), e288–e299. https://doi.org/10.3109/0142159X.2012.668637

CHAPTER 22

Key Components of Program Evaluation

For program evaluation efforts to be effective, it is important for faculty to adopt a systematic approach to evaluating program outcomes. A systematic approach to program evaluation ensures that all program elements are evaluated using ongoing strategies, thus allowing for continuous data collection. When data are systematically and consistently gathered and analyzed, it is easier for faculty to detect trends in program outcomes. Having a systematic program evaluation process in place also greatly enhances the program's ability to achieve accreditation and maintain compliance with accreditation standards, and to publicly demonstrate to stakeholders that a quality education is being provided to students. When faculty have a systematic evaluation plan (SEP) to follow, they will be able to collect and analyze data that will assist them in making timely decisions about what changes the program should make to better serve the learning needs of students and support faculty in their roles.

This chapter discusses how the process of systematic program evaluation can be used to measure a program's outcomes achievement and the faculty role in evaluating program outcomes. As you read this chapter you will learn how various program elements impact your ability to carry out your faculty responsibilities, and how being able to systematically evaluate those elements is key to promoting a culture of continuous quality improvement within the organization.

Evaluating Program Outcomes

A health professions education program must be responsive to factors in its internal and external environment to stay up to date and relevant to how health care is being practiced. Emerging trends in society, health care, higher education, the professional discipline, and student demographics are a few examples of factors that need to be continually monitored so that the program's curriculum can be updated to provide students with pertinent learning experiences. The program's continuing relevance is directly related to how willing the program's faculty are to monitor trends in program outcome data and measure achievement of program outcomes on an ongoing basis. Frye and Hemmer (2012) make a point of stating that educational programs are complex, with many interactions occurring between the program and its environment, and that educational programs are inevitably all about change. This is especially true of health professions programs, which are attempting to prepare graduates for practice in a health care system that frequently presents as chaotic and ever changing.

Frye and Hemmer (2012) further assert that program changes can be either intentional or unintentional, and that program evaluation should be used to detect if changes have occurred. The relationship between program elements tends to be complex and nonlinear and can be difficult to detect lacking a program evaluation plan. The plan should be robust and flexible enough to systematically capture the data needed to guide faculty in their decision making about program effectiveness. For this reason, systems theory and complexity theory can be useful to understanding the program evaluation process (Frye & Hemmer, 2012).

Given the complexity of education programs, especially those that are focused on health professions education, you can understand why program evaluation cannot be overlooked, haphazard, or episodic. To do so is to place the program in jeopardy of providing substandard education and its students in jeopardy of not being successful in achieving the desired learning outcomes. Systematic program evaluation is the most effective and efficient means of measuring program outcomes on an ongoing basis.

For the purposes of this discussion, systematic program evaluation is the systematic assessment of all elements of an educational program using appropriate evaluation strategies (Fig. 22.1). This assessment leads to the analysis of the data obtained with the goal of measuring the program's effectiveness in achieving program outcomes and making changes as needed to improve performance.

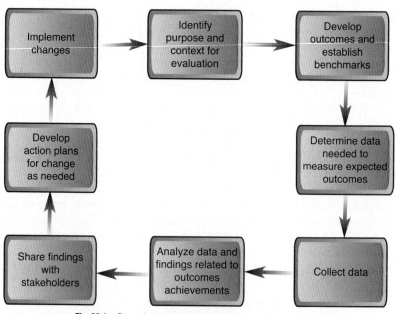

Fig. 22.1   Steps in systematic program evaluation process.

Program outcomes are the results achieved by the program, in response to established goals that are meant to indicate program quality. Program outcomes can be established for all program elements; for example, outcomes may be established for student learning and achievement, the curriculum, faculty accomplishments; student support services; instructional resources; program governance; and any other element the faculty determine to be important to evaluate. You will find that most accreditation agencies have standards that address each of these elements. Accreditation standards can be a helpful guide to developing your program's own evaluation plan. Chapter 23 further describes the accreditation process.

IMPORTANCE OF STAKEHOLDER FEEDBACK

While not immediately evident, systematic program evaluation is an important contributor to the program's development and nurturing of strong relationships with its stakeholders, including accreditors. A well-developed systematic program evaluation plan ensures that the perspective of multiple stakeholders is sought when determining if the program is achieving its desired outcomes. The perspectives of students, faculty, clinical partners, alumni, community members, and others should be reflected in the plan, and the plan should only be considered complete if feedback mechanisms are embedded, thus ensuring that stakeholders receive the results of data findings and faculty decisions on relevant program issues. Programs that have strong SEPs and consistently demonstrate attentiveness to what the data are telling them about program performance will be much more inclined to develop strong partnerships within the community and with their clinical partners, as well as attract the resources needed to fund future program growth.

Developing the Systematic Evaluation Plan

As your program develops its approach to systematic program evaluation, careful thought must be given to how this plan is operationalized. This is accomplished through the development of a written SEP. This section of this chapter describes what typically constitutes a SEP and how faculty can work together to craft a meaningful and useful document to guide their evaluation efforts.

For a program's systematic plan of evaluation to be successfully implemented, it must be committed to writing, and every faculty and staff member should have access to the document. Having a program evaluation plan in place carries such significance for the program's success that most health professions accrediting agencies have an evaluation criterion addressing this requirement (Table 22.1). Review the accreditation criteria for your own health professions discipline paying close attention to any standards related to program assessment and evaluation, and the accompanying criteria that detail the accrediting agency's expectations in this area.

It is very common for programs to choose to organize the SEP so that it is aligned with the accrediting agency's accreditation standards (Ellis, 2020); you

TABLE 22.1 ■ **Examples of Health Professions Accrediting Agencies Criteria Related to Systematic Program Evaluation**

Accrediting Agency	Website	Criterion
Commission on Accreditation in Physical Therapy Education (CAPTE)	https://www.capteonline.org/globalassets/capte-docs/capte-pt-standards-required-elements.pdf	Standard 2: The program is engaged in effective, ongoing, formal, comprehensive processes for self-assessment and planning for the purpose of program improvement.
Commission on Collegiate Nursing Education (CCNE)	https://www.aacnnursing.org/Portals/42/CCNE/PDF/Standards-Final-2018.pdf	IV-A: A systematic process is used to determine program effectiveness.
Joint Review Committee on Education in Radiologic Technology (JRCERT)	https://www.jrcert.org/wp-content/uploads/Documents/Resources/Standards-PDFs/2021-Radiation-Therapy-Standards.pdf	Standard Six: Programmatic Effectiveness and Assessment: Using Data for Sustained Improvement— The extent of a program's effectiveness is linked to the ability to meet its mission, goals, and student learning outcomes. A systematic, ongoing assessment process provides credible evidence that enables analysis and critical discussions to foster ongoing program improvement.
Commission on Dental Accreditation (CODA)	https://coda.ada.org/standards	Standard I Institutional Effectiveness: 1-1 The program must demonstrate its effectiveness using a formal and ongoing planning and assessment process that is systematically documented by (a) developing a plan addressing teaching, patient care, research and service which are consistent with the goals of the sponsoring institution and appropriate to dental hygiene education; (b) implementing the plan; (c) assessing the outcomes, including measures of student achievement; (d) using the results for program improvement.

may find that your program has chosen this approach as well. Your program may have also chosen to reference standards from regulatory bodies and professional organizations. Familiarize yourself with the criteria that your program has decided to reference in the SEP.

Creating a SEP document that is essentially a how-to guide to your program's evaluation plan is the responsibility of the faculty in collaboration with administration. Frequently a committee of faculty or possibly an administrator will provide the lead in developing the plan. You can think of the written plan as a blueprint or roadmap to the timelines, strategies, and dissemination plan the faculty are committing to when implementing the plan. Box 22.1 provides a list of categories that are commonly found in most SEPs. Fig. 22.2 provides an example of an SEP template.

BOX 22.1 ■ Written Systematic Evaluation Plan Categories

Outcomes: What does the program want to accomplish in each area of accomplishment?
Benchmarks: How will the program know if it has met its expected accomplishment?
Timeline for data gathering: At what time intervals will data be collected?
Data collection: What data will be gathered to measure the outcome achievement and what
   strategies will be used by which to gather it?
Responsibility for data collection: Who or what entity will be responsible for data collection
   and analysis?
Dissemination of findings: How will results of data analysis be shared with stakeholders?
Decision making and documentation: How will decisions be made based on the data? How
   and where will those decisions be documented?

Outcomes	Benchmark to be achieved	Timeline	Data to be collected	Evaluation strategies	Who is responsible	Stakeholder dissemination	Documetation of actions (decisions)

Fig. 22.2   Systematic evaluation plan template.

SETTING BENCHMARKS FOR THE SYSTEMATIC EVALUATION PLAN

A benchmark is a set standard by which faculty measure program performance. Benson (1994) defined the activity of benchmarking as "a continuous process by which an organization can measure and compare its own processes with those of organizations that are leaders in a particular area" (p. 35). A SEP that does not contain benchmarks is incomplete. Without benchmarks the faculty are unable to determine if the program is achieving its expected outcomes at an acceptable level.

One important aspect of developing the SEP is determining the benchmarks for each identified program outcome. What is the expected benchmark that will measure satisfactory achievement of the outcome? For example, if your health professions program leads to licensure or certification for the graduates to practice, what is the acceptable licensure or certification pass rate for your graduates when they take the required examination?

Factors to Consider When Selecting Benchmarks

Selecting benchmarks by which to measure performance is an important decision, and faculty need to consider what is a reasonable benchmark for each selected program outcome. Box 22.2 provides examples of program outcomes that are commonly benchmarked by programs. Your program may choose to include additional program outcomes that are specific to your individual program's mission and goals.

BOX 22.2 ■ Examples of Program Outcomes Commonly Benchmarked

- Licensure and certification pass rates
- Completion and graduation rates
- Employment rates
- Retention rates
- Aggregate student learning outcomes achievement
- Program satisfaction as measured by students, alumni, employers
- Faculty teaching evaluations
- Faculty accomplishments in scholarship/research
- Course evaluations
- Preceptor evaluations

There are several factors for faculty to consider when choosing benchmarks for the program. In higher education, institutions and programs often choose peer institutions and programs that are similar in mission and size and use them to benchmark performance. Ask your program administrator for the names of peer institutions and health education programs that have been chosen by your institution and program. Additionally, your accrediting agency or regulatory body may have set benchmarks in selected program outcomes, such as licensure/certification rates, employment rates, and completion rates. You will want to verify if that is the case for your program. In public universities or colleges, state legislatures may set expected benchmarks for institutions as well.

Institutions themselves may set internal benchmarks for performance in selected performance indicators. If that is the case, the program will need to remain aligned with those established benchmarks. However, when benchmarks have not been preset by another entity, the faculty are responsible for selecting reasonable benchmarks for the program outcomes they are evaluating. Box 22.3 provides a list of questions that faculty can use to determine how to set benchmarks for the program. These questions can be applied to any aspect of the program's expected outcomes, even your own courses and teaching performance. Once a benchmark is set, progress toward achieving the benchmark can be evaluated on a regular schedule with adjustments made as appropriate as indicated by the data. Box 22.4 provides some examples of program outcome benchmarks.

BOX 22.3 ■ Factors to Consider When Selecting Program Benchmarks

Consider these program factors when determining how to select program outcomes to benchmark and measure:

- Does your program have a strategic plan with set goals that would benefit from benchmarking?
- What program outcomes are you expected to benchmark by accrediting agencies, regulatory bodies, institution, or other external stakeholders?
- What are your program's priorities, concerns, challenges? What is your program's performance now in relation to these areas and to what extent do you want your program's performance to improve?
- What are your program's areas for growth?

BOX 22.4 ■ Examples of Program Outcome Benchmarks

- 85% of the faculty will achieve an annual teaching rating of 3.5 or higher for each course taught.
- 75% of all full-time faculty will annually demonstrate service on a program or institution committee.
- 90% of the graduates will achieve a first-time passing rate on the licensure examination.
- 85% of the students will complete the program within 150% of expected degree completion time.
- 95% of graduates will be employed within their field of preparation within 12 months of graduation.
- 75% of alumni will rate their satisfaction with the program as either very high or high within 12 months postgraduation.

Evaluating the Program Elements in a Comprehensive Systematic Evaluation Plan

Developing a comprehensive SEP requires that faculty carefully consider each program element, establishing outcomes and benchmarks and completing the SEP template for each outcome being measured (see Box 22.1 and Fig. 22.2). Box 20.1 in Chapter 20 identified the typical program elements evaluated through a systematic plan. This list is not exhaustive, and the faculty can identify any additional elements they wish to measure. The SEP should also be reviewed annually and adjusted as needed as new priorities emerge for the program to address. This section briefly addresses the various program elements, the types of outcomes the faculty may wish to measure for each element, and the significance these various program elements have for your faculty role. You will want to review your own discipline's specific accreditation standards for additional information on program evaluation expectations.

REQUIRED PROGRAM OUTCOMES

While faculty have considerable freedom in determining the outcomes that the program measures and evaluates, there are selected outcomes that the program will be required to evaluate by their accrediting agency. These program outcomes include student completion rates, licensure and certification rates (if required for your graduates to practice), and employment rates of your graduates in the field for which they have been educated. If your health professions accrediting agency is recognized by the US Department of Education (USDE), they are required by the federal government rules and regulations for accrediting bodies to evaluate these outcomes for all programs that they accredit.

The USDE expectation that accrediting agencies evaluate program outcomes related to completion rates, licensure/certification, and employment rates is related to program quality, protection of the public from ineffective programs, and student financial loans and indebtedness. Many students take out a considerable amount of loans to finance their education. It is very important that the programs they choose to attend are quality programs capable of producing well-prepared graduates. When students do not complete programs in a timely manner, fail their licensing or certification examinations, or cannot find employment in the field they were educated for, they are still responsible for repaying any student loans they may have received. If they cannot graduate or become licensed and employed, their ability to repay the student loans is jeopardized, creating further financial stressors for the students. Poor program outcomes in any of these three areas (completion rates, licensure/certification rates, and employment rates) serve as potential red flags to accreditors, demanding a closer examination of the program's curriculum, faculty qualifications, resources, and academic policies.

You can always anticipate that your program will carefully monitor these areas, collecting and analyzing data to ensure program performance remains strong and meets established benchmarks. It is essential that the program can reliably collect and annually report this data to the accrediting agency and any other external stakeholders, such as licensing boards. Any emerging trends that indicate performance is trending downward or not meeting benchmarks will require faculty to consider factors contributing to the poor outcomes and implement an action plan for improvement. Such action plans may require faculty to implement changes in the curriculum, ultimately impacting your courses and teaching strategies to achieve better outcomes for students.

Programs also commonly measure program satisfaction relying on feedback from current students, alumni, and employers. Program satisfaction data may be measured qualitatively in the form of focus group discussions or open-ended questions or quantitatively using surveys. Some programs may elect to use surveys that are electronically administered by a third-party vendor who works with the program to individualize the survey to the program's stated curriculum end-of-program outcomes and any other variables they choose to measure. Essentially the survey questions are related to how well the program is supporting the students' learning needs, how well the alumni think they were prepared for their role, and how well employers think the graduates are performing in their position within 1 year postgraduation. Collecting and analyzing data from multiple perspectives allows faculty to adjust as needed to improve satisfaction levels. This data will also be very helpful to you in your teaching role.

MISSION AND GOVERNANCE OUTCOMES

The program's ability to meet its mission and the governance structure that is used to provide faculty, students, and other stakeholders with opportunity to have input into program decision making are often addressed in the program's SEP. The program's mission is expected to be aligned with the institution's mission, providing the program with purpose and direction. Faculty use the program's mission statement to guide their decisions when identifying program goals, designing a strategic plan, and pursuing growth opportunities. The program may also have a philosophy statement that further expresses faculty beliefs and values about their discipline and the teaching-learning process. The program's mission statement is typically evaluated for its fit with the parent institution's stated mission (Ellis, 2020), how well it is communicated internally and externally to stakeholders, and its usefulness in guiding faculty's decision making.

BOX 22.5 ■ Examples of Areas to Evaluate Related to Program Governance

Governance Structure
- Bylaws
- Committee structure
- Opportunities for faculty and student participation in program and institution governance
- Opportunities for stakeholders to provide input and feedback to program

Published Documents
- Academic policies
- Faculty and student handbooks
- Accessibility of academic policies
- Bulletins, catalogs, website
- Currency and accuracy of all published documents

Program governance is related to the processes in place that allow for stakeholder input into the program and institution's operations. That faculty and students have the opportunity to participate in program governance is a valued expectation of those stakeholder groups. The governance of the program is also made visible through the quality and accuracy of its published policies and other program documents. Box 22.5 lists the program elements related to governance that the faculty may choose to regularly review to determine if outcomes are being met.

PROGRAM RESOURCE OUTCOMES

The adequacy of resources to support the program in achieving its mission and goals is another program element deserving careful review by faculty. How well you fulfill the expectations of your faculty role and meet the learning needs of your students can be directly related to the quantity and quality of resources made available to the program. Therefore you can expect the SEP to address outcomes that are related to the adequacy of resources needed to meet the needs faculty, staff, and students. Box 22.6 outlines the resource categories that are typically included in a program's SEP with relevant outcomes being established to address the adequacy of resources, the effectiveness of the resources provided, and stakeholder (faculty, staff, and students) satisfaction with the resources provided.

FACULTY OUTCOMES

Program outcomes related to faculty most commonly focus on faculty qualifications, composition, and accomplishments in areas deemed meaningful by the program and institution. The outcomes and evaluation of faculty role expectations will vary depending on the mission of your institution and the criteria that has been set forth according to faculty rank, including promotion and tenure as applicable. Depending on your institution and program's mission, you can expect the SEP to include faculty outcomes related to teaching, research/scholarship, practice, and service expectations. The faculty outcomes

---

BOX 22.6 ■ Examples of Areas to Evaluate Related to Program Resources

Physical Facilities

- Classrooms
- Learning resource centers/simulation facilities
- Study space for students
- Office space for faculty
- Conference rooms
- Libraries

Fiscal

- Faculty input into the budget process
- Annual budget allocation

Technology

- Computer hardware, network stability
- Support for distance education delivery
- Faculty support for teaching, scholarship
- Student support
- Electronic databases

Instructional

- Equipment for learning resource centers/simulation facilities
- Computer software to support learning
- Learning management systems
- Clinical facilities
- Remediation support

Personnel (Relevant to Program Mission)

- Faculty numbers
- Administrative support
- Instructional support
- Technology support
- Distance learning support
- Research support

BOX 22.7 ■ Examples of Areas to Evaluate Related to Faculty

- Faculty may be expected to hold specific academic qualifications, such as a terminal degree or specialty certification, or be working toward achievement of such a credential
- Faculty/student ratios in classroom and clinical settings
- Professional experiences and contributions to discipline
- Faculty composition representing diversity
- Success at recruitment and retention of faculty
- Teaching, scholarship/research, service, practice accomplishments relevant to program mission
- Adequate faculty development support
- Faculty performance evaluation process

---

described in your program's SEP have particular significance for you as you can make note of the benchmarks associated with the expected faculty outcomes and develop a plan for meeting those benchmark goals for your own professional development. Box 22.7 identifies areas in which faculty outcome statements may be written.

STUDENT OUTCOMES

When we refer to student outcomes we most often think of students' achievement of learning outcomes. These are of paramount importance when measuring program effectiveness, and faculty expend considerable thought on how best to support student learning through their teaching. However, besides faculty teaching, there are other factors that influence and support the students' achievement of learning outcomes, and this discussion focuses on those factors. Achievement of student learning outcomes is further addressed in the section on evaluating curriculum outcomes.

As a faculty member, it is important that you have a good understanding of the demographic profile of the students represented in your classroom and their unique learning needs. You should also be aware of the support services available to students so that you can most appropriately refer students to them as the need arises. Student support services need to be accessible to students and successful in providing their services to students.

The clarity of student policies and the way they are implemented also serve to foster a learning environment conducive to student success. Your program may create special support initiatives for your students, such as peer mentoring and tutoring programs, that faculty will want to evaluate to determine if the initiatives are producing the outcomes envisioned when they were designed. You may have the need for student support services specific to courses you teach that you will want to evaluate for effectiveness (e.g., math tutoring to assist with calculation of drug dosages).

Student satisfaction with support services and the learning environment are other key factors that deserve regular evaluation. Box 22.8 identifies areas in which student outcome statements may be written and benchmarks set for evaluation.

BOX 22.8 ▪ Examples of Areas to Evaluate Related to Students

- Support services: academic advising, tutoring, financial aid, counseling, accommodations (Americans with Disabilities Act), English as an additional language
- Student admission criteria
- Student demographics, diversity, and inclusion
- Student policies are accessible, current, and fairly administered (i.e., admission, progression, graduation, grievance and appeal policies)
- Student recruitment and retention
- Student satisfaction with support services
- Record of formal complaints, resolution, and emerging themes

---

CURRICULUM OUTCOMES

It can probably be stated that the evaluation of the curriculum demands the most time and attention of faculty. When program outcomes in the areas of student achievement of learning outcomes, licensure/certification pass rates, completion rates, and employment rates are not meeting established bench-marks, the first program element to be considered as a contributing factor to this lack of success is usually the curriculum. You can expect the SEP to have a section devoted to the evaluation of the curriculum. Your initial exposure to curriculum evaluation will be at the course level, as you will be responsible for evaluating your courses and your students' achievement of the learning out-comes expected of your course.

Evaluating the curriculum is a complex task, one that is never ending for fac-ulty. The curriculum requires evaluation at the course level as well as the broader program outcome level. In addition to the curriculum evaluation that the faculty conduct internally at the program level, if teaching undergraduate education your institution may also have evaluation expectations of the general education curriculum required of all students in which faculty and students will be ex-pected to participate. A review of the effectiveness of any prerequisite courses taken prior to admission to the professional program may also be conducted.

A robust SEP will have evaluation criteria that are discrete enough to evalu-ate all components of the curriculum on a clearly defined timeline and with data collection strategies that allow for aggregation of trending data. Familiar-ize yourself with the evaluation expectations of faculty at the course level, as you will be expected to carry out those responsibilities beginning with your first semester of teaching.

While curriculum evaluation is a complex activity requiring the input and participation of all faculty, the process can be broken down into three concep-tual areas, making it more manageable to set measurable outcomes and bench-marks. These three areas are (1) curriculum design and elements, (2) teaching and learning strategies, and (3) evaluation strategies. Box 22.9 illustrates the various curricular elements that require regular evaluation.

Using Data to Support Program Decisions

A comprehensive SEP is only helpful if the evaluation data collected are ana-lyzed and ultimately used to support faculty decision making about program changes. Chapter 24 details the impact of the ineffective use of data and steps that can be taken to ensure that data are collected, analyzed, and used to benefit the program.

The evaluation process outlined by the SEP is not complete until the feed-back loop is closed on the process. The evaluation feedback loop consists of compiling the analyzed data, disseminating it to the relevant stakeholders who are impacted by the findings for further review and discussion, and using the data to make informed decisions about program outcomes. The final step in the process includes documenting the findings, discussion, and decisions typically in committee meeting minutes. Stakeholders in the process should be informed of final decisions that are made through the appropriate program mechanisms. The SEP identifies who is responsible for overseeing data collection and its analysis, as well as to whom the findings are to be disseminated and where the discussions and actions taken are to be documented.

> **BOX 22.9 ■ Examples of Areas to Evaluate Related to Curriculum**
>
> **Curriculum Elements**
>
> - Achievement of end-of-program curriculum outcomes
> - Congruence of mission to program outcomes
> - Integration of major concepts, professional standards
> - Design and sequencing of curriculum
> - Review of competencies with links to program outcomes
> - Review of course outcomes with links to competencies and program outcomes
> - Achievement of student learning outcomes in the aggregate
> - Achievement of general education goals
> - Effectiveness of required science courses
>
> **Teaching-Learning Strategies**
>
> - Effectiveness of teaching-learning strategies in classroom and clinical settings
> - Student evaluation of teaching-learning strategies
> - Peer evaluation of teaching-learning strategies
> - Use of a variety of teaching-learning strategies
> - Integration of technology into learning environments, including distance learning
> - Effectiveness of learning materials
>
> **Effectiveness of Evaluation Strategies**
>
> - Evidence of regular assessment of student learning with feedback
> - Review of evaluation strategies used in the classroom setting to measure achievement of student learning outcomes
> - Review of evaluation of strategies used in the clinical setting to measure achievement of student learning outcomes

Your responsibility as a faculty is to review findings that are made available and participate in related decision making as guided by the findings. There will be times that data will be made available to you that are directly related to your own teaching practices (e.g., data from your course and teaching evaluations). You will most likely receive this data annually or even each semester. As you review evaluation data that are related to your teaching practices, you may find it helpful to discuss the data with your mentor or more experienced peers to help you process the findings and decide how to best utilize the data as part of a continuous quality improvement plan. You may use the findings to set goals for further developing your teaching practices. Additionally, you will want to consider how you will share relevant data findings from student evaluations with your students. It is always beneficial to let students know that you have thoughtfully considered feedback and share any changes you have made in your courses because of their feedback. This, too, is an example of closing the feedback loop for all stakeholders and an example of an effective evaluation plan.

Chapter Summary

In this chapter you were introduced to the process of systematic program evaluation and how to develop and implement an effective SEP. Here are some key points to consider about your role in participating in the program evaluation process:

- The process of systematic program evaluation can be used by the program to demonstrate to public stakeholders its commitment to quality education.
- Having a systematic program evaluation process in place enhances the program's ability to achieve accreditation and maintain compliance with accreditation standards.
- Programs that consistently demonstrate their attentiveness to the data collected from their stakeholders through the systematic evaluation process are much more inclined to develop strong partnerships within their community and with their clinical partners, as well as attract resources to fund future program growth.
- It is a common requirement of health professions programs' accrediting agencies to have standards requiring programs to provide evidence of having a systematic and ongoing process to evaluate program outcomes.
- Developing the written SEP is a faculty responsibility in collaboration with program administration.
- The SEP contains the following elements: expected outcomes and related benchmarks, timeline for data gathering, data to be collected, collection strategies, responsibility for data collection and analysis, dissemination plan for findings, and documentation of decision making.
- Program elements that are typically included for evaluation purposes in the SEP are mission and governance, resources, faculty, students, curriculum, and outcomes related to completion rates, licensure and certification rates, and employment rates.
- Closing the feedback loop in the evaluation process is a critical final step in the program evaluation process, where the analyzed data are shared with appropriate stakeholders and used to inform faculty decision making about program changes.

References

Benson, H. R. (1994). An introduction to benchmarking in healthcare. *Radiology Management, 16*(4), 35–39. https://pubmed.ncbi.nlm.nih.gov/10139084/

Ellis, P. (2020). Systematic program evaluation. In D. Billings & J. Halstead (Eds.), *Teaching in nursing: A guide for faculty* (6th ed., pp. 514–557). Elsevier.

Frye, A. W., & Hemmer, P. A. (2012). Program evaluation models and related theories: AMEE guide 67. *Medical Teacher, 34*(5), e288–e299. https://doi.org/10.3109/0142159X.2012.668637

CHAPTER 23

The Accreditation Process

As a health care professional you are probably very familiar with the accreditation and certification of health care agencies through organizations such as The Joint Commission. Achieving such institutional designations is an external mark of quality and serves to notify the public that the institution has met professional standards indicating a high degree of quality and safety in the delivery of health care. Institutions of higher education also pursue the similar process of accreditation to publicly attest to the quality of education occurring within the institution and its academic programs.

Accreditation standards have significant influence over the development of a program's curriculum and the processes and procedures faculty use to implement the program. This is especially true in professions that require licensure or certification for employment upon graduation, such as the health professions. As a new educator you will want to familiarize yourself with the accreditation process and the accreditation standards of your discipline so that you understand what your program is expected to do to maintain accreditation and how the accreditation process affects your practice as an educator. This chapter is designed to introduce you to the accreditation process, the faculty role in the process, and how to prepare to participate in an actual accreditation visit. By increasing your fundamental understanding of the accreditation process you will be able to prepare for and participate in the process knowledgeably and confidently.

Overview of the Accreditation Process

Accreditation has been defined as a "standards-based, evidence-based, judgement-based, peer-based process" (Eaton, 2012a, p. 14). Accreditation is not a new process; it has been in existence within US educational institutions for over 100 years (Eaton, 2012b). The primary purpose of accreditation is to protect the public, serving to ensure prospective and current students that the institution and program offer quality education to help them meet their education and career goals (Halstead, 2017a). In the health professions, many employers require students to graduate from accredited programs as one eligibility criterion to be hired.

In the United States there are two types of accreditation: (1) institutional accreditation, in which the accrediting body evaluates the entire college/university for compliance to accreditation standards; and (2) programmatic accreditation, which is specific to programs and academic disciplines. While you may be

---

BOX 23.1 ■ Roles and Benefits of Accreditation

- Provides the public, students, and other stakeholders with evidence of quality assurance
- Bestows eligibility on institutions and programs to seek federal and state funding, such as student financial aid, grants, etc.
- Facilitates the transfer of academic credit between accredited institutions
- Serves as a public mark of quality to the community such as prospective donors, employers, etc.

Adapted from Eaton, J. S. (2012b). *An overview of US accreditation.* Council for Higher Education Accreditation.

---

involved in both types of accreditation as faculty in an institution of higher education, you will work most closely with your program accreditors. This chapter focuses on the process of programmatic accreditation. See Appendix F for a partial listing of health professions program accrediting agencies and their websites. Visit the website of your discipline's accreditor to review current accreditation standards and policies.

US accreditation has four primary roles (Box 23.1) in the regulation of institutions of higher education and academic programs that ultimately benefit students. Students benefit from attending accredited institutions and programs as it increases their ability to access federal student financial aid, transfer academic credits they have earned from one accredited college or university to another, and find employment opportunities after graduation. Attending an accredited program also enhances students' future educational mobility options if they choose to advance their degree later. While seeking accreditation has historically been a voluntary activity for institutions and programs, in many health professions disciplines there is increasing momentum toward requiring program accreditation so that students can fully benefit from attending accredited programs. You can see from this discussion how important accreditation is to your program's reputation and why there is so much emphasis on achieving and maintaining accreditation. Institutions and programs seek out accreditation to benefit their students and demonstrate their commitment to providing quality education.

The accreditation process requires considerable preparation time and effort on the part of faculty and administrators. The process requires the program to conduct a self-assessment, identifying strengths and areas for improvement, and to undergo a peer review process by a team of evaluators (Hanna et al., 2016). As discussed in Chapter 22, a systematic process of data collection and analysis needs to be in place to ensure program evaluation is ongoing. It is important that faculty be engaged in all aspects of the accreditation process to ensure program quality.

THE US DEPARTMENT OF EDUCATION AND ACCREDITATION

The US Department of Education (USDE) has a role in the accreditation process that affects postsecondary education in both institutions and programs. The

USDE's interest in accreditation stems from the federal government's use of the accreditation process to determine the quality of education delivered in post-secondary education institutions that seek federal funding. If institutions or programs want to be eligible to receive Title IV student financial aid funds or federal grant money, they are required to be accredited by an agency that has been recognized by the USDE.

The USDE reviews and grants recognition to institution and program accrediting agencies that meet a published set of USDE criteria, thus ensuring quality and relatively standardized policies and practices among all federally recognized accrediting agencies. While the federal government is not directly involved in the accreditation of institutions and programs, the USDE can use its role in recognizing accrediting agencies to drive changes in US postsecondary education by stipulating changes in the criteria the USDE uses to recognize accrediting agencies.

GOVERNANCE STRUCTURE OF ACCREDITATION AGENCIES

The USDE regulations for accrediting agencies include criteria that address the governance of all accrediting agencies and the policies to be used for making accreditation decisions. All accrediting agencies have elected or appointed boards that make accreditation decisions. Such boards are composed of individuals who are discipline-specific academic educators and practice experts. Additionally, most boards have members who represent the public.

The accrediting agency's board is responsible for developing professional accreditation standards that are discipline specific and indicative of quality education within the discipline. The board is also responsible for conducting program reviews and making accreditation decisions, based on data collected by teams of evaluators who are assigned to conduct a site visit for a specific program. The team consists of peer evaluators who typically have experience in higher education and relevant teaching experience. During the site visit the team reviews data, program reports, and records; conducts interviews; and documents findings in a written report that is shared with the program and accrediting agency's board. Programs are scheduled to undergo continuing accreditation reviews at regular intervals on a timeline that is established by the accreditation agency.

ACCREDITING AGENCIES AND STANDARDS IN THE HEALTH PROFESSIONS

All accrediting agencies that are recognized by the USDE, including those that accredit health professions programs, must address certain program elements in their accreditation standards. Those elements include the following: curriculum, faculty, resources, budget and administrative capacity, student support services, record of student complaints, and policies related to advertising and publications (USDE, 2019). The USDE also expects accrediting agencies to collect data on student achievement of selected program outcomes: completion rates, licensure and certification pass rates, and employment rates. Therefore health professions accreditation standards will, at a minimum, address these program elements.

You can anticipate that to be compliant with the standards, your program has developed and implemented an internal systematic evaluation plan to systematically review these program elements (see Chapter 22). Table 23.1 provides some examples of health profession standards categories that speak to these program elements. Appendix F contains a partial listing of health professions accrediting agencies that are recognized by the USDE; you can locate the standards for your professional discipline on the relevant website.

In addition to the USDE-mandated general program elements, accrediting agencies must include in their accreditation standards that accreditors need to be responsive to emerging professional issues that are discipline specific. As a result, all accreditation standards will contain criteria that are unique to the discipline, especially in the areas of curriculum and clinical field experiences. Accreditation standards will also be periodically revised to keep relevant professional issues in the forefront.

TABLE 23.1 ■ Examples of Health Professions Accreditation Standards Categories

Accreditation Standards for Dental Education Programs—Pre-doc (CODA)	Commission on Accreditation for Respiratory Care—Entry into Practice (COARC)	Radiography Standards (JRCERT)	Accreditation Commission for Midwifery Education (ACME)	National League for Nursing Commission for Nursing Education Accreditation (CNEA)
I. Institutional Effectiveness	I. Program Administration and Sponsorship	I. Accountability, Fair Practices, and Public Information	I. Organization and Administration	I. Program Outcomes
II. Educational Program	II. Institutional and Personnel Resources	II. Institutional Commitment and Resources	II. Faculty	II. Mission, Governance, and Resources
III. Faculty and Staff	III. Program Goals, Outcomes and Assessment	III. Faculty and Staff	III. Students	III. Faculty
IV. Educational Support Services	IV. Curriculum	IV. Curriculum and Academic Practices	IV. Curriculum	IV. Students
V. Patient Services	V. Fair Practices and Record-keeping	V. Health and Safety	V. Resources	V. Curriculum and Evaluation Processes
VI. Research Programs		VI. Program Effectiveness and Assessment: Using Data for Sustained Improvement	VI. Assessment and Outcomes	

IMPACT OF ACCREDITATION ON THE FACULTY ROLE

So, how does the accreditation process impact your faculty role? From this brief overview of the accreditation process and the purpose that accreditation plays in education, you can see that there are many external factors that have the potential to influence your program's curriculum and the outcomes that stakeholders may expect the program to achieve. As a result, there will be expectations of you in your faculty role.

When a program participates in the accreditation process, it will be evaluated on how and to what extent it meets the accreditation standards set forth by the accrediting agency. These standards will require program administration and faculty to design processes to collect and analyze program data and to report the findings to the accreditors in the form of annual and self-study reports that are written as part of the accreditation process. In turn, these expectations require faculty to commit to participating in the data collection and analysis process, and the use of data to identify program strengths and areas for improvement. The value of participating in the accreditation process is that it encourages you to engage in continuous quality improvement and reflect on how you can best create a learning environment in your courses that will facilitate students' success (Halstead, 2017b). Review a current copy of your discipline's accrediting standards and familiarize yourself with what is expected of your program to demonstrate compliance with the standards.

Additionally, the various factors that can influence accreditation standards and processes for health professions programs include emerging discipline-specific professional issues as well as trends in higher education and health care. Educational issues can also emerge nationally through federal policy changes that will influence accrediting agency policies and procedures. As an individual faculty, staying abreast of emerging trends in your discipline, education, and healthcare will help you to be an informed faculty when considering potential program changes.

Finally, accreditation is a peer review–driven process. There are opportunities for faculty to participate in accreditation by serving as program evaluators on accreditation teams. As you gain further experience in the faculty role, you may decide to set a professional goal to become a program evaluator for an accrediting agency.

The Faculty Role in Accreditation

Even as a new health professions educator you can expect to have the opportunity to be involved in accreditation activities. This will be especially true if your program is scheduled to undergo an accreditation review within the first 2 to 3 years of your faculty appointment. If you are on the faculty of a relatively small program you will undoubtedly be involved in preparing for the accreditation review despite having limited teaching experience. Due to the increasing shortage of health professions educators and loss of expertise due to retirement from the profession, you may also find yourself in a leadership role as the program prepares to host the evaluation team. Many faculty who are new to the accreditation experience are nervous and somewhat apprehensive about their role in the process, fearing that they may say or do something that casts an unfavorable light on the program. However, by taking the time to develop an understanding of accreditation and program evaluation, and being an engaged participant in the process, you will find that you are prepared to interact with the evaluation team and respond to their questions.

A program may begin preparation for a scheduled accreditation review and the accompanying visit anywhere from 12 to 18 months before the actual review is scheduled.

Administration, faculty, and staff will be involved in the preparations. Students and other stakeholders will also need to be prepared for their role in the process. An accreditation review involves several steps: (1) preparation and submission of the self-study report, (2) hosting an onsite visit by a team of program evaluators, and (3) accrediting agency's review process of program documents culminating with board's accreditation decision.

Preparing for an accreditation visit requires organization and attention to detail. Box 23.2 provides a list of preparatory activities that the program must engage in prior to hosting an onsite evaluation visit. Attention to these activities will allow the faculty to conduct a self-assessment of the program's strengths and areas for improvement in preparation for writing the self-study report.

BOX 23.2 ■ Program Preparatory Activities for an Accreditation Review

Governance Documentation

Gather, review, and organize the following documents, ensuring that they are accurate, current, and readily accessible in hard copy and/or electronically:
- Program's systematic evaluation plan
- Academic policies for students and faculty
- Institution and program organizational charts
- Institution and program mission statements, goals, and values
- Relevant bylaws, union contracts (if applicable)
- Clinical agency affiliation contracts
- Faculty committee meeting minutes from the previous 3–5 years
- Institution and program catalogs, faculty handbooks, student handbooks, and other similar documents specific to program
- Faculty documents: promotion and tenure guidelines; faculty role expectations for teaching, scholarship, practice, and service; workload policies; professional development opportunities and support
- Faculty curriculum vitae
- Table of faculty (full and part time), including their credentials and teaching assignments
- Formal complaint/grievance policies
- Recruitment and marketing materials for prospective students
- Reports and any other relevant communications related to accrediting body, certification agencies, licensing boards
- Fiscal reports (program budget) covering last 3 years

BOX 23.2 ■ **Program Preparatory Activities for an Accreditation Review** (Continued)

Curriculum Documentation

Gather, review, and organize in hard copy and/or electronic, the following documents related to curriculum implementation and evaluation:
- Curriculum plans depicting curriculum design
- Most recent copy of course syllabi for all required and elective nursing courses
- Course evaluation documents
- Student clinical performance evaluation tools
- Student assignments or examinations used to evaluate student achievement of expected learning outcomes
- Documentation related to preceptor roles and responsibilities, orientation programs, and evaluation
- Copies of all professional standards used to guide curriculum development
- Curriculum mappings demonstrating integration professional standards and guidelines
- Examples of student work demonstrating their ability to meet course and program expected learning outcomes
- Examples of teaching-learning strategies utilized by faculty across the curriculum
- Documentation of adequacy of instructional learning resources
- Grading policies and scales
- Curriculum evaluation plan (end-of-program outcomes, course, faculty, clinical sites, preceptors)
- Copies of curriculum committee minutes documenting faculty decision-making process based on data analysis
- Program curriculum data demonstrating ongoing collection and analysis processes

Program Outcomes Documentation

Gather and analyze the following for the period required by the accrediting agency:
- Trended completion rate data for each program under review
- Trended licensure and certification pass rates for each program under review
- Employment rates of graduates for each program under review
- Aggregated data demonstrating student achievement of program curriculum outcomes
- Documented evidence of data analysis for each program outcome element to determine if benchmarks are met; if not met, evidence of action plans addressing the benchmark deficit

---

WRITING THE SELF-STUDY REPORT

In addition to the preparatory activities mentioned, the program must also prepare a self-study report that will be submitted to the accrediting agency several weeks before the onsite visit. The accreditation process requires the program to conduct a self-assessment of compliance with the accreditation standards and write a report that addresses each standard and its criteria. This report, commonly called a self-study report, serves several purposes (Box 23.3). It is submitted to the accreditation agency several weeks prior to the visit for the program evaluators to read in preparation for their visit to the program. They will use the information in the self-study report to begin their review of the program before arriving on campus for the onsite visit. The self-study report is a documentation of the program's compliance with the accreditation standards, and it is important that it be organized, concisely written, and accurate in details. The accreditation agency usually provides a report template and detailed instructions of how to prepare the report.

> **BOX 23.3 ▪ Purposes of the Self-Study Report**
>
> - Engages faculty in reflection and self-assessment of the program's accomplishments and areas for improvement
> - Documents the program's compliance with accreditation standards
> - Provides a comprehensive, organized narrative that presents data and evidence for evaluators to use to guide to their peer review of the program

> **BOX 23.4 ▪ Activities Related to Preparing the Self-Study Report**
>
> - Collecting and assembling evidence documents for appendices
> - Drafting wording related to standards' criteria
> - Identifying program strengths and areas for improvement based on data
> - Contributing data and information for charts, tables, crosswalks
> - Reading drafts of self-study report, providing feedback

It is desirable that faculty and staff be involved in the development of the self-study report and knowledgeable about its contents. As self-study reports can be lengthy documents requiring numerous data tables and multiple appendices, many individuals are usually involved in compiling evidence and preparing the report. For example, it is common to divide up the writing of the report by standards or criteria, with various individuals and groups assuming responsibility for drafting the narrative for a specific standard. You may wish to volunteer to write a portion of the report, choosing an area that you have experience with. Participating in the preparation of the report is a particularly good way to prepare yourself for the onsite evaluation visit and any discussions you may have with the program evaluators.

Besides writing portions of the report's narrative, there are numerous other ways for you to assist in preparing the self-study report. Examples of such activities can be found in Box 23.4. With the coordinated efforts of many, a comprehensive self-study report will be prepared. The finished report will be made available to program stakeholders to help them prepare for the actual onsite visit, as the evaluation team will likely cite portions of the report as they conduct interviews. It is an expectation for faculty, staff, and other stakeholders to be familiar with sections of the report relevant to their responsibilities (Halstead & Frank, 2018).

PREPARING FOR AND PARTICIPATING IN ONSITE VISITS

In addition to writing the self-study report, there are numerous other preparations that you may be involved in before and during the scheduled onsite visit. These preparations may be related to the courses you teach, your own personal documentation of your teaching activities, faculty interviews with the evaluation team, clinical partners and students, and gathering of onsite resources for the evaluation team's review.

You can expect these preparations to be ongoing until the time the evaluation team arrives for the scheduled onsite visit. The length of the visit varies depending on the number, nature, and size of the programs under review, but that information will be clearly communicated to your program's administration well in advance of the visit. The onsite visit will most likely take place on campus with a team of evaluators physically present for a specified number of days; however, in recent years due to the COVID pandemic, accrediting agencies conducted their accreditation visits virtually, using teleconferencing technology. Whether your program's visit is an on-campus one or a virtual one mediated through technology, the overall evaluation process remains unchanged.

Team composition will vary as well, depending on the discretion and policies of your accreditation agency. However, teams usually include a minimum of three evaluators with the number of evaluators increasing based on the number of programs under review and their complexity. Most evaluation teams will consist of academic educators familiar with the type of program being reviewed as well as an evaluator who will represent practice in your discipline. The team will follow an agreed upon agenda that is prepared before the visit.

Site Visit Agenda

The evaluation team will follow a set agenda during the site visit. The agenda will be developed in consultation with program administrators and publicly shared prior to the visit. The team will interview many different stakeholders each of whom will be given specific times to meet with the evaluators. Faculty will have their own assigned time to meet with the evaluation team. Box 23.5 lists individuals who will likely be scheduled to meet with the accreditation team members.

BOX 23.5 ■ Individuals Likely to Be Interviewed by Program Evaluation Team

Institution Level

President (CEO)
Academic Provost or Vice President of Academic Affairs
Chief Financial Officer
Student Support Services Administrators
Instructional Technology/Distance Education Administrators
Librarians
Chief of Compliance
Administrators of Faculty Development Departments (teaching and learning centers; scholarship and grant support, etc.)

School/Program Level

School dean/director
Program dean/director
Department Chairs
Faculty
Students (representative of all programs under review)
Advisory Committee members
Clinical Agency Partners
Community members
Support staff
Clinical coordinators
Simulation/Learning Resources staff
Alumni

In addition to participating in the faculty interview, you can also anticipate that the evaluation team may choose to visit your classroom, laboratory, or simulation setting while class is in session. They may also visit clinical sites to interact with students and staff in the clinical setting. Remember that when the team visits those settings they are there to observe the teaching-learning strategies and note physical and instructional resources that are available for use. They will also inquire of clinical staff and preceptors about their role in the clinical education of the students. While the team may observe classes in session, they do not evaluate the teaching performance of individual faculty and they will not interrupt class sessions; they will be silent, unobtrusive observers of the teaching-learning environment.

The evaluation team will use their visit to verify that what has been written in the self-study report is accurate, clarify any questions they may have, and gather additional data to supplement the self-study report. They are primarily interested in hearing the perspective of the program's various stakeholders so they can compare themes that emerge in the interviews among the different groups.

You can prepare for the site visit in several ways. First, be sure to read the self-study report and be familiar with its contents. You will also want to ensure that your students are prepared to interact with the team if asked to do so. Box 23.6 provides additional tips on how to personally prepare yourself and your courses

---

BOX 23.6 ■ Tips for Preparing Yourself for Participating in Accreditation Review

- Familiarize yourself with the accreditation standards
- Read the self-study report
- Ensure the current version of your course syllabi are up to date and in the approved format
- Review the program's systematic evaluation plan
- Have copies of course evaluation instruments available for review
- Be prepared to cite examples of how your courses address expected program outcomes
- Have copies of all course examination materials and student assignments available for review
- Update your curriculum vitae
- Be prepared to cite how your faculty workload is calculated and your understanding of the faculty expectations for promotion and tenure, as appropriate to your institution
- Consider faculty development opportunities offered by the institution or program and be prepared to provide examples of how you have utilized such support
- Anticipate being asked to describe the faculty role in collecting and analyzing data related to program outcomes and provide examples of how faculty use the data to make program decisions
- Be familiar with any action plans the program may have in place to address any areas needing improvement
- Familiarize your students with the purpose of accreditation and their role in the process
- If you teach a clinical course, be prepared to answer questions about how you communicate course objectives to clinical staff and interact with preceptors, set student learning outcomes and make assignments for clinical experiences, and evaluate student clinical performance
- Be able to identify examples of the adequacy of institution and program resources used to meet faculty role expectations in teaching, scholarship, and service
- Participate in any mock interviews your program may conduct in preparation for the onsite visit; be sure to speak up and answer questions!

for the site visit. This will help decrease any anxiety or uncertainty you or your students may feel about the accreditation review.

Preparing for Interviews

A key part of the onsite evaluation visit is the interviews that the evaluation team will conduct with many different stakeholders (see Box 23.5). They may ask similar questions of multiple stakeholders as they seek the perspective of those who hold differing roles within the institution and program. By asking similar questions of multiple stakeholders, the program evaluators are seeking confirmation of themes that may be emerging in the visit. For example, if the institution's president asserts that budgetary resources are adequate to support the program's outcome achievement and describes the process used to determine the program's budget, do the program administrators and faculty hold similar viewpoints and understanding of the process?

You can anticipate being expected to participate in the faculty interview. The length of and the manner in which the interviews are conducted are at the discretion of the evaluation team, but you can expect the faculty interview session to last at least 1 hour or longer. The team uses the interview process to validate and expand upon what has been written in the self-study report, and they will be particularly interested in eliciting specific examples of faculty's lived experiences in their faculty role. Common areas of questioning dwell on faculty's understanding of their role expectations; adequacy of resources; faculty workload; faculty role in curriculum development, implementation, and evaluation; faculty development support; and use of the systematic evaluation plan and data to make program decisions, to cite a few examples. The team members will ask questions, typically taking copious notes of responses for later reference, and faculty are expected to respond extemporaneously.

Some programs choose to conduct mock interviews to prepare faculty for the site visit, using a consultant who is familiar with the accreditation process to pose questions for faculty to respond to. This allows faculty a chance to practice the process. Be sure to participate in any such activities and practice speaking up to answer questions. It will be important for multiple faculty to respond to the evaluation team's interview questions, and to not rely on just a few faculty to speak up. The evaluation team will want to be assured that the faculty as a whole are familiar with the program's processes. Box 23.6 provides further information to help you prepare for the interview experience.

Onsite Resources

Typically the accreditation visit requires the program to gather and organize many resources for the evaluation team to review. Preparing these resources can be a monumental undertaking. This is one area that you can contribute to the preparations for the site visit, even as a relatively new faculty member. Resources may be physically gathered in a resource room, or increasingly the resources are organized in an electronic repository to which the evaluation team is given access. Regardless of the method by which the resources are shared it is very important that the evaluation team have access to the information they need as they conduct their review of the program.

Accreditation standards often cite the data that they expect the programs to make available to the evaluation team. Programs can also choose to make available additional resource materials as they desire. Box 23.2 provides a comprehensive listing of the resource materials commonly requested by accrediting agencies. A careful review of your discipline's accreditation standards will reveal what data resources they will expect to have access to during the evaluation team visit.

Chapter Summary

In this chapter you were introduced to the accreditation process and your role as faculty in preparing for and participating in the accreditation process. Here are some key points about faculty's role in the accreditation process:

- The process of accreditation in your health professions discipline will have considerable influence over curriculum development, program outcomes, and other program elements, including your faculty role.
- Achieving and maintaining accreditation is an external mark of program quality and a form of quality assurance for prospective and current students.
- Participating in the accreditation process requires you to engage in continuous quality improvement efforts in your teaching role, ultimately facilitating your students' successful achievement of expected learning outcomes.
- Familiarizing yourself with your discipline's accreditation standards is a core faculty responsibility.
- Your program's commitment to the accreditation process requires faculty to participate in ongoing data collection and analysis, with documented use of the data to guide faculty decision making in the evaluation of program outcomes.
- The program's self-study report is a self-assessment of the program's strengths and areas for improvement; you will want to be sure to read the report in anticipation of the team's visit.
- Participation in the accreditation process will require you to prepare for the faculty interview. You can anticipate questions related to the following areas: your understanding of your faculty role expectations; adequacy of resources; faculty workload; faculty role in curriculum development, implementation, and evaluation; faculty development support; and use of the systematic evaluation plan and data to make program decisions.
- Even as a new faculty, you will be expected to be familiar with your program's policies and procedures; addressing the items listed in Box 23.6 will help ensure that you are prepared to participate in the accreditation process with confidence.

References

Eaton, J. S. (2012a). *Accreditation and recognition in the United States.* Council for Higher Education Accreditation.

Eaton, J. S. (2012b). *An overview of US accreditation.* Council for Higher Education Accreditation.

Halstead, J. A. (2017a). The accreditation process in nursing education. In M. Oermann (Ed.), *A systematic approach to assessment and evaluations of nursing programs* (pp. 79–91). National League for Nursing.

Halstead, J. A. (2017b). The value of nursing program accreditation. *Teaching and Learning in Nursing, 12*(3), 182–183.

Halstead, J. A., & Frank, B. (2018). Preparing to interact with the on-site program evaluation team. *Teaching and Learning in Nursing, 13,* 193–194.

Hanna, K., Duvall, J., Turpin, R., Pendleton-Romig, K., & Parker, S. (2016). Mastering the journey to continuous compliance: Process improvements for excelling at CCNE accreditation. *Sage Open,* 1–5. https://doi.org/10.1177/2158244016656231

US Department of Education. (2019). Regulations of the Offices of the Department of Education, Postsecondary Education, Department of Education Code of Federal Regulations (ch. 6). https://www.ecfr.gov/current/title-34/subtitle-B/chapter- VI/part-602

Common Issues Related to Program Evaluation

Many faculty find participating in program evaluation efforts challenging. This may be because they don't have a good understanding of the program evaluation process, don't understand their individual role in the process, or they may lack trust in the process and have concerns about how evaluation data will be used. Faculty also sometimes consider the evaluation process to be time consuming and distracting from their primary teaching responsibilities. As a novice faculty, you may have experienced some of these feelings and be reluctant to participate in the process. However, the ability of any program to successfully meet program outcomes and produce graduates qualified to enter the health care workforce is highly dependent on the effectiveness of the program's implementation of its systematic evaluation plan (SEP), and faculty understanding of and participation in the process is crucial.

There are several common issues programs must address with faculty when designing and implementing their program evaluation plan. These issues include lacking a systematic approach to program evaluation, ineffectively analyzing and using data to improve program operations, and lacking faculty participation and shared responsibility in the process (Halstead, 2019). In this chapter we will discuss strategies that can be used to ensure that all faculty are encouraged to participate in the process and how you can become an informed participant in the program evaluation process.

Lack of A Systematic Approach to Program Evaluation

In Chapter 22 we discussed the importance of systematic program evaluation and having a SEP that enables the program to evaluate the expected outcomes established for the program. A challenge many programs face, however, is implementing the written evaluation plan that has been committed to paper. When the SEP is not regularly consulted and used as intended, it leads to inconsistent data collection and faulty data analysis. Faculty cannot use incomplete data to identify trends and make informed decisions about the program (Halstead, 2019). When faculty do not have access to reliable program data to inform decision making, they begin to rely on their intuition and biases to make program decisions. Such an approach is ineffective and may lead faculty to overlook critical information about their program's performance.

As an individual faculty member, what is your role in implementing the SEP and ensuring that data collection is timely, complete, and accurate? Your primary responsibility is to familiarize yourself with the SEP document and note any areas in which you will have responsibility for collecting data. Note the type of data that will need to be collected, the instruments to be used, and the timeline that has been established. You will find that individual faculty responses are most often sought in areas related to curriculum mapping of content relevant to your courses and course evaluations, faculty productivity and performance evaluations, and adequacy of teaching-learning resources.

Additional responsibilities include participating in the review of any data findings and using those findings to inform decision making about your courses' effectiveness and other aspects of your teaching role. Sometimes the feedback may not be what you anticipated, and you may wish to seek input from more experienced faculty to assist you in deciphering the feedback.

As a member of the faculty, you also have the responsibility to be an informed participant in any faculty discussions about the implementation of the SEP and how the data are used to make decisions about program outcomes. Based on data review, faculty will need to determine if outcome benchmarks are being met, and if not, what action plans need to be developed to address the situation. By being knowledgeable about the SEP and the data being collected, you will be well positioned to contribute to the discussions.

Ineffective Use of Data

Another common issue to effective program evaluation is the ineffective use of data. In some cases, data are collected but not analyzed for a variety of reasons, leaving faculty unable to use the data to make program decisions. Box 24.1 identifies some common examples of ineffective use of data by program faculty (Halstead, 2019). These examples are discussed further in the following paragraphs.

BOX 24.1 ■ Examples of Ineffective Data Use

- Disorganized records or data
- Inability to identify program trends
- Lack of data sharing with stakeholders

DISORGANIZED DATA RECORDS

Disorganized data records can lead to inaccurate analysis and the overlooking of meaningful trends in program performance. Disorganized data can also camouflage gaps in the data collection process, making it difficult for faculty to draw any meaningful conclusions from the data. To address this issue the program should adopt a system for maintaining the program's records in an easily accessible manner that leads to prompt data retrieval as needed.

Identifying the program's data needs and setting up an organized, systematic approach to collecting and analyzing the desired data requires the thoughtful consideration of faculty. This is also true about evaluation data that you may be collecting about your courses and your students' learning. There should be a clear purpose and identified use for any data collected. What questions do faculty have about their program's expected outcomes and effectiveness in meeting those outcomes? What questions do you have about your teaching and courses' effectiveness? What data do you need to gather to answer these questions? Without clarifying the questions you want to have answered and the reason for collecting the data, the likelihood of being able to analyze the data diminishes.

Once a clear purpose for data collection has been established, you will want to identify all the types and sources of data to be collected and who is responsible for managing the data collection, as well as how it will be stored for future access and analysis. By clarifying purpose, data type and source, responsibility, and the process to be used for storing and retrieving data the program will be able to organize and store data for future reference. Having these data collection processes in place will also help ensure that data are gathered on a regular, ongoing basis, even over a period of years. See Chapter 22 for further discussion of developing a SEP.

INABILITY TO IDENTIFY PROGRAM TRENDS

Disorganized and inconsistent data collection poses a threat to being able to identify trends in the program's effectiveness in achieving established outcomes. Data need to be reliable and valid for faculty to make decisions about future program efforts and take action to improve program outcomes as indicated by data findings. It is also important, however, for faculty to proactively identify the program areas that will most benefit from trended data analysis. Without those determinations it is very likely that the needed data will not be available for faculty to analyze and identify trends. It often takes a minimum of 3 years of data to detect program trends.

Box 24.2 provides examples of common program outcomes in the health professions that would benefit from trended data collection. It is often the expectation of health professions accrediting bodies that programs will collect

---

BOX 24.2 ■ Examples of Program Outcomes Benefitting From Trended Data Analysis

- Licensure or certification pass rates
- Completion rates/graduation rates
- Employment rates
- Attrition rates
- Achievement of student learning outcomes in the aggregate
- Employer satisfaction with graduates

and analyze such data. Your discipline's accrediting agency may also stipulate how many years of data to report to provide evidence of effective evaluation of program outcomes. Data collection efforts to measure these and other program outcomes are sophisticated and require the planned input of multiple stake-holders. Such data collection often needs to occur over a period of years to produce enough evidence to detect trends. Without advanced planning, data collection will be inadequate, and faculty will not be able to effectively measure program outcomes. Like the previous discussion about disorganized data, the first step toward trend identification is for faculty to determine what questions they have about program effectiveness in meeting outcomes, and what data are needed to answer those questions.

At the course level, you may also have the need to collect trended data re-garding your teaching effectiveness, as well as your courses' effectiveness in helping students meet established learning outcomes. Proactively consider which aspects of your course and your teaching performance may benefit from trended evaluation data and put a plan in place to collect this data.

LACK OF DATA SHARING WITH STAKEHOLDERS

In another example of ineffective data use, program data are collected and ana-lyzed, but the resulting findings are not shared with appropriate stakeholders, and thus the feedback loop of the evaluation process is not closed. Stakeholders who would benefit from receiving the findings may be faculty, students, clinical partners, alumni, institution administration, regulatory bodies, and others who are vested in the success of the program.

Sharing the data results with those who are potentially affected by the find-ings and demonstrating that program decisions are made based on data is a critical step in the success of the evaluation process. It inspires confidence in program decisions and encourages stakeholders to willingly participate in the evaluation process. When data are not shared, stakeholders may express con-cerns about what is happening to feedback they have given to the program and if it is being used for continuous quality improvement. Every effort should be made by those who are engaged in data collection to establish an understand-ing with stakeholders that findings will be shared as appropriate, the results will be used to improve program outcomes, and the evaluation process will be conducted with transparency.

Lack Of Participation In The Evaluation Process

All faculty have a responsibility to participate in the evaluation process and to commit to using data to support decisions made to improve program outcomes. Program evaluation is a collaborative process, one that requires collective decision making among faculty and program administration to be successful (Halstead, 2019). Sometimes faculty may be reluctant to participate in evaluation activities as they fear the data may be used to find fault with their teaching performance or how they conduct their courses.

With any evaluation activity there should always be a clarity of purpose established as to why the evaluation is being conducted and how the findings will be used. As previously stated, transparency serves to build trusting relationships with stakeholders and encourages participation. The organizational culture of the institution and program must be one that values and demonstrates that the evaluation process will be respectfully conducted (Halstead, 2019). Stavropoulou and Stroubouki (2014) stated that participants in the evaluation of educational programs needed to possess several qualities, including openness and commitment, willingness to change, teamwork, administrative support, resources and infrastructure, vision, and optimism, among other attributes. These characteristics speak directly to the importance of the organizational culture and its willingness to embrace continuous quality improvement. When a culture of mutual support and trust has been established with stakeholders, program administrators and faculty can have increased confidence that stakeholder participation in the process will increase, and the program outcome data being collected will more likely be reliable and valid.

Chapter Summary

In this chapter you were introduced to the common challenges associated with program evaluation and strategies designed to minimize these challenges. Here are some key points to consider as you prepare yourself to be a knowledgeable participant in the program evaluation process:

- Many faculty find program evaluation to be a time-consuming and challenging process because they do not have a full understanding of the process. Allow time to familiarize yourself with the program evaluation process in place within your program and any program evaluation expectations that are specific to your health profession discipline.
- Faculty have a shared responsibility to participate in program evaluation activities and commit to collecting and using valid and reliable data upon which to base program decision making. Familiarize yourself with evaluation instruments that are used within your program to collect data on program outcomes.
- Common issues related to program evaluation include lacking a systematic approach to program evaluation, analyzing and using data ineffectively to improve program operations, and lacking faculty participation in the process due to concerns about how data will be used. Make note of any questions regarding your program's evaluation process so that you can ask them of your mentor, supervisor, and others as appropriate.
- Familiarizing yourself with your program's SEP and your role in its implementation will help you become an informed participant of the evaluation process.
- Clarify the purpose, data type and source, and the process to be used for storing and retrieving data for all data that you are responsible for collecting as a means to ensure data are gathered on a regular, ongoing basis.

References

Halstead, J. A. (2019). Program evaluation: Common challenges to data collection. *Teaching and Learning in Nursing, 14*(3), A6–A7. https://doi.org/10.1016/j.teln.2019.04.001

Stavropoulou, A., & Stroubouki, T. (2014). Evaluation of educational programmes—the contribution of history to modern evaluation thinking. *Health Sciences Journal, 8*(2), 193–204.

CHAPTER 25

Evaluating Effectiveness of Program Evaluation

The purpose of Part V of this book was to provide you with an introduction to the fundamental concepts of program evaluation and accreditation, emphasizing the importance and the integral role that evaluation will play in shaping your faculty practice. The evaluation process will be a consistent and daily presence throughout your faculty career, and it is well worth the investment of your time to grow in your understanding of how to best integrate evaluation principles into the various aspects of your faculty role. Whether you are implementing a new curriculum, developing new lesson plans and teaching strategies, choosing new instructional materials, or striving to increase your teaching skills in the classroom and clinical settings, how you will evaluate the success of those changes will be an important consideration. The strategies you choose to measure your teaching effectiveness will be guided, in part, by the evaluation plan developed by your program. Your ability to evaluate students' success at achieving learning outcomes is directly related to understanding how to effectively evaluate not only your students' performance, but all the program elements that potentially can influence the learning environment created within your program.

A considerable amount of effort goes into the development and implementation of any program's systematic evaluation plan (SEP). How do faculty know that their evaluation plans are effective and providing them with reliable and valid data upon which to base decisions? How can program leaders and faculty be assured that the findings will be trusted and acted upon as indicated to improve program quality? The systematic program evaluation process itself requires periodic review and updating to remain relevant (Lewallen, 2015). This final chapter briefly summarizes steps that can be taken to help ensure that your program's evaluation plan is one that will be a useful guide to faculty as they make important decisions that will influence the program's future success.

Evaluation: A Collaborative Process

As previously discussed, evaluation is a complex process that requires the input and perspective of multiple stakeholders to be effective. Program evaluation is especially complex as it is unique and context specific to the program being evaluated (Ellis, 2020), and it needs to include the interplay between multiple internal and external factors that can affect how well the program

---

BOX 25.1 ■ Features of a Comprehensive Program Evaluation Process

- Select evaluation strategies that demonstrate reliability and validity.
- Ensure that data collected are meaningful to the program and can be used to guide program improvement efforts.
- Review the SEP periodically and revise as needed to improve relevance and effectiveness.
- Ensure that the evaluation plan is consistently implemented as intended.
- Document any decisions and changes made relative to data collected and analyzed.

Adapted from Ellis, P. (2020). Systematic program evaluation. In D. Billings & J. Halstead (Eds.), *Teaching in nursing: A guide for faculty* (6th ed., pp. 514–557). Elsevier.

---

achieves its mission and stated outcomes. Hatry et al. (2015) explicitly state that "evaluation requires a team rather than a single individual" (p. 817).

In an organizational environment that truly epitomizes a commitment to continuous quality improvement, the development and implementation of the program's SEP will involve all key contributors to the program's success. These individuals will need to bring to the process an understanding of the context within which the program operates (Ellis, 2020; Hatry et al., 2015) to develop an evaluation plan that will produce meaningful data to evaluate the program's outcomes. Hatry et al. (2015) suggest that peer review of the evaluation plan by others who are expert in evaluation design can be beneficial to ensuring the quality of the plan. Ellis (2020) also identifies features of a comprehensive program evaluation process (Box 25.1) that help ensure the effectiveness and quality of the process.

COLLABORATING TO EVALUATE YOUR TEACHING PRACTICES

While the strategies referenced earlier are recommended for program evaluation efforts, they can also be useful as you evaluate your courses and teaching practices. You do not need to work in isolation as you consider which elements of your course or teaching practices you want to evaluate and how to best select appropriate evaluation strategies. In addition to having the program's SEP to guide you, it can be helpful to seek the feedback of your peers, mentors, and others who are experienced in evaluation to assist you in designing evaluation strategies that will be reliable and valid. If your institution has a department dedicated to the assessment and evaluation of learning, be sure to contact them for advice and access to evaluation resources they may have. Conducting literature reviews may also uncover evaluation methods and instruments that others have used and found to be reliable and valid, thus possibly increasing the reliability and validity of your own findings. Be willing to venture outside of your discipline to find evaluation tools that may be relevant to your teaching.

Learn to consider the evaluation process to be critically important to the success of any change that is undertaken by the program or that you undertake as an individual faculty. Be proactive in determining what aspects of the change will need to be evaluated, what questions you will want to have answered, what data you will collect, and how the data will be used. A proactive approach to evaluation will allow you to build evaluation steps into the change process, collecting and analyzing data during the implementation phase, instead of viewing evaluation as an afterthought.

Responsible Use of Evaluation Data

Demonstrating the responsible use of evaluation data to the program's stakeholders is key to establishing the effectiveness of the program's evaluation plan and trust in the resultant findings. As discussed in Chapter 24, faculty and other stakeholders may be reluctant to participate in the evaluation process for fear of fault finding. These fears can be minimized with the appropriate use of data findings, starting with understanding and appreciating the stakeholder's perspectives on how the data findings will be communicated and shared with others (Newcomer et al., 2015). When analyzed program evaluation data reveal program deficiencies, it is especially important for program leaders to model a sensitivity to how the data will be disseminated and used to guide program improvements. The emphasis should always be on a collective and collaborative approach to addressing any areas requiring improvement and knowledge that the data will be used to improve program outcomes. Before any finding reports are made public it is important that the dissemination plan allows time for the affected stakeholders to review and provide feedback.

The ethical use of data requires that anonymity and confidentiality of all participants providing data should be protected (Hatry et al., 2015). When participating in data collection efforts, the respondents should always be made aware of how the data will be used and reported. This is also a consideration for you in your faculty role when you ask students to provide evaluation data related to your courses and teaching performance. Most institutions have processes in place that provide students with the ability to provide evaluation feedback in a confidential manner. It is important that you reinforce with your students that you value their feedback, that you will not have access to the aggregated findings until after the course is completed and grades submitted, and that you will carefully review and consider their feedback, using it to improve the course and your teaching.

Harty et al. (2015) assert that programs need to engage in "capacity-building... to support learning and using information to improve program performance" (p. 821). In other words, using evaluation data effectively to improve program outcomes requires a specific skill set, one that needs to be intentionally developed and nurtured, on the part of program leaders, faculty, and staff. There needs to be a fervent and ongoing commitment by all to using data findings for the continued quality improvement of the program.

In your faculty role, what can you do to commit to developing your own evaluation skill set and using data effectively? Box 25.2 provides a list of tips for the responsible use of data that you can incorporate into any evaluation strategies utilized to improve your courses and teaching practices. As you continue to develop expertise in your faculty role there will be many opportunities to incorporate these tips into your evaluation strategies and develop an evidence-based practice as a health professions educator.

BOX 25.2 ■ Tips for Using Data Effectively in Your Teaching Practices

- Be clear about the intent of your evaluation strategies and how the data obtained will be used.
- Ensure evaluation criteria are relevant to the expected outcome that you are evaluating.
- Select evaluation strategies that will allow you to detect trends in the outcomes you are measuring.
- Ensure that your evaluation strategies allow for obtaining the differing perspectives of relevant stakeholders.
- Review data findings in a timely manner, considering potential changes in response to the feedback.
- Document any changes you make and implement an evaluation plan to evaluate the effectiveness of the changes.
- Share feedback and resulting actions as appropriate with relevant stakeholders.

Chapter Summary

In this chapter measures that can be used to evaluate the effectiveness of the program's evaluation plan are addressed. Here are some key points to consider when determining the effectiveness of your program's evaluation process:

- Evaluation is a complex process that requires the input and perspective of multiple stakeholders to be effective.
- Effective implementation of the program's evaluation plan is not the responsibility of any single individual; rather it requires a team effort.
- Evaluation should be proactively considered for any program, project, initiative, or change that is being implemented
- Developing an evaluation plan that will produce meaningful data to evaluate program outcomes requires an understanding of the context within which the program operates.
- Program leadership should model a commitment to using data to improve program outcomes.
- The ethical use of data requires that anonymity and confidentiality of participants providing data should be protected.
- Using evaluation data effectively to improve program outcomes requires a specific skill set, one that needs to be intentionally developed and nurtured. Use the tips in Box 25.2 to help you develop effective evaluation strategies to measure outcomes related to your teaching practices.

References

Ellis, P. (2020). Systematic program evaluation. In D. Billings & J. Halstead (Eds.), *Teaching in nursing: A guide for faculty* (6th ed., pp. 514–557). Elsevier.

Hatry, H. P., Newcomer, K. E., & Wholey, J. (2015). Evaluation challenges, issues, and trends. In K. E. Newcomer, H. P. Hatry, & J. Wholey (Eds.), *Handbook of practical program evaluation* (4th ed., pp. 816–832). Jossey-Bass.

Lewallen, L. P. (2015). Practical strategies for nursing education program evaluation. *Journal of Professional Nursing, 31*(2), 133–114. https://doi.org/10.1016/j.profnurs.2014.09.002

Newcomer, K. E., Hatry, H. P., & Wholey, J. (2015). Planning and designing useful evaluations. In K. E. Newcomer, H. P. Hatry, & J. Wholey (Eds.), *Handbook of practical program evaluation* (4th ed., pp. 7–35). Jossey-Bass.

Documents and Policies to Review Before Getting Started With Curriculum Development Activities

- Mission and vision statements of institution and program
- Philosophy statement of program
- Conceptual (organizing) framework
- End-of-program outcomes and competency statements
- Curriculum sequencing plan
- Course syllabi of required discipline-specific courses
- Curriculum evaluation plan for program
- General education requirements for institution
- Curriculum review policies of institution and program
- Academic policies related to admission, progression, and graduation
- Curriculum committee reports
- Curriculum evaluation reports

Documents and Policies to Review Before Getting Started With Teaching in the Classroom

- Course syllabus
- Student/faculty handbook for school and college/university
- Student accommodation process
- Student appeal process
- Organizational chart for school and campus
- Student, faculty, peer, administrator evaluation instruments used to evaluate course and teaching effectiveness
- Self-evaluation of the course/teaching for your portfolio

Documents and Policies to Review Before Getting Started With Teaching in the Clinical Setting

- Course syllabus
- Student/faculty handbook for school and college/university
- Student accommodation process
- Student appeal process
- Organizational chart for school, campus, and clinical agency
- Policy manual for the clinical agency
- School of nursing contract for student placement at the clinical agency
- Preceptor contract/role description
- Evaluation of student clinical performance form—used to assign grade
- Clinical course evaluation form—student's evaluation of course and instruction
- Evaluation of clinical agency, staff, and preceptor from (student form, faculty form)
- Self-evaluation of the course/teaching for your portfolio

Documents and Policies to Review Before Getting Started With Using Learning Technology

Academic Institution Technology Policies Related to:

- Confidentiality and privacy of e-communications
- IT security, password protection
- Fair use and open access policies of educational materials
- Access to student academic records
- Use of institution or program owned hardware and software
- Intellectual property guidelines related to digital materials
- Common Creative Attribution licensure arrangements
- Copyright laws
- Proctoring guidelines for distance enrolled students
- Library policies for accessing online databases and resources
- Student use of social media in clinical care settings and patient care

Clinical Agency Technology Policies Related to:

- Regulating use of social media in protection of patient confidentiality
- Use of mobile devices in patient care settings
- Access to clinical information systems such as electronic health records

Documents and Policies to Review Before Getting Started With Program Evaluation

- Relevant accrediting agency's accreditation standards
- Relevant regulatory body rules and regulations
- Program's systematic evaluation plan
- Student course evaluation tools
- Faculty course evaluation tools
- Clinical agency evaluation tools (for clinical courses)
- Preceptor evaluation tools (for clinical courses)
- Faculty performance evaluation tools
- Institutional and program policies related to course evaluation process
- Institutional and program policies related to faculty evaluation process

Health Professions Accreditation Agencies Recognized by the US Department of Education*

Accreditation Commission for Education in Nursing (ACEN): www.acenursing.org

Accreditation Commission for Midwifery Education (ACME): www.acnm.org

Accreditation Council for Pharmacy Education (ACPE): www.acpe-accredit.org

American Dental Association, Commission on Dental Accreditation: http://www.ada.org/coda

American Occupational Therapy Association, Accreditation Council for Occupational Therapy Education (ACOTE): www.acoteonline.org

American Physical Therapy Association, Commission on Accreditation in Physical Therapy Education (CAPTE): capteonline.org

American Speech-Language-Hearing Association, Council on Academic Accreditation in Audiology and Speech-Language Pathology: caa.asha.org

Commission on Collegiate Nursing Education (CCNE): www.ccneaccreditation.org

Council on Accreditation of Nurse Anesthesia Educational Programs (COA): https://www.coacrna.org/about-coa/

Council on Education for Public Health (CEPH): www.ceph.org

Joint Review Committee on Education in Radiologic Technology (JRCET): www.jrcert.org

National League for Nursing Commission for Nursing Education Accreditation (NLN CNEA): cnea.nln.org

---

*This is a partial listing. The complete listing can be accessed at https://www2.ed.gov/print/admins/finaid/accred/accreditation.html#health.

Accommodations: Adjustments or modifications to learning assignments/experiences that allow students with disabilities to demonstrate expected student learning outcomes. Examples of reasonable accommodations include extra time to take a test or write a paper, an adaptation of a stethoscope, computer text-to-speech, or large-print learning materials. Student service offices at colleges and universities facilitate implementation of accommodations once the students' health care provider has provided the information for the student to request the accommodations.

American Disability Act (ADA): The Americans with Disabilities Act (1990) prohibits discrimination based on disabilities and provides opportunities for those individuals with documented disabilities (physical or mental) to participate in education and employment activities. In the education setting, the ADA requires institutions to provide reasonable accommodations for students to allow them to demonstrate achievement of expected student learning outcomes in all learning environments: classroom, clinical, learning resource centers, etc.

Assessment vs. Evaluation: Assessment of student learning is formative and provides students with information about their progress toward attaining learning outcomes; the faculty role is to use assessment techniques that give students an opportunity to practice in the way they will be evaluated and provide feedback and coaching. Evaluation is summative and provides judgment about the extent to which students met learning outcomes. Evaluation results in a grade.

Blended courses: Courses that are delivered through a combination of in-classroom presence and online learning activities.

Case studies: Teaching strategy that provides students with a real-life scenario, allowing them to apply theory to practice in the analysis of the situation presented in the case. Case studies may be written to be unfolding, in which they progress over time as the students work through the situation that has been presented. Case studies work well for group work, interprofessional collaborative team learning experiences, and can be used in classroom settings or online.

Classroom assessment techniques (CAT): Brief, formative evaluation tools that educators can quickly use to assess student learning, to determine need for further instruction. CATs are informal and nongraded, providing educators with feedback used solely to further facilitate student achievement of expected student outcomes.

Classroom response systems: Also known as clickers, is a set of hardware and software that facilitates activities such as responding to polling questions or test questions. In the classroom, each student is assigned to a transmitter (clicker), and the software will record the response and display results to individuals (student or teacher) or the group. Response systems are also embedded in learning management systems or digital meeting programs.

Clinical setting: Refers to the location in which the student is having a clinical learning experience. The location may be the patient's home, a telehealth interaction, or hospitals and health care facilities. May also be called clinical site, clinical environment, clinical agency, clinical placement, or clinical practicum.

Competencies: Competency statements are foundational to the curriculum in that they identify the behaviors (knowledge, skills, and attributes/values) that students need to acquire to achieve expected curriculum end-of-program outcomes. Competency statements are progressively leveled throughout the curriculum leading students to gradually acquire deeper understanding of curriculum concepts in various contexts.

Conceptual framework: Organizing framework of the curriculum identifying major concepts relevant to a discipline's practice and the interrelationships of the concepts, structuring knowledge in a meaningful way for both faculty and students in the teaching-learning process. Frequently, concepts are derived from theories that have meaning for health professionals' practice (e.g., health, wellness-illness, health care systems, caring, environment, social structure, society, communities, culture, population, social justice).

Course outcomes: The knowledge, skills, and attributes/values learners are expected to achieve at the completion of a course (student learning outcomes); course learning experiences and assignments are designed by faculty to facilitate student achievement of course outcomes as measured by evaluation strategies and valid and reliable evaluation instruments. Course outcomes should be linked to curriculum competency statements, ultimately leading to the achievement of end-of-program curriculum outcomes.

Curriculum: Multiple definitions of curriculum exist; most commonly curriculum is broadly defined as all the educational experiences learners have in a program of study, progressively leading to the achievement of preestablished goals. Educational experiences may occur within coursework, extracurricular activities, support services, and are influenced by the nature of interpersonal relationships that are present in the teaching-learning process.

Curriculum outcomes: The all-encompassing characteristics that learners should be able to demonstrate at the completion of the curriculum (end of program), representative of the role the learners have been prepared to assume upon graduation. Curriculum outcomes are brought to fruition as they are linked to the multiple competencies students are expected to acquire through the curriculum's designed learning experiences.

Digital whiteboard: Software that is a component of a learning management system or digital meeting programs that enables students to brainstorm or collaborate by writing, typing, or posting sticky note comments on the digital white board.

Due process: A requirement that legal and academic matters be resolved according to established rules and principles, and that individuals be treated fairly. Health professions schools have policies and procedures for advising students of their rights to due process as it pertains to teaching, learning, and evaluation and implementing the process as described in the procedures.

Evidence-based teaching: Using research findings as a foundation upon which to base one's teaching practices and teaching-learning strategies.

Expected program outcomes: Anticipated program outcomes and benchmarks established by faculty to measure program effectiveness in achieving goals.

Experiential learning: Learning experiences that are designed to facilitate learners' application of theoretical knowledge to practice, focusing on hands-on learning and opportunities for students to engage in critical inquiry and reflective practices.

Extended reality (ER), virtual reality (VR), augmented reality (AR): ER is an umbrella term for VR, use of technology in a three-dimensional environment, and AR, the projection of digital content in an environment in which the student can interact with the setting, patient, and equipment. Mixed reality is the combination of digital content and the students' environment.

Family Educational Rights and Privacy Act (FERPA): Federal law enacted in 1974 to protect students' right to privacy in relation to educational records. After the age of 18 or when attending a school beyond the level of high school, students must grant permission for education institutions to release student records to others, including parents.

Learning community: A cohort of learners who come together with others (teachers, preceptors, practitioners, etc.) in a supportive learning environment for the purpose of achieving expected student learning outcomes.

Learning domains: Knowledge can be categorized by domains of learning: affective (attitudes, feelings), cognitive (retention and application of information), and psychomotor (skills and procedures). Each domain can be further described by levels of complexity and expected behavior. Knowledge domains are used in courses to specific levels of learning outcomes and evaluation criteria.

Learning management system (LMS): Course management software that provides a framework for supporting multiple course functions. LMS are used to deliver online courses but are also used in traditional courses to provide learning resources and facilitate course interactions. Examples of course functions facilitated by LMS include delivery of course content (syllabus, course calendar, learning modules, etc.), submission of course assignments, administration of exams, facilitation of course communication, maintaining of grade records, and integration of links to other learning resources.

Mannikin, high-fidelity mannikin: A full-body representation of a body or body part that is used for students to practice clinical skills. Manikins are described by their fidelity. Low fidelity, or static manikins/partial task trainers, are body parts such as an arm to practice starting an intravenous infusion or a head/throat to practice intubation; medium-fidelity manikins offer more realism such as breath sounds and pulses; high-fidelity manikins most realistically represent the human body and can breathe, talk, blink, and respond.

Mission statement: A brief statement that describes an institution's or program's goal and reason (purpose) for existence.

Mobile health (M-health): Refers to the use of technology to track and monitor patient's health. The technology uses wearable devices such as an insulin pump or cardiac monitoring and digital record keeping such as dietary history or tracking blood pressure over time.

Objective Structured Clinical Examination (OSCE): The use of a standardized patient (actors, volunteers) playing the role of a patient in a structured scenario to test students' clinical abilities to communicate appropriately, obtain health histories, perform physical assessment and psychomotor skills, and make clinical judgments. Because the task is structured, and each student interacts with the same patient, bias and subjectivity is minimized from evaluation and grading.

Philosophy statement: Used to convey faculty beliefs and values about concepts pertinent to the practice of nursing and other health profession disciplines. Concepts that are usually addressed in a program's philosophy statement include the faculty's beliefs and values related to human beings, health, society, environment, the role of the professional discipline, education, and the teaching-learning process. The philosophy statement serves as the philosophical foundation for the curriculum and guides the integration of the faculty's beliefs and values into the curriculum.

Prebriefing and debriefing: Prebriefing occurs prior to a learning event (classroom activity, pre/postconference, simulation) to set the stage for learning by identifying learning outcomes or expectations. Debriefing is used following the learning event to help the student connect the event to course content and reflect on actions and experience. Guidelines and models for facilitating the pre/debrief guide the discussion and reflection.

Preceptor: An experienced health care practitioner who provides supervision and coaching to students to whom they have been assigned during the students' clinical experience. Preceptors have a collaborative relationship with the faculty and student and are oriented to the expectations of the course and the role. State legislation may dictate who can serve as a preceptor; experience and degrees are among criteria.

Presentation software: Software that creates images that can be projected in a classroom or viewed on a digital device. PowerPoint is an example of presentation software.

Program outcomes: Results attained by the program with the intention of meeting program goals. Outcomes may be identified for any program element deemed necessary to ensure program success (i.e., curriculum, resources, faculty, student learning, and any other program element faculty deem important to measure).

Rubric: An assessment and evaluation tool that defines expectations for performance at various levels that relate to a score or grade for the assignment. Using descriptive criteria for each level, rubrics identify the task or learning outcome, a scoring scale, descriptive dimension of the performance, and quality for each level. Rubrics can be used to assess/evaluate/grade oral presentations, written work, and clinical performance.

Screen capture recordings: A digital record of the entire screen in a video and audio recording. The software is used by students and faculty to record presentations, lectures, webinars.

Standardized patients: Individuals (often volunteers) who have been trained to portray a specific clinical condition for the purposes of simulating learning experiences for health professions students to practice their assessment and diagnostic skills.

Student-centered (learner-centered) environment: A learning environment that is focused on facilitating student learning needs and empowering students to have input into the learning process.

Student learning outcomes: The knowledge, skills, and attributes/values that students are expected to demonstrate at specific times within a curriculum (e.g., completion of learning module, a course or program level, end of program).

Teaching prompts (teaching questions): Posed by the faculty to elicit a response to the question. Prompts/questions are used for teaching and assessment and to engage the student in developing thinking and clinical judgment skills.

Telehealth: The use of telecommunications technology to deliver health care from a distance.

Universal design: The design of an environment so that all individuals can access it to their fullest extent regardless of capability. In education, universal design is applied to the learning environment so that all students have an equal opportunity to learn successfully.

INDEX

Page numbers followed by *"f"* indicate figures, *"t"* indicate tables, and *"b"* indicate boxes.